# NAIL IT!

Wendell Cole MD

Spencer Woolwine MD

ISBN: 978-1-7323843-3-0

Dedicated to all of the orthopods out there!

Correspondence:

Nailed It Ortho Podcast

naileditortho@gmail.com

www.naileditortho.com

Facebook/Instagram/Twitter: @naileditortho

Authors

Wendell W. Cole III, MD

Spencer Woolwine, MD

Illustrations

Wendell W. Cole III, MD

Acknowledgements:

Jamal Fitts, MD

# CONTENTS


**PREFACE** **6**

**CHAPTER 1 - TRAUMA** **9**

GENERAL PRINCIPLES 9

**UPPER EXTREMITY** **13**

STERNOCLAVICULAR JOINT 13

CLAVICLE FRACTURES 13

ACROMIOCLAVICULAR JOINT 15

SCAPULA FRACTURES 16

SHOULDER DISLOCATIONS 17

PROXIMAL HUMERUS FRACTURES 18

HUMERAL SHAFT FRACTURES 21

DISTAL HUMERUS FRACTURES 23

OLECRANON 25

CORONOID FRACTURES 25

RADIAL HEAD FRACTURES 26

ELBOW DISLOCATIONS 27

PELVIS FRACTURES 29

ACETABULUM FRACTURES 34

**LOWER EXTREMITY** **39**

HIP DISLOCATIONS 39

FEMORAL HEAD 39

FEMORAL NECK 40

INTERTROCHANTERIC FEMUR FRACTURES 42

SUBTROCHANTERIC FEMUR FRACTURES 44

FEMORAL SHAFT FRACTURES 45

DISTAL FEMUR FRACTURES 46

KNEE DISLOCATIONS 47

PATELLA FRACTURES 48

TIBIA PLATEAU FRACTURES 49

TIBIA SHAFT FRACTURES 51

PILON FRACTURES 53

**CHAPTER 2 - SPORTS** **61**

GENERAL SPORTS 61

**HIP** **64**

**KNEE** **69**

KNEE LIGAMENT INJURIES 73

PATELLO-FEMORAL JOINT 77

FOOT/SPORTS INJURIES 79

SHOULDER 81

SHOULDER PHYSICAL EXAM 82

SHOULDER PATHOLOGY 84

SHOULDER INSTABILITY 85

SHOULDER IMPINGEMENT 86

ROTATOR CUFF TEARS 87

THROWING/ OVERHEAD ATHLETES 89

OTHER SHOULDER CONDITIONS 92

SHOULDER ARTHRITIS 94

SOME ELBOW CONDITIONS 97

**CHAPTER 3 - BASIC SCIENCE** **105**

ORTHOPAEDIC TISSUES 115

ARTHRITIS 120

MOLECULAR BIOLOGY 124

GENETICS 126

INFECTIONS 128

BIOMATERIALS 131

PERIOPERATIVE STUFF 139

**CHAPTER 4 - SPINE** **147**

RHEUMATOID 154

ANKYLOSING SPONDYLITIS 155

C-SPINE TRAUMA 157

**LUMBAR SPINE** **162**

ADULT SPINAL DEFORMITY 168

TRAUMA 170

INFECTIONS 173

**CHAPTER 5 - FOOT & ANKLE** **179**

ANATOMY 179

ANKLE ARTHRITIS 180

FIRST RAY + TOES 181

ANKLE + FOOT TRAUMA 188

OTHER FOOT CONDITIONS 198

**CHAPTER 6 - ADULT RECONSTRUCTION** **209**

**KNEE** **209**

KNEE ARTHRITIS 209

TKA IMPLANTS 101 211

TKA PRINCIPLES 213

TKA COMPLICATIONS 218

REVISION TKA 219

TKA INFECTION 221

**HIP** **224**

HIP ARTHRITIS 224

HIP BIOMECHANICS/ TEMPLATING 226
THA/ IMPLANTS 101 228
THA WEAR 232
THA COMPLICATIONS/ REVISION 235
THA INFECTION 239

**CHAPTER 7 - HAND 245**
WRIST + HAND ANATOMY 245
WRIST + HAND TRAUMA 247
CARPAL FRACTURES 250
WRIST LIGAMENT INJURIES 253
HAND FRACTURES 255
THUMB INJURIES 257
TENDON INJURIES 258
NAIL/FINGERTIP INJURIES 260
NERVE INJURIES 261
TENDON TRANSFERS 264
TENDONOPATHY 265
HAND INFECTIONS 266
ARTHRITIS 266
RHEUMATOID 267
DUPURTYEN 268

**CHAPTER 8 - PEDIATRICS 275**
UPPER EXTREMITY PEDS 275
LOWER EXTREMITY PEDS 279
PEDIATRIC SPINE 282
PEDIATRIC HIP 287
PEDIATRIC FOOT 290
INFECTIONS 291
NEUROMUSCULAR DISEASE 293
LIMB GROWTH + CONGENITAL DEFORMITIES 296
UPPER EXTREMITY DEFORMITIES 299
SYNDROMES & DYSPLASIAS 300

**CHAPTER 9 - PATHOLOGY 305**
OVERVIEW + TREATMENT PRINCIPLES 305
BENIGN BONE FORMING LESIONS 309
MALIGNANT BONE FORMING TUMORS 310
BENIGN CARTILAGE FORMING LESIONS 313
MALIGNANT CARTILAGE FORMING TUMORS 314
BENIGN FIBROUS/ HISTIOCYTIC TUMORS 315
CYSTIC/OTHER BENIGN BONE TUMORS 317
OTHER MALIGNANT BONE TUMORS 318
HEMATOPOIETIC BONE TUMORS 319
SMALL ROUND BLUE CELL TUMORS 320
BENIGN SOFT TISSUE TUMORS 321
SOFT TISSUE SARCOMAS 322
SYNOVIAL PROLIFERATIVE DISORDERS 325

**CHAPTER 10 - STATISTICS 329**

# PREFACE

**These notes are notes that we've made throughout the years while studying for the OITE and board exam, as well as for everyday duties. These are notes that we've taken from doing questions, listening to lectures, preparing for podcast episodes, studying powerpoints, doing review courses, and reading other review books. These are the same notes that the Nailed it Ortho podcast review series is based on. When you listen to the podcast, you'll notice these are the same questions.**

## What is this book?

- It's the companion book to the Nailed it Ortho OITE podcast review series. We aim to deliver high yield information that is concise and to the point

## How to use this book

- This book is not to be intended as your sole resource for OITE studying, but it is to help reinforce the material we covered in the podcast. This is an extra tool to have in your toolbox for studying. We all know repetition is the father of learning, so we recommend after listening to an episode, that you review that same section in the book. That's two forms of learning: audio + visual.
- Throughout this companion book, there will be time marks to specific times in an episode where we mention the topic, in case you'd like to go and listen to it again. You will see this icon next to the information
- We've organized the material in this book in a similar order as the Miller's Review book, for ease of studying/flow since many of you all use that for review (including us!).
- We try to make sure all of the information is accurate, but if there are mistakes feel free to reach out to us via email and let us know. Some of the information that we state we will also put the article that we read, where we got the information. You will see this icon and the name + year of the article next to the information.
- If you want a deeper dive into some topics that we cover in the review, but have done an entire podcast episode on before, you'll see this icon and we'll put the episode you can listen to for a more in depth conversation.
- You should study year round for this exam! Knowing this information will not only help you on the exam, but help you in real life as well. Also, there may be some references in this text that were mentioned in the podcast to help jog your memory or commit things to memory.
- This book is not medical advice, it is purely educational in nature.

## How NOT to use this book

- Again, this should not be your sole study guide. This will contain quick bullet points and questions to help assist with learning. For a deeper dive into any of these topics, we suggest reading a book specific to that topic!

## Last words

- Listen to the podcast board/OITE review series! More than once! It will help you remember certain things.
- DO QUESTIONS, nothing beats cranking out a lot of questions to help reinforce and test your knowledge. Utilize your question banks. ResStudy has great questions. Orthobullets as well!
- Study, prepare for your exam, and do the best you can. You got this! CRUSH it! We hope you enjoy these illustrations that go along with this too!

## Abbreviations Commonly Used

ATLS: Advanced Trauma Life Support
Abx- Antibiotics
BP- Blood pressure
CT: Computerized tomography scan
Dec: Decrease
Ex-Fix: External fixation
ER: External rotation
FFP- Fresh frozen plasma
Fx: Fracture
IMN:- Intramedullary nailing
IR: Internal rotation
Inc: Increase
L- liter
ORIF: Open reduction internal fixation
Non-op: Non-operative
NS: Normal saline
Pt- Patient
Pts: Patients
RB: Red blood cells

## How NOT to use this book

## Last words

## Abbreviations Commonly Used

ATLS: Advanced Trauma Life Support
BP: Blood pressure
CT: Computerized tomography scan
Dx: Diagnosis
ExFix: External fixation
ER: External rotation
FFP: Fresh frozen plasma
Fx: Fracture
IMN: Intramedullary nailing
IR: Internal rotation
Inc: Incorporated
L: liter
ORIF: Open reduction internal fixation
Post-Op: Postoperatively
NS: Normal saline
Pt: Patient
Pts: Patients
RBC: Red blood cells

# TRAUMA

# CHAPTER 1

## General Principles

**What does the primary assessment of a polytrauma patient consist of?**

- ABCDE
- Airway- Are they talking? Intubated? C-Spine stabilization
- Breathing- Pneumothorax present?
- Circulation - Pulses present?
- Disability - Neuro exam, assess level of consciousness
- Exposure - Expose skin, keep patient warm
  - *ATLS protocol improves outcomes & decreased errors*

**What does fluid resuscitation consist of?**

- 2 large bore catheter placement, 2L infusion of NS
- If no response after 2L crystalloid > 2 units PRBCs
  - *1:1:1 ratio of PRBC, FFP, and platelets* (Coagulopathy w/ just RBC's)

**What are the complications seen with massive blood transfusions?**

- Dilutional thrombocytopenia > hypothermia > metabolic alkalosis
- Hypocalcemia (from citrate in RBC binding to Ca2+)

**Trauma 1: 9:05**

**What is the best measure of adequate resuscitation?**

- Base deficit, measured by lactate level (<2.5 considered adequate)
- Others: Urine output >1mL/kg/hr, stable hemodynamics, normal coagulation

**What classes of hemorrhagic shock require blood product administration (+crystalloid)?**

- Class III/IV

**What's the difference between class II/III shock**

- Class III shock: ~30% blood loss, HR>120, BP decreased, respirations 30-40, urinary output 5-15mL/hr
- Class II shock: Tachycardia <120, blood pressure normal

**What's class IV shock?**

- >40% blood loss, >140HR, dec BP, negligible urine output

**What is SIRS?**

- Systemic inflammatory response syndrome
- Increase in cytokines, complement, + hormones
- HR >90, WBC>12 or<4, RR>20/min, T<36° or >38°

**What is Damage Control Orthopaedics (DCO)?**

- Staging definitive care of the patient to avoid adding to overall trauma
- After trauma there is a surge of inflammatory mediators > ARDS/SIRS

Trauma 1: 19:18

**What are some conditions that should be treated in the severely injured polytrauma patient?**

- Compartment syndrome, open fx, unstable spine fx, unreduced dislocations
- Temporary stabilization (ex fix)

(Vallier, 2013)

**What is early appropriate care (EAC)?**

- Definitive management of unstable fx of the: pelvis, acetabulum, prox femur, femoral shaft + spine within 36 hours if pts demonstrate response to resuscitation w/ lactate <4, pH>7.25, base excess <25.5mmol/L

**What does EAC lead to?**

- Fewer ICU days stay, fewer complications, less costs, shorter hospital stay & time to surgery

**What position should a pregnant pt >20 weeks gestation be placed into?**

- Left lateral decubitus (relieve pressure off IVC)

**In polytrauma, are women or men more affected psychologically?**

- Women show higher rates of PTSD and take more sick leave time at 10 years after traumatic event

**What is the treatment for snake bites?**

- Antivenom

**What is the initial treatment of chemical burns?**

- Irrigation > debridement

Trauma 2: 4:47

**What is the gustillo anderson classification for open fractures?**

- Type I - <1cm
- Type II- 1-10cm
- Type III- >10cm
    - A- Periosteal stripping
    - B- Soft tissue flap required, extensive periosteal stripping
    - C- Vascular repair required

**What antibiotics (abx) should you give for an open fracture?**

- Type I and II- 1st generation cephalosporin
- Type III- 1st generation cephalosporin and aminoglycoside or fluoroquinolone
    - + updated tetanus

**What abx to give if there is a farm injury?**

- Penicillin to cover clostridium

**What abx to give if there is exposure to saltwater/brackish water?**

- Broad spectrum cephalosporin + tetracycline or fluoroquinolone
    - *Higher contamination with vibrio, pseudomonas, and mycobacterium

**What abx to give if there is exposure to an open wound with freshwater?**
- Fluoroquinolone or 3rd or 4th generation cephalosporin

**What abx to give if there is an open pelvic fx w/ bowel injury?**
- 3rd generation cephalosporin (ex: cefotetan)

**Is a delay in abx associated with infection?**
- YES

**What is the general treatment for open fractures?**
- **Antibiotics**, Irrigation & debridement (I&D), + bony stabilization
- Urgent thorough I&D is important to decrease infection risk

**Trauma 2: 14:00**

**When should an I&D be performed in patients w/ open fx?**
- Within 12-24 hours is appropriate, is what most evidence supports

**Is there any benefit to irrigating with pulsatile lavage in open fx?**
- No. Saline is typically used
- Soap in the irrigation fluid leads to a higher re-operation rate

**Should you get primary wound cultures at first I&D for an open fx?**
- No, they have no value in managing patients who have an infection after an open long bone fx

**Should the wound coverage for an open fx goal be late coverage (>10 days) or early coverage (<5 days)?**
- Early coverage <5 days, once zone of injury is defined

**What type of soft tissue flap is typically used for wound coverage in proximal ⅓ tibia shaft fractures?**
- Gastrocnemius flap
- Soleus flap—for middle ⅓
- Fasciculo cutaneous flap or free tissue transfer- distal ⅓

**How can you manage an open fx w/ bone defects?**
- Masquelet (induced membrane technique), distraction osteogenesis, bone transport

**What is the induced membrane technique?**
- 2 stage technique to handle defects up to >20cm
- Stage 1: polymethylmethacrylate spacer placed in defect - produces bioactive membrane
- Stage 2- spacer removal + cancellous autograft placement Membrane prevents resorption

**Trauma 2: 21:42**

**What is the pathophysiology of Compartment syndrome?**
- Traumatic insult > muscle swelling > increased (inc) compartment pressures > inc venous pressure > ***decreased venous outflow***,
  - The arterial flow is unchanged > dec tissue perfusion > continued muscle injury

**What are some symptoms of compartment syndrome?**

- *Clinical diagnosis*
- Pain out of proportion, pain w/ PROM, paresthesias -later, motor deficits- later, pulseless is very late

**How do you test for compartment syndrome in the polytrauma obtunded patient?**

- Intracompartmental pressure within 30mmHg from diastolic
- Diastolic pressure can be lower under anesthesia (avg 18mmHg)

(Richardson, 2012), (Stannard, 2012)

**How does negative pressure wound therapy work?**

- Removes excess interstitial fluid > promotes local vascularity > inc granulation tissue formation
- Reduces deep infection in open tibia fx
- Higher rate of wound closure w/ use in fasciotomy + inc wound perfusion
- Dec wound dehiscence and infection w/ use in high risk surgery (pilon/plateau/calc)
- It does NOT decrease bacteria

# UPPER EXTREMITY

## Sternoclavicular Joint

**What's the best view to see a SC joint dislocation?**

- Serendipity xray view (40 degree cephalic tilt), or CT scan

**Is anterior or posterior SC dislocation more common?**

- Anterior, likely to be unstable but also asymptomatic
    - Tx non op w/ closed reduction + figure 8 brace if stable

Trauma 3: 3:54

**What are some possible symptoms of a posterior SC dislocation?**

- Dysphagia, difficulty breathing, throat fullness
- 30% have compressive dysfunction

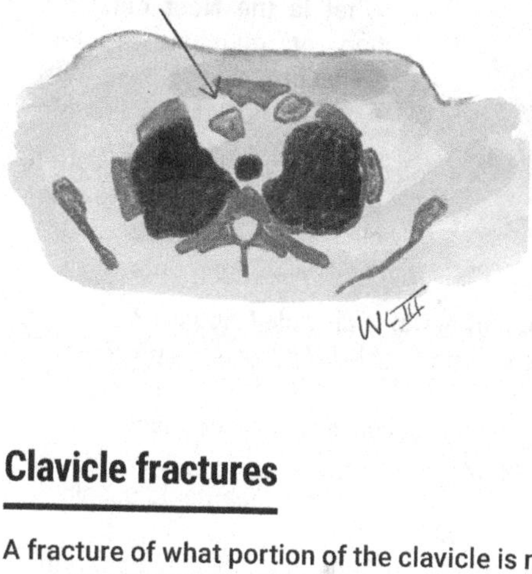


**Figure 1.1: Axial cut of a CT scan showing a posterior sternoclavicular joint dislocation. The arrow is pointing to where the clavicle should be and you can note the displacement.**

**What's the treatment of posterior SC joint dislocation?**

- In OR under anesthesia
- Closed v open reduction w/ towel clip or fingers
- Thoracic surgeon on standby- may not be needed

## Clavicle fractures

**A fracture of what portion of the clavicle is most common?**

- Midshaft 80%, 15% distal ⅓, 5% medial

**What other injuries are OPEN clavicle fractures associated with?**

- Pulmonary + closed head injuries

**What are risks for non-union (~15%) in midshaft clavicle fractures?**

- Female
- Elderly
- Comminution
- Shortening >2cm
- Displacement

**What are the typical non-operative indications and treatment for midshaft clavicle fractures?**

- <2cm shortening/displacement, <100% displacement

- Figure of 8 brace and sling are equivalent
- Decreased shoulder endurance/strength with healed fracture >2cm shortened

**What are some absolute indications for operative treatment of midshaft clavicle fractures?**

- Open fracture, impending open fracture, associated neurovascular injury

**What are some relative indications for operative treatment of midshaft clavicle fractures?**

- Floating shoulder, shortening >2cm, complete displacement, comminution, symptomatic nonunion

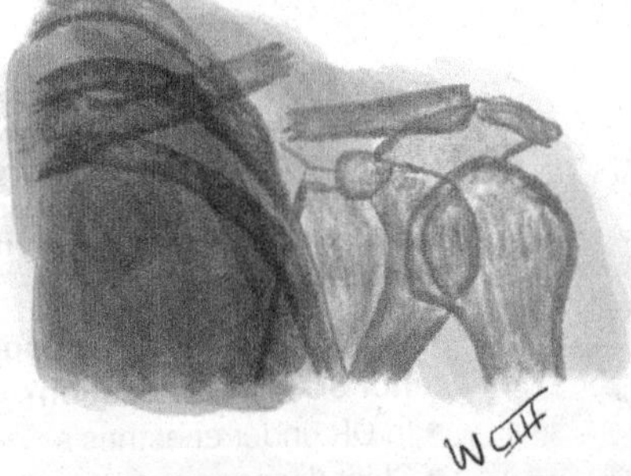

**Figure 1.2: AP of the shoulder showing a completely displaced midshaft clavicle fracture.**

**What is the Neer classification of midshaft fractures based on?**

- > or < 100% displacement

**What structures contribute to the stability of distal ⅓ clavicle fractures?**

- AC + CC ligaments

Trauma 3: 17:37

**What is the Neer classification of distal ⅓ clavicle fractures?**

- Type 1: Lateral to CC ligaments- stable w/ minimal displacement- tx: non op
- Type 2A: Medial to CC ligaments- usually displaced- assoc w/ >50 % nonunion rate if non-op tx
- Type 2B: Between or lateral to CC ligaments- ligaments usually torn- unstable- typically operative
- Type 3: Lateral to CC ligaments- extends to AC joint- usually non-op- high risk arthritis
- Type 4: Pediatric distal ⅓ physeal fracture, usually non-op
- Type 5: comminuted with displacement, CC ligaments usually intact but comminution warrants ORIF

**What is the operative decision for distal clavicle fx based on?**

- Amount of displacement + patient demands
- In elderly w/ displaced fx: sling + early ROM is typically first tx

(Wilkerson, 2017)

**When undergoing operative tx for clavicle fx, what's the difference w/ anterior vs superior plating? (using a 3.5 LC-DCP plate)**

- Anterior plating-superior strength and durability (based on a cadaver study)
  - BUT other studies show higher load to failure w/ superior plating- so it's debatable

- Superior plating- assoc w/ more plate prominence + higher removal rates. Also assoc w/ inc subclavian penetration + shorter screw lengths
- Similar union rates between anterior/superior plating

**What is the usual post-op rehab (for ORIF clavicle fx)?**
- Strengthening at 6 weeks, return to sport at about 3 months

## Acromioclavicular Joint

**What is the best view to visualize an AC joint injury?**
- Zanca view (10 deg cephalic tilt)

**What part of the AC joint capsule is the strongest?**
- Posterior + superior (resist posterior displacement)

**What ligaments are typically disrupted in AC joints injuries?**
- AC & CC (conoid + trapezoid) ligaments

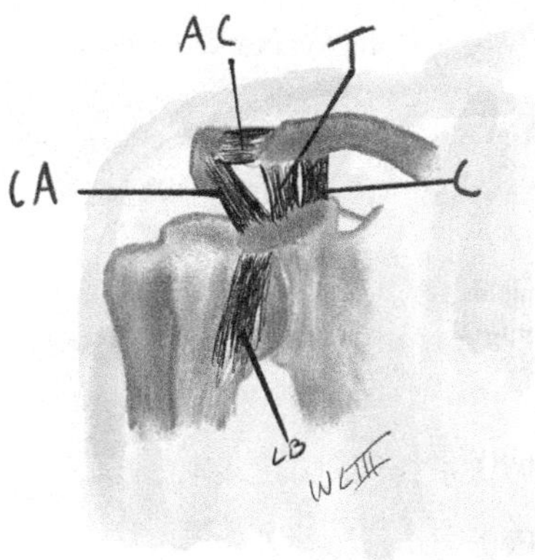


**Figure 1.3: Photo of a shoulder showing the ligament in the shoulder. T- trapezoid ligament, C-conoid ligament, AC- acromio-clavicular ligaments, CA- coracoacromial ligament, CB- coracobrachialis tendon**

**What type of injury occurs when both ligaments are torn?**
- *Type III*
- Type II-AC ligaments ruptured, CC sprained
- Type I- AC joint sprain
- Type IV-VI (PSI- posterior, superior, inferior)

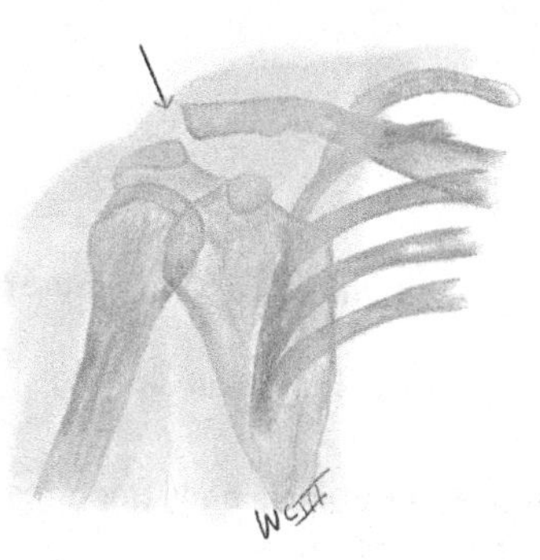


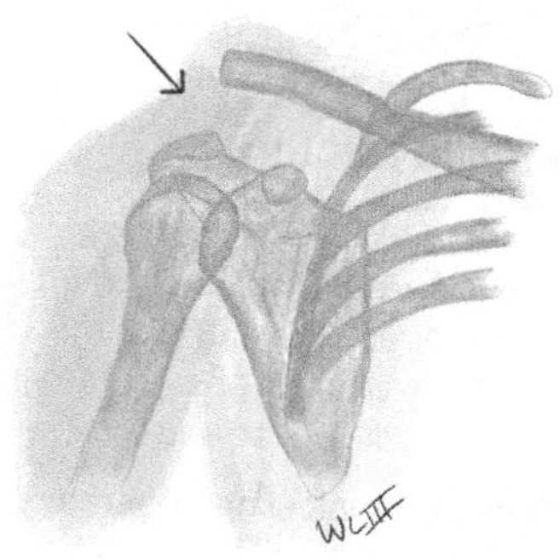


**Figure(s) 1.4 & 1.5: AP of the shoulder showing an AC joint injury with partial (1.4) and complete (1.5) displacement.**

**What is the typical treatment for type I-II AC joint injuries?**

- Non-op w/ sling 7-10 days then early ROM

**What is the treatment for type III injuries?**

- Controversial, start w/ non-op

(Petri, 2016)

**Are there any differences in operative v non-op management in type III injuries?**

- Operative group- better cosmesis + greater duration sick leave
- Non-op group- return to work quicker
- No difference in strength, pain, ability to throw overhead, or AC joint arthritis

**What type AC injuries are usually treated operatively?**

- IV-VI, however some studies show similar outcomes between op vs non-op

(Society, 2015)

**What are some fixation options for AC injuries?**

- CC fixation: type of suspensory fixation (numerous available options)
- AC fixation: hook plate
- Some combine the two. CC fixation only leads to anterior clavicle translation
- Modified weaver dunn- (CA ligament transfer to distal clavicle + augmented)

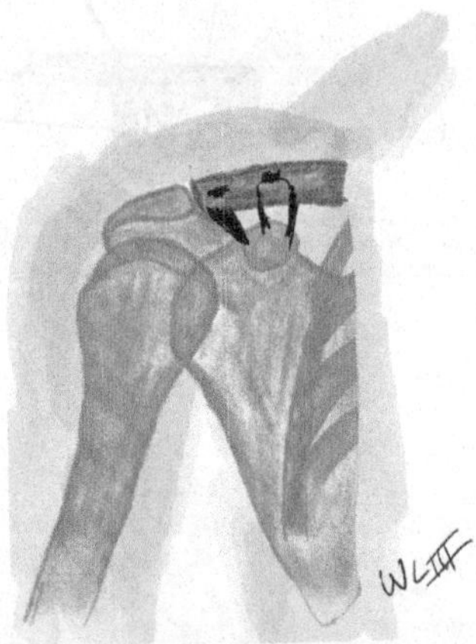

**Figure 1.6: AP of the shoulder showing an example of the modified weaver dunn procedure. The CA ligament has been transferred to the distal clavicle and augmented.**

**Should you operate on a Type IV AC injury in a skeletally immature patient?**

- No, it's likely a distal clavicle fx. Periosteal sleeve is intact and ligaments remain attached

## Scapula fractures

**What is the most common fracture associated with a scapula fracture?**

- Rib fractures ~53 % of the time
- Other injuries: pneumothorax, clavicle fx/AC separation (floating shoulder), head and brachial plexus injuries

**What is the typical non-operative treatment for scapula body fractures?**

- Sling immobilization for 7-10 days followed by ROM

**What are the indications to operate on a scapular body fracture?**

- Medial/lateral displacement >20mm, glenopolar angle <20 degrees (normal ~40), body angulation >45 degrees

(Schroder, 2016)

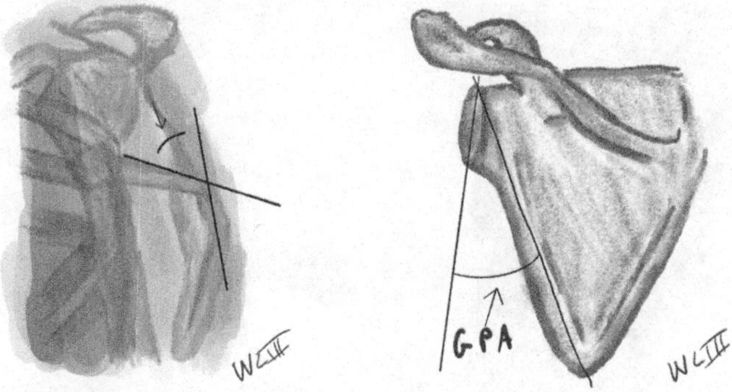


**Figure(s) 1.7 & 1.8: Scapular-Y film (1.7) showing the degrees of scapula sagittal plane deformity along with AP of the scapula (1.8) showing the glenopolar angle (GPA).**

**What is the interval used in the posterior Judet approach for scapula fx?**

**Trauma 4: 5:00**

- Infraspinatus and teres minor (Suprascapular nerve & axillary nerve)
- Circumflex artery at risk during approach

**What are the operative indications for glenoid fractures?**

- Intra articular step off >3-10mm, involvement of 20-30%+ of articular surface, glenohumeral joint instability (persistent HH subluxation)

**What injuries are associated with scapulothoracic dissociation?**

- Brachial plexus avulsion, subclavian/axillary artery injury, clavicle fracture, AC/SC dislocation
- 10% mortality rate

**What is the functional outcome of scapulothoracic dissociation based on?**

- Severity of neurological injury

**What should you look for on CXR in cases of scapulothoracic dissociation?**

- Distance from spinous process to medial scapula border, compare both sides

## Shoulder dislocations

**What is the most common position the arm is in when there is an anterior shoulder dislocation?**

- Arm abduction and external rotation

**What xray view can help diagnose an anterior shoulder dislocation?**

- Axillary

**What is the most common neuropraxia seen with anterior shoulder dislocation?**

- Axillary n

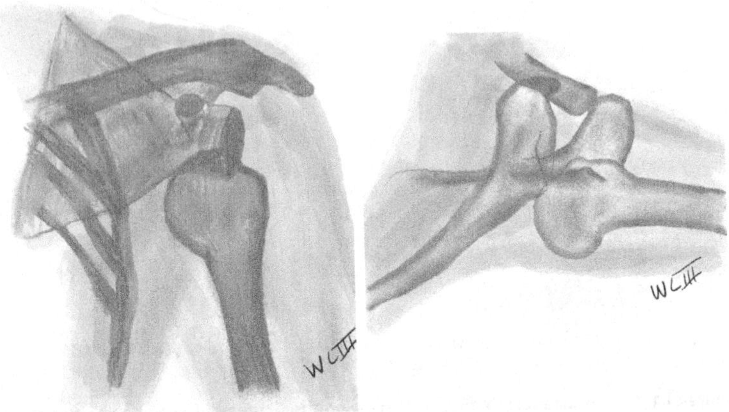

**Figure(s) 1.9 & 1.10: Figure 1.9 shows an AP of the shoulder with an anterior-inferior shoulder dislocation. Figure 1.10 is an axial view showing a posterior shoulder dislocation.**

**What is the most common injury after acute anterior shoulder dislocation in a young pt?**

- Anterior labral tear > anterior capsular insufficiency + hill sachs lesion

**What is a common injury seen in older patients (>50 y/o) after acute shoulder dislocation?**

- Rotator cuff tear

**What is the treatment for an acute shoulder dislocation?**

- Reduce + sling for 2-4 weeks followed by PT

**What is an important PE finding in posterior shoulder dislocations?**

- Lack of ER

**What key components of the history are common in patients with posterior dislocations?**

- Seizures or electrical shock

Trauma 4: 18:30

**What are some associated bony lesions that can be seen in posterior shoulder dislocations?**

- Lesser tuberosity fracture or reverse hill sachs lesion
- Soft tissue lesions: Posterior labral tears

**What is the typical position of the arm seen in inferior shoulder dislocations? (Luxatio erecta)**

- Arm abduction 100-160 degrees
- Assoc w/ neurovascular injury

## Proximal Humerus fractures

**What are the four parts of a proximal humerus fracture ? (Neer)**

- Articular surface, shaft, greater tuberosity, lesser tuberosity
- Displacement >1cm, >45 degrees

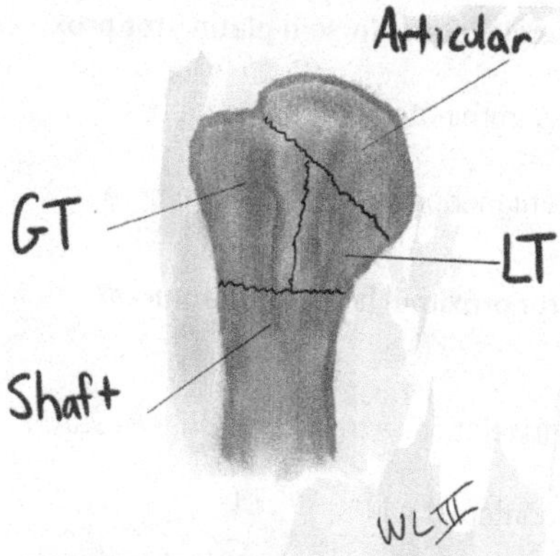


**Figure 1.11: The four parts to a proximal humerus, the greater tuberosity (GT), lesser tuberosity (LT), shaft, and articular segment.**

**What are the factors associated with humeral head ischemia? (Hertel criteria)**

- Medial periosteal hinge disruption
- Medial metadiaphyseal extension <8mm
- 4 part fracture
- Increasing complexity pattern
- >1cm displacement & angulation >45 degrees (less important)
- (they also noted posterior circumflex vessels alone may be sufficient for head survival)

**(Hertel, 2004)**

**What is the single greatest predictor of humeral head AVN after proximal humerus fracture?**

- Calcar length <8mm

**What is the tx for a one part (humeral neck, minimal displacement) fx?**

- Sling + early ROM

**What is the tx of an isolated greater tuberosity fracture w/ >5-10mm displacement?**

- ORIF (young), nonabsorbable sutures in older pts

**What motion is blocked in isolated GT fractures, and why?**

- ER and abduction
- Fx is displaced superior + posterior due to RTC

**Trauma 5: 1:26**

**What is the treatment for stable (<50% displaced or impacted) 2 part proximal humerus fractures?**

- Sling followed by PT
- Early rehab > inc outcomes and dec pain

**When would you consider operative tx for a 2 part proximal humerus fracture?**

- Considerable displacement, block to ROM, anatomical neck involvement

**What are some surgical options for displaced 2 part proximal humerus fxs in the young pt?**

- CRPP (less common), ORIF w/ locked plating, IMN (medial entry v straight nail)

**What are two things you should consider when fixing proximal humerus fractures?**

- Bone stock + blood supply

**What is an advantage to using fixed angle lateral locked plating for proximal humerus fractures?**
- It allows more secure fixation in comminuted/osteoporitic bone
- ORIF in physiologically young
- *Better functional outcomes and higher patient satisfaction compared w/ hemiarthroplasty*

**What are some key points with ORIF for proximal humerus fractures?**
- Reduce the tuberosities
- Avoid varus malreduction
- Anatomic reduction of the head in relation to the shaft- reduces varus malalignment
- Medial cortical buttress helps counteract varus*

**What are some risk factors for loss of reduction in proximal humerus fractures?**
- Humeral head varus, varus malreduction, lack of medial cortical support, osteoporosis, local BMD, age

**What are some options to help with preventing varus collapse in pts w/ high comminution?**
- Fibula allograft - also helps restore medial cortical support

**What is a surgical option for patients w/ a varus malunion w/o GH degenerative joint changes?**
- Valgus producing osteotomy

**What neurovascular structures are at risk with the lateral and deltopectoral approaches?**
- Lateral- axillary nerve
- Deltopec approach- Cephalic vein, musculocutaneous nerve (medially)

**What are some key points w/ plating for proximal humerus fractures?**
- Place plate lateral to biceps tuberosity
- Use calcar screws for medial support

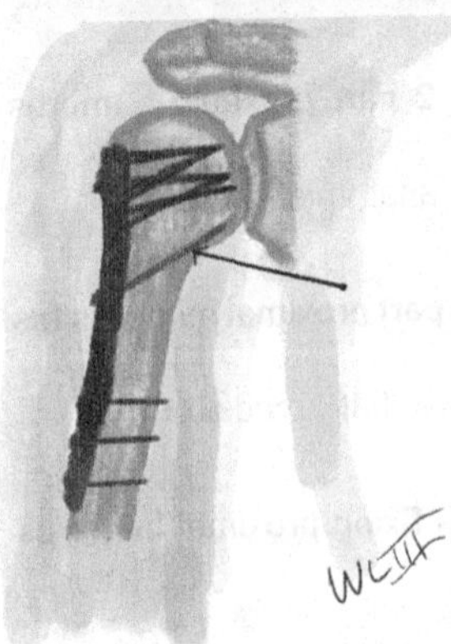


**Figure 1.12: AP of the shoulder showing lateral locked plating of a previous proximal humeral shaft fracture. The arrow is pointing to a screw placed along the calcar to help with medial cortical support.**

**What are common complications after plating proximal humerus fx?**
- Screw cutout, osteonecrosis

**What are common complications after IMN for proximal humerus fx?**
- Shoulder pain (RTC violation), rod migration, nonunion, malunion
- IMN found to be equivalent to locked plating

**Do all 3 and 4 part proximal humerus fractures need operative tx?**
- No, elderly patients/low demand can be treated non-op
- Similar outcomes between op v non-op tx of displaced prox humerus fx
- Young healthy patients w/ good bone stock- ORIF

**What is a surgical tx option in the eldery pt w/ 3 or 4 part proximal humerus fx?**
- Hemiarthroplasty (need a functioning RTC, + healed anatomically reduced tuberosities)

**Why is it important that the tuberosities be healed in proximal humerus fx for hemiarthroplasty?**
- Motion is restricted w/ nonunion
- Component too high- dec abduction and elevation
- Component too lateral- inhibits ER

**How can you judge humeral height in shoulder arthroplasty?**
- Superior border of pec major tendon, HH is 5.6cm proximal

**Trauma 5: 18:25**

**What are the indications for reverse TSA?**
- Old patients w/ 3 or 4 part fx w/ comminuted tuberosities, revision of failed fixation, sequelae of fracture (nonunion/malunion) rotator cuff arthropathy,

**What are the mechanics of R-TSA, that makes it usable in pts w/ comminuted tuberosities/RTC incompetence?**
- RTSA medializes the glenohumeral center of rotation & increases the deltoid level arm (Grammont Style)

## Humeral Shaft fractures

**What is the acceptable alignment for good function for humeral shaft fractures?**
- 30 deg varus/valgus, 20 deg anterior angulation, 15 degrees malrotation, 3cm shortening (after reduction)

**What is the treatment of choice for a closed humeral shaft fx within acceptable alignment?**
- Coaptation splint followed by functional bracing (sarmiento)
- Excellent outcomes- up to 90% union
- Secondary bone healing

**What is the most common reason for conversion from non-op to op tx for humeral shaft fx?**
- Nonunion (around 6 weeks, movement at fx site)

**What are the contraindications for functional bracing for humeral shaft fractures?**

**(Rämö, 2020)**

- Brachial plexus injury
- Severe soft tissue injury / bony loss

- Vascular injury requiring repair
- Inability to maintain reduction
- NOT comminution
- NOT radial nerve palsy

Trauma 5: 27:30

**What are the absolute indications for operative intervention of humeral shaft fractures?**
- Open fracture, intra-articular extension, vascular injury, floating elbow

**What are some relative indications for operative intervention of humeral shaft fractures?**
- Impending pathologic fracture, failure of closed management (not tolerated or reduction not held), polytrauma (allows WB), bilateral humerus fractures

**Is there any advantage to using a 4.5mm DCP plate for humeral shaft fx in the polytrauma patient?**
- Yes, it allows early safe weight bearing through the extremity

**What are some approaches and uses for humeral shaft fractures?**
- Anterolateral approach- proximal ⅔ fx
- Anterior- Biceps is medial- brachialis is split deep (innervated by MC nerve + radial N)
- Lateral- useful in distal ⅓- Radial n at risk
- Posterior- Triceps split v sparing- axillary nerve is proximal limit

**What is the typical treatment for ORIF of a humeral shaft fx?**
- 4.5 DCP plate w/ 3-4 screw on each side (8 cortices)- used as neutralization
- Lag screw if fx line is amenable to primary bone healing
- Bridge fx if comminuted

**What are the IMN options for humeral shaft fractures, and structures at risk during distal interlock screw placement?**
- Anterograde - Shoulder issues - Entry is through RTC, alternative approach through rotator interval
- Retrograde - Entry is proximal to olecranon fossa
- Radial nerve - lateral to medial screw
- Musculocutaneous nerve - A-P screws
  - *decreased sensation in volar lateral forearm*

Trauma 6: 4:59

**What is the difference in outcomes and union rates for plating vs intramedullary nailing for humeral shaft fractures?**
- Similar union + functional outcomes between the two
- Some studies show IMN associated w/ shoulder impingement & need for reoperation (IMN removal)
- ORIF may be the gold standard? Some conflicting studies

(Bhandari, 2006)
(Kurup, 2011)

**In patients w/ radial nerve palsy (occurs around 22% of the time) and an associated humeral shaft fx, how long does it take for nerve function to return?**

- 3-6 months, 92% resolve
- EMG at 6 weeks (controversial)

**What are the first and last muscles to return in cases of radial n palsy?**

- Brachioradialis - returns first
- EPL + EIP- returns last

**What are indications to acutely explore a radial nerve ?**

- Open fx, vascular injury, high velocity gunshot or penetrating wound
- Nerve deficit after closed reduction and distal ⅓ fractures (controversial)

**How often do you find a radial n palsy in distal ⅓ humerus fractures?**

- ~20% of the time

**How do you treat humeral shaft nonunion?**

- 1st determine nonunion type (atrophic, hypertrophic, oligotrophic)
- Atrophic- Plate + graft (needs stability + biology)
- Hypertrophic- Plate (needs stability)

## Distal Humerus fractures

**What are the groups of different distal humerus fractures?**

- Supracondylar, distal single column fractures, distal bicolumnal fractures

**What imaging can be used to assist with pre-op planning in comminuted, displaced intra-articular distal humerus fractures?**

- Xray: traction views
- CT scan

**What is the classification system for single column (condyle) distal humerus fx?**

- Milch, for both medial and lateral column fractures
- Milch I: trochlear ridge intact
- Milch II: trochlear ridge not intact (elbow stability compromised)

**What is the treatment for single column fractures?**

- Milch I- non displaced: immobilization (in supination for lateral column, pronation for medial)
- Milch I- displaced- ORIF v CRPP
- Milch II- ORIF

**What is the goal of treatment in intra-articular distal humerus fractures?**

- Early ROM w/ <3 weeks of immobilization

**In the plating of intra articular distal humerus fractures, what plate configuration has been shown to be biomechanically strongest?**

- Parallel plating- in comparison to orthogonal (90-90)

- Literature supports use of both

**What are some of the different options for the posterior approach for distal humerus fractures?**

- Triceps on (para tricipital, splitting)
- Triceps off (reflecting, tongue)
- Olecranon osteotomy (provides the best visualization of the distal humerus)

**When performing an olecranon osteotomy, which type of cut provides the most stability?**

- Chevron osteotomy (more stable than transverse or oblique osteotomy)
- Perform cut at least 2cm distal to triceps insertion **

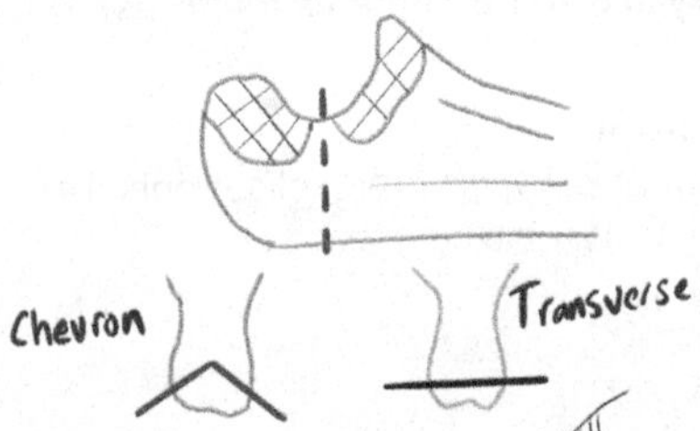


**Figure 1.13: Chevron v transverse cut orientation when performing an olecranon osteotomy. Chevron osteotomy offers more stability, and the cut should be in the articular bare area (dashed line).**

**Is there any benefit from ulnar nerve transposition during ORIF?**

- No

Trauma 6: 18:50

**What's the difference between TEA and ORIF for comminuted intra-articular distal humerus fractures in the elderly, low demand patient?**

- TEA has improved function and decreased re-operation rates

(Mckee, 2009)

**Should you do an olecranon osteotomy in the elderly patient you are considering doing a TEA on?**

- No, you will have issues with component fixation
- Preserve the proximal ulna- triceps sparing approach ok

**What is the most common complication following distal humerus ORIF?**

- Stiffness

**What is the classification system for fractures of the capitellum?**

- Bryan Morrey
  - Type I - complete capitellum fx
  - Type II- shear fracture of articular cartilage
  - Type III- comminuted capitellum fx
  - Type IV- coronal shear including capitellum and trochlea

**What is the treatment for capitellum fractures?**

- Nondisplaced- splint
- Displaced >2mm- ORIF
- Comminuted- fragment excision

**What is the recommended approach for type IV capitellum fractures?**

- Lateral approach, +/- osteotomy

## Olecranon

**What is the treatment of a non-displaced olecranon fracture?**

- Rare, splint at 60-90 deg flexion for 7-10 days, then ROM

**What is the treatment of a displaced, non-comminuted olecranon fracture?**

- Tension band wiring (tensile forces > compressive)
- Plate

**What's the difference between K-wires placed in the medullary canal vs penetrate the cortex in olecranon fx?**

- K wires that penetrate cortex assoc w/ risk for diminished rotation + AIN injury
    - They are less likely to back out though

**In older, low demand patients with displaced olecranon fx, is operative tx better than non-op?**

- No, satisfactory short and long term outcomes were noted in patients treated operatively and non-operatively

**What is a surgical option for proximal olecranon fractures that are not reconstructable in a low demand patient?**

- Fragment excision w/ triceps advancement
- Attaching tendon close to articular surface helps w/ stability

**(Duckworth, 2014)**

**What are some complications after ORIF of olecranon fx?**

- Decreased ROM
- Some patients have hardware prominence that require re-operation

## Coronoid fractures

**What are 2 classification systems for coronoid process fractures?**

- Regan & Morrey: Type 1- Tip fx (shear), Type 2- <50% coronoid, Type 3- >50% coronoid
- O' Driscoll: Tip, anteromedial process, basal

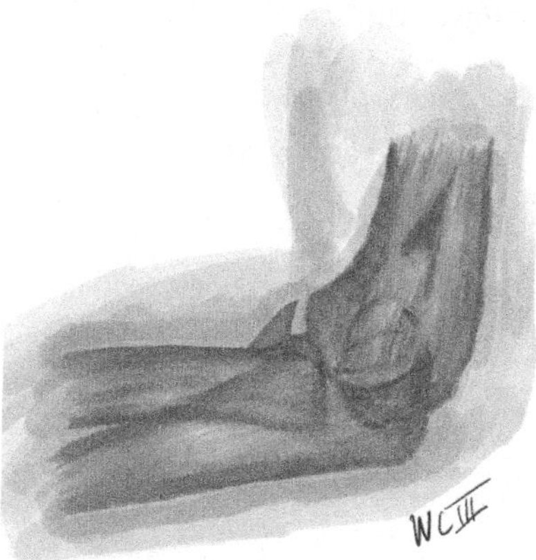

**Figure 1.14: Lateral film of the elbow showing a coronoid process fracture. The coronoid process serves as an attachment site for the anterior capsule and contributes to elbow stability.**

**Why are coronoid process fx important?**

- Assists w/ anterior stability
- Anterior bundle of MCL + anterior capsule attachment site

Trauma 7: 2:25

**What type of instability is associated with anteromedial process fractures?**

- Posteromedial instability (injury due to a varus + PM force)
- Injury is where Anterior bundle of MCL

**What should you consider when considering operative intervention for coronoid process fractures?**

- Elbow stability
- If elbow instability in Type 1 fx- fix (sutures through drill holes, many techniques)
- Type 2 + 3- ORIF for elbow stability

## Radial Head fractures

**What is the classification + associated treatment for radial head fractures?**

- Mason 1- nondisplaced - Tx w/ early ROM
- Mason 2- partial articulation w/ displacement >2mm- Tx non Op w/ ROM unless block to ROM + instability > ORIF
- Mason 3- Comminuted fractures involving head/neck- ORIF if <3 pieces, if severe comminution do radial head arthroplasty (most use metal), excision in low demand elderly patients
- Mason 4- Radial head + monteggia variant- Same as 3

**What are common approaches used for ORIF of radial head fx and their intervals?**

- Kocher- ECU/Anconeus- more risk LUCL injury than Kaplan
- Kaplan- ECRL/ECRB- more anterior- less risk LUCL
- Pronation during approach protects PIN

**What are some predictors of worse patient outcomes in patients w/ radial head fractures?**

- Displacement >4mm (worse DASH scores)
- Socioeconomic deprivation, Increasing age, numerous comorbidities, active Workers Compensation

(Duckworth, 2014)

**What is the safe zone for radial head/neck ORIF?**

- Posterolateral area- between radial styloid and longitudinal line along lister's tubercle ~ 110 degree area of non articulation

**What is a common complication with radial head arthroplasty?**

- Overstuffing the joint

**What is an essex-lopresti lesion?**

- Radial head fx/ DRUJ dislocation/ interosseous membrane rupture
- Due to an axial load on the limb

**What should you do with the radial head fx in an Essex-Lopresti injury?**

- ORIF v arthroplasty
- +/- DRUJ fixation

# Elbow dislocations

### What is the classification of elbow dislocations based on?
- Direction of dislocation
- Posterolateral dislocation most common (80%), anterior, medial, posterior, lateral, and divergent are less common

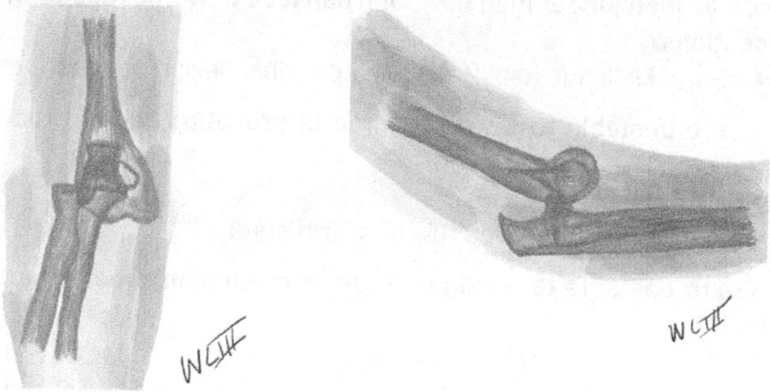

**Figure 1.15 & 1.16: AP and Lateral films of an elbow showing a postero-lateral elbow dislocation. This is the most common dislocation direction.**

### What is the mechanism of injury in elbow dislocation?
- Circle of horii disruption, begins laterally and progresses medially in 3 stages

### What are the 3 stages of collapse in elbow dislocations?
- Stage 1- PLRI instability- complete/partial LCL disruption
- Stage 2- Perched ulna- anterior/posterior capsule disruption
- Stage 3- Dislocation- complete/partial tear of MCL anterior band

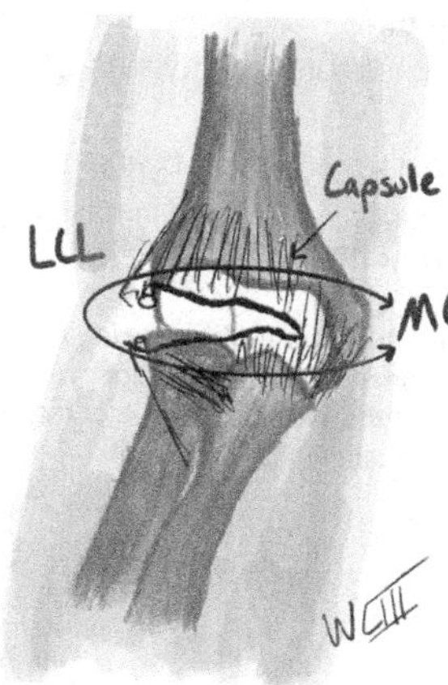


**Figure 1.17: Image showing the circle of horii disruption, with the injury beginning laterally with LCL disruption, followed by capsule disruption and then eventual MCL disruption.**

### What are some important things to note about the anterior band of the MCL?
- Primary medial stabilizer from 20-120 degrees, resists valgus stress
- Insertion is on the sublime tubercle

### What are some important things to note about the posterior band of the MCL?
- Problems with flexion occur if the posterior band is contracted

**Trauma 7: 19:28**

**What is the treatment for an elbow dislocation?**

- Acute reduction + splint application
- Short period (~7 days) of immobilization followed by ROM for stable dislocations
- Longer period of immobilization followed by ROM in hinged brace for unstable dislocations

**Immobilization longer than how long can lead to worse results with elbow dislocations?**

- >3 weeks- leads to stiffness and possible flexion contractures

**If you are unstable to a valgus force in pronation, what structures are injured?**

- MCL + LUCL
- Pronation- tightens lateral sided structures

**If you are unstable to a valgus force in supination, what structures are injured?**

- LUCL, with a possible MCL injury

**What forces will aggravate a patient with post-traumatic PLRI?**

- Valgus, supination + axial load (sitting up from a chair)
- Tx w/ LUCL reconstruction

**What consists of a terrible triad injury?**

- Elbow dislocation + radial head fx + coronoid process fx
- Operative tx is indicated

**What is a common approach for fixing terrible triad injuries?**

- Start medial + work lateral
- Fix coronoid > radial head > LUCL repair/reconstruct
    - If continued instability > MCL repair

**Ep 35**
**w/ Dr. Mauricio**

**What is a transolecranon fracture dislocation?**

- Anterior elbow dislocation where distal humerus is driven through olecranon (PRUJ intact)
- Fix the proximal ulna fx and restore contour + dimensions of trochlear notch > good results

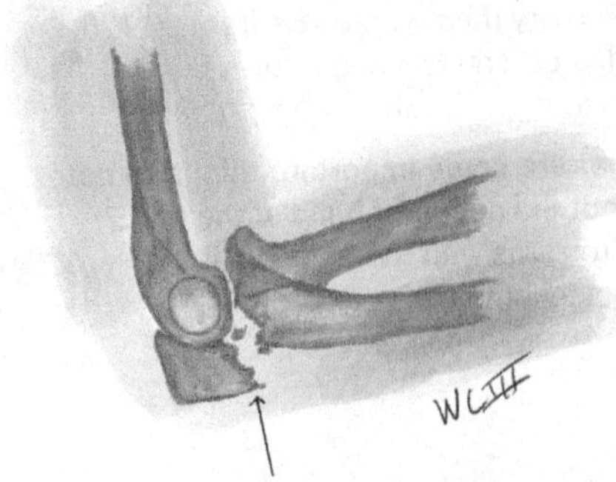

**Figure 1.18: Lateral film showing a transolecranon fracture dislocation. You can note that the PRUJ is still intact but the radiocapitellar joint is dislocated.**

## Forearm fractures

**What is a Monteggia fracture?**
- Radial head dislocation w/ proximal ulna fx

**What is a Monteggia variant or equivalent?**
- Radial head fx- instead/in addition to dislocation

**If the radial head does not reduce when fixing a monteggia fracture, what is a likely problem?**
- Malreduction of the ulna

**What is a Galeazzi fracture?**
- Radius fracture w/ DRUJ disruption
- Tx: ORIF radius +/- DRUJ fixation

**What is the treatment for an adult BBFA?**
- ORIF w/ 3.5 LC-DCP plate
- +/- grafting for significant bone loss
- 4.5 LC-DCP plate assoc w/ refracture after removal

**What are some complications seen w/ BBFA?**
- Malunion + Loss of rotation - restoration of radial bow is essential
- Nonunion- tx w/ ORIF + bone graft
- Refracture after plate removal (seen when plate is removed before 12-18mo have passed)
  - Brace after plate removal
- Synostosis- tx w/ excision, radiation + indomethacin. Assoc w/ a single approach for both radius and ulna

Trauma 8: 5:45

**When is ORIF indicated for isolated ulna shaft (nightstick) fractures?**
- Proximal ⅓, >10 degrees angulation, over 50% displacement

## Pelvis fractures

**What are the ligamentous connections that stabilize the pelvis?**
- Posterior SI complex: Interosseous SI ligaments, Anterior/Posterior SI ligaments, iliolumbar ligaments
  - Posterior SI ligaments- strongest
- Together they resist rotational and vertical forces
- Sacrospinous ligament (transverse band from lateral sacrum to ischial spine)
- Sacrotuberous ligament (dorsal sacrum to ischial tuberosity)
  - External and vertical shear forces

**What images are necessary for evaluation?**
- AP

- Inlet: Eval AP displacement of SI joint + pelvis ER/IR
  - Used intraop for AP placement of SI screws
- Outlet: Eval vertical displacement + hemipelvis flexion
  - Used intraop for Sup/Inf placement of SI screws
- CT scan (helps classify & eval SI complex)

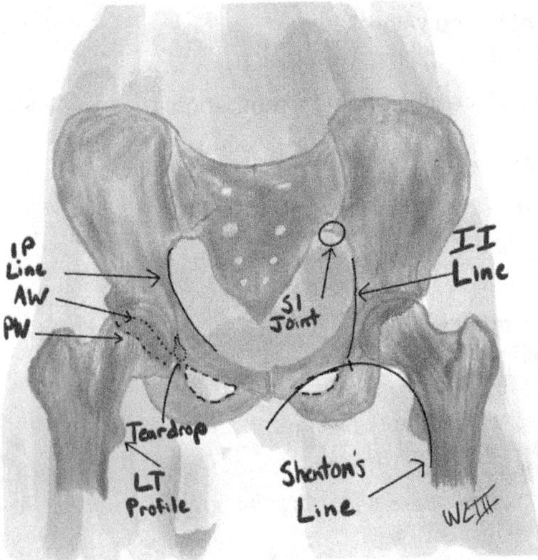


**Figure 1.19: AP of the pelvis. Symmetry of the obturator foramen (dashed lines) can be evaluated. The iliopectineal (IP) and ilioischial (II) lines can be evaluated for any discontinuity. Shenton's line can be used to help evaluate any frank hip dislocations. The anterior wall (AW) and posterior wall (PW) of the acetabulum can be assessed for any fractures. The sacroiliac joints (SI) can be evaluated for any SI dislocations of subluxations. The lesser trochanter (LT) profile can be assessed for rotation of the limb as well.**

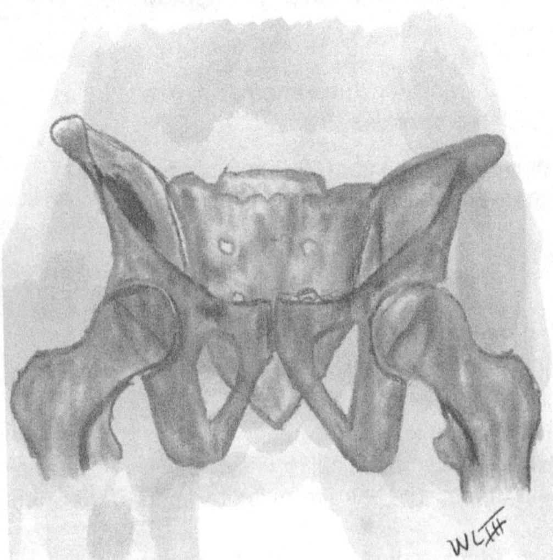

**Figure 1.20: Outlet view of the pelvis. This can help evaluate any vertical displacement of the hemipelvis. Sacral dysmorphism can also be evaluated on the outlet.**

**What is the obturator outlet view used for in pelvic fixation?**

- Supra-acetabular column screws

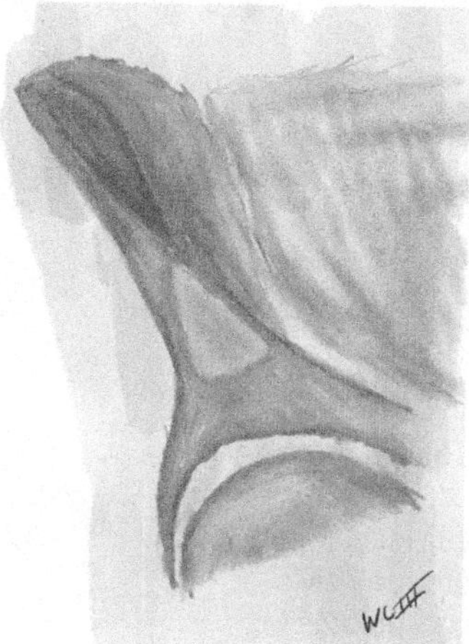


**Figure 1.21: Obturator outlet view of the pelvis.**

**What is the obturator inlet view used for in pelvic fixation?**

- Confirm pins are within inner/outer tables

**What are some things you should look for on CT scan?**

**Trauma 9: 8:05**

- SI complex
- Look for 2 areas of disruption.
  - Pelvis is a ring structure so a disruption in one area is accompanied by a disruption in another area
- Sagittal recons- Eval for kyphosis, U shaped fx, spine/pelvic dissociation
- Contrast extravasation - arterial bleed

**What are signs of sacral dysmorphism seen on AP pelvis xrays?**

- Upper sacrum is at the level of L5 disk is collinear with iliac crests

**What are signs of sacral dysmorphism seen on outlet pelvic xrays?**

- Residual mammillary process in sacral ala region
- Large, irregular sacral neural foramen
- Residual disk space between upper and 2nd sacral segment

**What are signs of sacral dysmorphism seen on the lateral of the sacrum?**

- Acute alar slope (less room for screws)

**What are signs of sacral dysmorphism seen on CT scan?**

- Tongue in groove articulations

**Why is identifying sacral dysmorphism important?**

- It may make placement of a S1 screw difficult

**What is the most likely cause of death overall in pelvic ring injuries?**

- Hemorrhage (the reason why immediate application of binder and external fixation is standard)

**What is the most likely cause of death in lateral compression pelvic ring injuries?**

- Closed head trauma

**What are the 6 factors that increase mortality in patients with pelvic ring injuries?**

- 1. Systolic BP < 90 on presentation
- 2. Age over 60
- 3. Increased ISS score
- 4. Need for transfusion > 4 units

- 5. Open fractures
- 6. APC 3 (windswept pelvis)

**What are the 2 main classification schemes for pelvic ring injuries?**
- Tile, Young & Burgess

**What is the Tile classification?**
- Based on ABC with
- A: stable (doesn't involve ring) - AIIS/ASIS avulsions, crest fx
- B: rotationally unstable/vertically stable
- C rotationally/ vertically unstable

**What is the Young Burgess classification based on?**
- Force dictates the fx pattern
- LC force: applies internal rotation force on pelvis
- AP force: applies external rotation force on pelvis
- Shear force: applies vertical displacement force

**What is the Young Burgess classification?**
- APC I: <2.5cm diastasis, APC II: >2.5cm diastasis + SI widening, APC III: APC II + SI joint disruption
- LC I: sacral (complete or incomplete) compression fx, LC II: LC1+ iliac wing fx, LC III: LC II+ contralateral external rotation injury (windswept pelvis)
- VS

**In which APC injuries are the posterior SI ligaments intact?**
- APC I and II (ruptured in III)

**What are some associated injuries w/ pelvic ring injuries?**
- APC: urethral/ bladder injuries
  - If repair is needed- prefer repair at same time or before hardware placed to reduce infection
- LC: Brain/head injuries > bowel injuries
- Women w/ pelvic fx have inc risk for C- section & dyspareunia

**What is a Morel- Lavallee lesion?**
- An internal degloving injury, leads to hematoma formation w/ inc risk of infection
- Treat in a staged fashion (ORIF + staged closure vs I&D w/ delayed ORIF)

**What are the most common causes of death with LC and APC injuries?**
- APC: shock, sepsis, ARDS
- LC: brain injuries

**What are some of the goals with the acute management of pelvic injuries?**
- Hemorrhage control + pelvic ring stabilization

**What are the critical factors in treating pelvic injuries?**
- Resuscitation blood:platelets:FFP (1:1:1 ratio)
  - Trend lactate, base deficit, hemoglobin

- Stabilization (binder placement/ ex fix)

**What source of bleeding is the most likely cause of hemorrhage?**

- Venous (85%), arterial (15%)
- Venous (posterior venous plexus), arterial (superior gluteal a is MC)

**What are the indications for angiography/embolization ?**

- Variable indications: unlikely to be tested (used in ~20% APC/ VS cases)
- Complications can include gluteal necrosis/ impotence

Trauma 10: 2:15

**What are some ways in the ED to acutely stabilize a patient w/ an unstable pelvic injury?**

- Wrapped sheet / pelvic binder
- Binder must be centered around the greater trochanters
  - This may help an unstable ER injury
- Pelvic packing (provides tamponade)
- Skeletal traction (vertically unstable fx)
- Ex fix

**What to do in a hemodynamically unstable patient with an ER (APC) injury?**

- Place pelvic binder/sheet

**Can use of a binder mask a pelvic ring injury on CT scan?**

- Yes

**When should an ex-fix ideally be applied if a patient is going to OR for hollow viscus/injury (ex lap)?**

- Ex fix should be applied before an ex lap ideally
- Abdominal packing in an unstable pelvis will contribute to instability, inability to pack against a closed volume pelvis

**What are common pin placements for ex-fix of pelvis?**

- Supra-acetabular pins
- Iliac crest pins

**What xray views can you utilize in the placement of supra-acetabular ex fix pins?**

- Supra-acetabular pins - obturator outlet for starting point
- Obturator inlet to ensure pin is within inner/outer tables
- Iliac oblique- pin above acetabulum

**What are some of the risks with ex-fix pin placement?**

- LFCN injury (thigh numbness)- most common
- Heterotopic ossification

**What are some other acute fixation options for pelvic ring injuries?**

- Subcutaneous anterior pelvic fixation (In-fix)
- Pelvic C clamp- helps w/ posterior ring injuries

**What are some complications seen with In-fix placement?**

- Heterotopic ossification (most common), femoral nerve palsy

**What are some predictors for mortality in patients with pelvic ring injuries?**
- Major hemorrhage, severe polytrauma, male, older age

**What fracture patterns are amenable to non-op tx?**
- APC I (<2.5cm displacement)
- Most LC I
  - incomplete sacral fx w/ ipsilateral rami fx - WB trial + repeat images
- *Complete sacral fx w/ ipsilateral or bilateral rami fx- controversial- some stabilize to improve pain

**What are some general surgical tx options for an APC II pelvic injury?**
- Anterior fixation +/- posterior screw fixation

**What about surgical tx options for APC III?**
- Anterior + posterior fixation

**What is the sacral fracture classification system?**
- Denis
- 1 lateral to neural foramen, 2 within neural foramen, 3 medial to neural foramen

**What is the rate of neurologic injury in sacral fractures based on location of fracture?**
- 5% for zone 1
- 20-30% for zone 2
- 60% for zone 3 (can be assoc w/ cauda equina)

**What sacral fractures are amenable to non-op treatment?**
- Stable, minimally displaced fractures, incomplete fx

**What sacral fractures are indicated for operative treatment?**
- Displaced sacral fx

**What nerve root is at risk during placement of a S1 screw?**
- L5 nerve root (Big toe)

**When can open foraminal decompression be used for sacral fx?**
- Zone II injuries

**What should be ruled out in a patient with bilateral sacral fractures?**
- Spinopelvic dissociation
- Treat with lumbopelvic fixation (triangular osteosynthesis)
  - Associated w/ high rate of hardware prominence and pain

**How do you diagnose persistent instability after pelvic fixation?**
- Diagnosed with single leg stance XR (also known as flamingo radiographs)

# Acetabulum fractures

**What makes up the posterior column?**

- Quadrilateral surface, posterior wall/dome, ischial tuberosity, greater and lesser sciatic notches

**What makes up the anterior column?**

- Anterior iliac wing (glut med tubercle), lateral superior pubic ramus, anterior wall/dome, iliopectineal eminence

**What pelvic views best show acetabular fractures?**

- AP, judet views which are termed depending on the side involved, obturator oblique and iliac oblique

**What does the obturator oblique of the RIGHT side show?**

- Obturator oblique recognized as seeing the obturator foramen en face and shows anterior column and posterior wall

**What does the iliac oblique of the RIGHT side show?**

- It's the inverse of the obturator oblique (ie, an iliac oblique of the RIGHT side is essentially the same as the obturator oblique of the LEFT side). It demonstrates anterior wall and posterior column fractures.

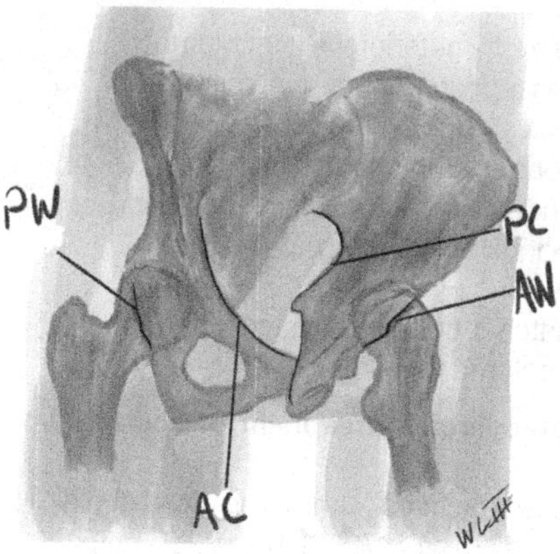


**Figure 1.22: Judet views showing an obturator oblique of the right side (obturator foramen is en face), and an iliac oblique of the left side (illium is seen en face). On the obturator oblique on the right side, the posterior wall (PW) and anterior column (AC) are evaluated. On the iliac oblique on the left, the anterior wall (AW) and posterior column (PC) are evaluated.**

**What are some things that you should look for on CT scan when evaluating acetabulum fractures?**

- Fracture pattern orientation
- Presence of intra-articular fragments
- Marginal impaction
- Articular step off
- Congruent articulation between acetabulum and femoral head

**What does a transverse acetabulum fracture look like on an axial CT cut?**

- A vertical line (T-type has a vertical line too)
- A horizontal line is assoc w/ column fractures

**What acetabular fracture is characterized as a dissociation of the articular surface from the intact ilium and axial skeleton?**

- Associated both column

Trauma 11: 8:40

**What is a spur sign and on what radiograph is it seen?**

- The intact portion of the ilium with associated both column acetabular fractures and is best seen on obturator oblique view
- The articular segment medializes

**What is a gull sign?**

- Fracture dislocation of the acetabulum. The posterior displaced acetabulum combines with rest of acetabulum, and on xray looks like flying seagull
- Seen in elderly fractures and is a poor prognostic sign

**What is the roof- arc angle?**

- Angle between vertical line through femoral head and fracture line (measured on AP + Judet views)
- It is considered stable if the line exits out of the WB dome (>45 degrees)
- Less predictive for 2 column injuries

**How can you classify acetabulum fx while evaluating x'rays systematically?**

- Look for breaks in iliopectineal + ilioischial lines
    - If intact > posterior wall fx
    - If only iliopectineal line disrupted > anterior wall or column
    - If only ilioischial line disrupted > posterior column, or posterior wall + column fx
    - If BOTH disrupted > look at obturator ring and see if intact
        - Obturator ring intact > transverse or transverse + posterior wall
        - Obturator ring not intact > look at iliac wing
            - Iliac wing intact > T-type
            - Iliac wing disrupted > anterior column +posterior hemitransverse, associated both column fx

**What are some indications for non-operative treatment of acetabulum fractures?**

- Non-displaced/minimally displaced fractures (<1mm step off, <2mm gap)
- Posterior wall fx w/o instability (~<20% of wall- debateable)
- Roof arc angle >45 degrees (on AP + Judets)
- Both column fx w/ secondary congruence
- Elderly w/ severe comminution where THA is planned

(Firoozabadi, 2015)

**Is it a hard rule that posterior wall fractures involving <20% of the wall on CT scan are stable?**

- No, you can consider the cranial exit point of the fx in relation to the acetabular dome as well
- Cranial exit point of the fx <5.0mm from the dome can be seen in unstable hips

- Exit point around 9.5mm can be seen in stable hips

**Which patients with posterior acetabular wall fx may be candidates to undergo EUA in the operating room?**

- Fx w/ a history of dislocation or impaction on CT

**What is the typical non-operative tx course for patients with acetabulum fx that meet non-op criteria?**

- PWB for 6-10 weeks

**What are some surgical indications for acetabulum fractures?**

- Dome displacement >2mm, roof angle <45 degrees, displaced fx
- Posterior wall fx > 20-30% OR hip instability
- Loose intra-articular fractures
- Irreducible fx dislocation

**Which type of acetabulum fracture has the worst prognosis?**

- T-Type (transverse fx w/ extension into obturator ring)

**Is early (<5days) or late (10-14 days) surgery associated with improved fracture reduction in acetabulum fractures?**

- Early

**Which patients with acetabulum fractures may benefit from tx w/ acute ORIF and THA?**

- Severe pre-existing arthritis
- Assoc displaced femoral neck fx

**What are some of the surgical approaches used for acetabulum fractures?**

- Posterior (Kocher Langenbeck):
- Anterior (ilioinguinal)
- Modified Stoppa
- Extensile approaches (extended iliofemoral, triradiate)
- Combined

**What acetabulum fractures are indicated for a posterior approach?**

- PW, PC, transverse, transverse PW, PC/PW, some T-type
- Posterior approach assoc w/ iatrogenic sciatic n injury + damage to femoral head

**Debridement of what structure decreases HO formation when performing a kocher-langenbeck?**

- Gluteus minimus debridement + a single dose of 700 cGy radiation within 72 hours of surgery will decrease rate of HO formation compared to gluteus minimus debridement alone

**What acetabulum fractures is an anterior ilioinguinal approach useful for?**

- AW, AC, ACPHT, both column, some T-types
- It is divided into three windows: medial (stoppa), middle (vascular), lateral (iliac)

**Injury to the obturator nerve will manifest as what?**

- Inner thigh numbness

Trauma 12: 2:40

**Injury to what structure causes lateral thigh numbness?**

- LFCN

**What is the modified stoppa approach?**

- An extraperitoneal, intrapelvic approach through rectus abdominis
- Less invasive than ilioinguinal

**What approach provides the best access to the quadrilateral surface?**

- Modified stoppa

**During a stoppa approach, what structure is encountered with lateral dissection over superior pubic ramus?**

- Corona mortis

**What structures make up the corona mortis?**

- Anastomosis of internal and external iliac arteries, more specifically, Inferior epigastric artery and obturator artery

**When are the extinsile approaches considered for acetabulum fractures?**

- Complex fractures + fracture >3 weeks old

**What approach is associated w/ the highest occurrence of HO?**

- Extended iliofemoral
- Some do ppx w/ indomethacin or radiation 600cGy within 48hrs of surgery

**What LE position reduces tension on the sciatic nerve?**

- Hip extension and knee flexion

Trauma 12: 7:37

**If DVT/PE is diagnosed pre-op in patients w/ acetabulum fx, what is a treatment option?**

- IVC filter

**Does the quality of reduction directly correlate with outcome in acetabulum fx?**

- Yes, also early surgery, + no femoral head damage, no comminution, + no acetabular impaction

# LOWER EXTREMITY

## Hip dislocations

**What is the usual mechanism of injury for a hip dislocation>?**
- Axial load + hip position determines dislocation direction
- Posterior hip dislocation is MC- hip is flexed, adducted+ IR
- Anterior dislocation- hip extended, abducted + ER

Trauma 13: 1:40

**Is AVN associated with a hip that is dislocated more than 12 hours?**
- Yes, 50% chance of AVN if hip is left dislocated >12 hrs
- AVN rate 2-6% if reduced within 6hrs (AVN appears within 2 years of nearly all cases)

(Foulk, 2010)

**What is the treatment of a hip dislocation?**
- Emergent closed reduction + stability assessment post-reduction

**What imaging should you get after a hip dislocation?**
- Xrays: AP + Judet view. CT scan

**What do you look for on post-reduction CT scans after a hip dislocation is reduced?**
- Concentric reduction
- Intra-articular loose bodies
- Femoral head fracture

**What may be used in unstable hips after reduction (ex: assoc posterior wall fx)?**
- Skeletal traction or abduction pillow

**What is the most common complication after a hip dislocation?**
- Post-traumatic arthritis (~16 %, can be as high as 70% for posterior fx dislocation)
- Other complications include sciatic nerve injury (peroneal division MC)

## Femoral head

**What is the Pipkin classification for femoral head fractures based on?**
- Fx location relative to fovea + assoc injuries (acetabulum + femoral neck fx)
- 1- below fovea, 2- above fovea, 3 + femoral neck fx, 4 + acetabulum fx

**What is the tx for a Pipkin 1 femoral head fx?**
- If non-displaced- non-op w/ PWB 4-6wks
- If displaced / comminuted w/ intra articular fragments present- excise

**What is the tx for a Pipkin 2 femoral head fx?**

- Nondisplaced- PWB 4-6 weeks with frequent radiographs v ORIF w/ countersunk screws

**What approach is typically used for operative tx of Pipkin 1 + 2 femoral head fx?**

- Anterior Smith-Peterson approach (sartorius + TFL)
- No inc AVN risk

**What is the tx for Pipkin 3 + 4?**

- Pipkin 3- ORIF head + neck, arthroplasty in elderly patient
- Pipkin 4- ORIF head + acetabulum

**What classification is associated w/ the highest rate of AVN?**

- Pipkin 3 (head + femoral neck)

**What artery contributes the most to the blood supply of the femoral head?**

- The lateral retinacular vessels of the MEDIAL femoral circumflex artery

## Femoral Neck

**What are the two commonly used classification systems for femoral neck fractures?**

- Pauwels + Garden classification

**What is the Pauwels classification system?**

- Based on fx line orientation
- Type I- transverse- 30 degrees or less
- Type II- oblique- 30-50
- Type III- vertical- greater than 50 (highest rate nonunion + AVN)

Trauma 13: 21:00

**What is the Garden classification system?**

- Judged by degree of displacement and trabecular lines
- Garden I/II (nondisplaced / stable)
    - I- valgus impacted, II- complete nondisplaced fx
- Garden III/IV (displaced - unstable)
- III- incomplete displacement, IV- complete displacement

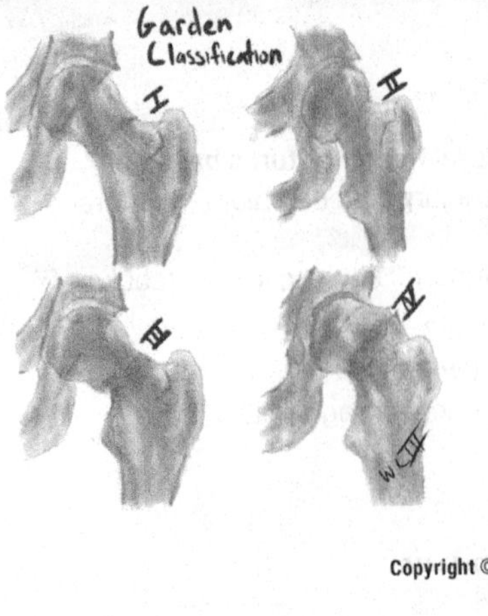


**Figure 1.23: The Garden classification of femoral neck fractures.**

**What is the most sensitive scan to rule out femoral neck fractures?**

- MRI

**What is important to discern regarding treatment of femoral neck fractures?**

- Patient functional status and physiological age

**When should surgery be performed to decrease mortality rates for femoral neck fx?**

- Within 48 hrs

**What femoral neck fx is non-operative tx indicated?**

- Non displaced fx, although most stabilize to prevent further displacement

**What patients with femoral neck fractures should undergo internal fixation?**

- Displaced fractures in the physiologically young + patients w/ non-displaced fractures

**What is the typical fixation for Garden I/II + occult femoral neck fx?**

- 3 parallel screw in an inverted triangle (V) orientation inserted at level of or above lesser trochanter
  - Screws placed below lesser troch are associated w/ peri-implant sub-troch fracture
- Improved fixation w/ screws against cortex posterior + inferiorly (esp in osteoporotic bone)

**What is the fixation choice commonly used for basicervical/Pauwels III (vertical orientation) femoral neck fx?**

- Sliding hip screw + derotation screw

**In young patients w/ comminuted femoral neck fx, where is the area of comminution most commonly seen?**

- Posterior + inferior

**Is there any difference in re-operation rates in patients fixed w/ sliding hip screw w/ cannulated screw fixation?**

- No significant differences
- Patients w/ displaced basicervical neck fx and current smokers may do better with sliding hip screw

**(Nauth, 2017)**

**What is associated w/ improved outcomes for young patients w/ displaced femoral neck fx?**

- Quality of reduction
- Separate anterior approach w/ capsulotomy may be needed for ORIF

**Trauma 14: 3:30**

**Is varus or valgus reduction associated w/ increased failure rates for femoral neck fx fixation?**

- Varus reduction

**What is a common complication after femoral neck ORIF?**

- AVN

**What is a surgical option for a femoral neck varus nonunion in a young, active patient?**

- Valgus intertrochanteric osteotomy

**In what patients w/ femoral neck fx is hemiarthroplasty indicated?**

- Displaced femoral neck fractures in patients w/ low demand/functional status
- Lower risk of dislocation compared w/ THA

**Is there any difference between bipolar v unipolar hemiarthroplasty for femoral neck fx?**

- Similar outcomes. Controversial results

**Is there any difference between cemented v non-cemented hemiarthroplasty for femoral neck fx?**

- Cemented > uncemented in pts w/ Door C/ Stove pipe type medullary canal
  - Assoc w/ higher cardiopulmonary complications

**What patients w/ femoral neck fx are total hip arthroplasty indicated?**

- Active older patients w/ displaced femoral neck fx + patients w/ prior OA
- Assoc w/ improved functional outcomes compared w/ hemiarthroplasty and internal fixation
- Assoc w/ in risk dislocation rate vs hemiarthroplasty

(Healy, 2004)

**What factors are associated w/ inc risk of osteonecrosis in femoral neck fx?**

- Anything that disrupts the blood supply
- Inc initial fx displacement, poor reduction

**What is the 1 year mortality rate in elderly patients w/ a femoral neck fx?**

- 30%

## Intertrochanteric femur fractures

**What timeframe is ideal for surgery in patients with intertrochanteric femur fractures?**

- Surgery within 48 hours
- Medical co-management improves outcomes
- Higher ASA level predicts mortality

**What are the characteristics of an unstable intertrochanteric femur fracture?**

- Lateral wall blowout, reverse obliquity, posterior-medial comminution, subtrochanteric extension
- (lesser + greater trochanteric fractures can also be markers of instability)

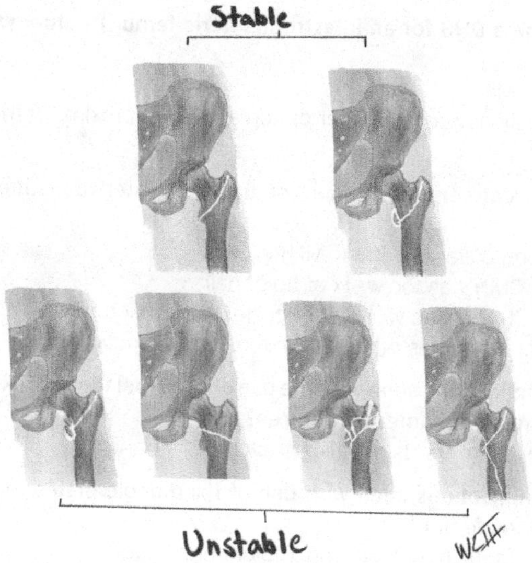


**Figure 1.24: Stable and unstable intertrochanteric femur fractures. Unstable intertrochanteric femur fractures can be characterized by posteromedial comminution, reverse obliquity, lateral wall blowout, subtrochanteric extension (from left to right).**

**What is the implant of choice for stable intertrochanteric femur fractures?**

- Dynamic sliding hip (DHS) screw (no difference between 2 and 4 hole plates)

**How is the tip apex distance measured?**

- # of millimeters on AP + lateral hip film (added together) from tip of screw to subchondral bone

**Where is the ideal placement of a DHS screw for tx of stable intertrochanteric femur fx?**

- Center - center
- Tip apex distance <25 assoc w/ lowest screw failure rate
  - TAD >25 is associated w/ implant failure/cutout

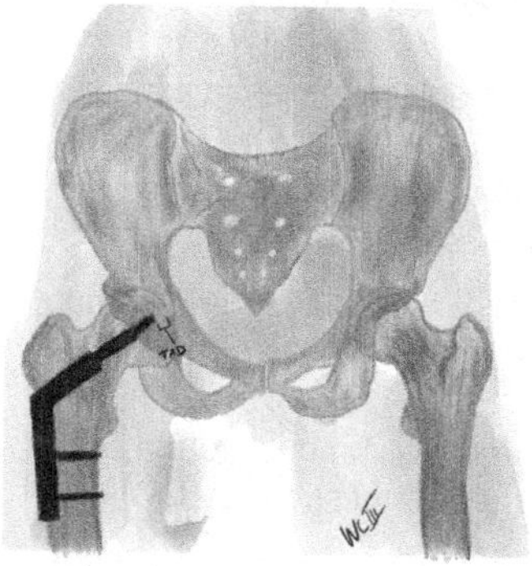


**Figure 1.25: Films showing an intertrochanteric femur fracture that was treated with a DHS construct. A tip apex distance (TAD) less than 25 is associated with the lowest screw failure rate.**

**If you fix an unstable intertrochanteric femur fx w/ a DHS screw, what are some common complications?**

- Shaft medialization (integrity of lateral femoral cortex is key)

**Should you use a DHS for an intertrochanteric femur fracture w/ reverse obliquity?**

- No, use CMN
- Fixed angle device is another option as well as proximal femur locking plate

**What is the treatment of choice for unstable intertrochanteric femur fractures?**

- Cephalomedullary nailing (CMN)
  - Short CMN's assoc w/ fx at tip of nail
  - Long CMN assoc w/ anterior cortex perforation
  - Similar outcomes otherwise in regards to function

**What are complications seen with the use of proximal femur locking plates for unstable intertrochanteric fractures?**

- Fixation failure, varus malalignment

**What are complications seen with use of fixed angle plates for unstable intertrochanteric femur fx?**

- Inc risk cutout, nonunion, and implant breakage

## Subtrochanteric femur fractures

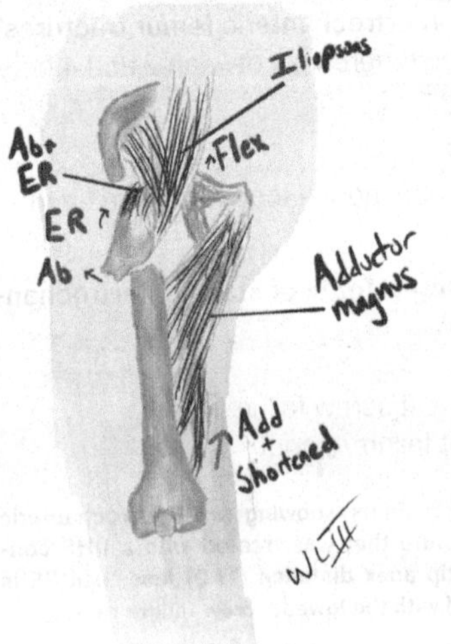


**What are the deforming forces on the proximal and distal fragment in subtrochanteric femur fractures?**

- Proximal fragment: flexion, abduction, external rotation
- Distal fragment: adduction +shortening

**Figure 1.26: The deforming forces on the femur in subtrochanteric femur fractures.**

**What is the fracture pattern seen in bisphosphonate associated subtrochanteric femur fractures?**

- Lateral cortex thickening with transverse orientation and a medial spike
- Prolonged healing times anticipated

**What is the typical treatment of choice for a subtrochanteric femur fracture?**

- CMN - open reduction often needed
- Apex anterior + varus angulation are the most common deformities
- Varus malreduction leads to increased mechanical stress on fixation construct

**Should you use a piriformis entry nail if the fracture extends into the piriformis fossa?**
- No

## Femoral shaft fractures

**What fractures are associated with femoral shaft fx that can be missed up to 50% of the time?**

Ep 4:
w/ Dr. Bernstein

- Femoral neck fractures. They are typically vertically oriented and mid-cervical due to the high energy. DHS plate w/ derotation screw may be beneficial in these patients. Fix the neck fx first

**What is early stabilization (24hrs) of femoral shaft fractures associated with?**
- Reduced systemic (pulmonary, TE) complications
- Dec hospital costs

**What is the treatment of choice for most femoral shaft fractures?**
- Intramedullary nailing (IMN)- statically, locked reamed nail inserted through piriformis fossa

**What are some differences between reamed and unreamed nailing?**
- Reamed- higher union rates
- Unreamed- decrease fat embolism (may not be clinically significant though?)

**What are some points to make with reaming technique?**
- Sharp reamer, fluted designs, slow advancement, less heat generation + less embolism generation

(Ricci, 2009)

**What muscles are weak after antegrade femur nailing?**
- Abductors and quadriceps

**Is knee or hip pain more common with retrograde femur nailing?**
- Knee pain

**What are some relative indications for retrograde femur nailing?**
- Bilateral femur fractures, obesity, pregnancy, ipsilateral tibial shaft fracture, ipsilateral acetabulum fracture, ipsilateral femoral neck fracture

Trauma 15:
9:25

**When is piriformis starting point contraindicated?**
- When the fracture line extends through the piriformis fossa

**What does a starting point too anterior in the piriformis fossa lead to?**
- Inc hoop stress + iatrogenic comminution

**What are some risks associated with a trochanteric starting point?**
- Varus malalignment + medial shaft comminution

**What is the starting point for a trochanteric entry nail?**
- Just lateral to long axis of femur

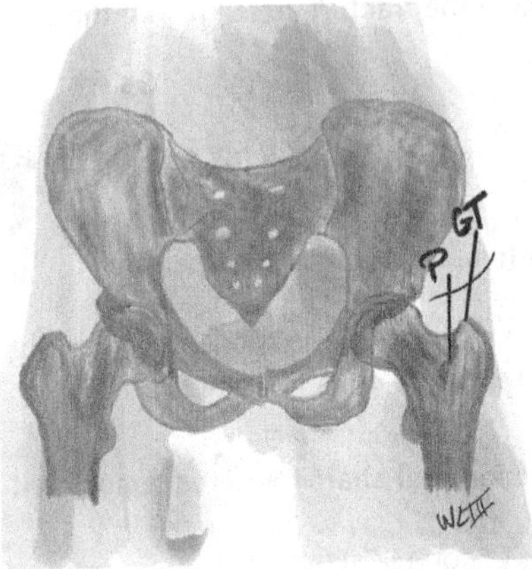


- Most nail designs have a proximal lateral bend to accommodate

**Figure 1.27: AP of the pelvis showing the starting points for a piriformis (P) and greater trochanteric (GT) intramedullary nail.**

**What are some indications for ex-fix use in femur fractures?**

- Polytrauma patient (DCO), severe open fx w/ contamination, vascular injury
- Safe to convert to IMN up to 3 weeks

**Is immediate IM nailing indicated in most open femoral shaft fractures?**

- Yes, unless there is evidence of severe contamination /canal contamination > serial debridements

**What is the most common complication after IMN of a comminuted femoral shaft fx?**

- Malrotation
  - Internal rotation more common in proximal femur fracture
  - External rotation- more common in distal femur fx

## Distal femur fractures

**Ep 30: w/ Dr. Spitler**

**In patients w/ distal femur fractures, what should you always look for when getting a CT scan?**

**Trauma 15: 23:15**

- A coronal plane fracture (Hoffa fragment) occurs up to 40% of the time
  - Lateral femoral condyle is most common ~80%

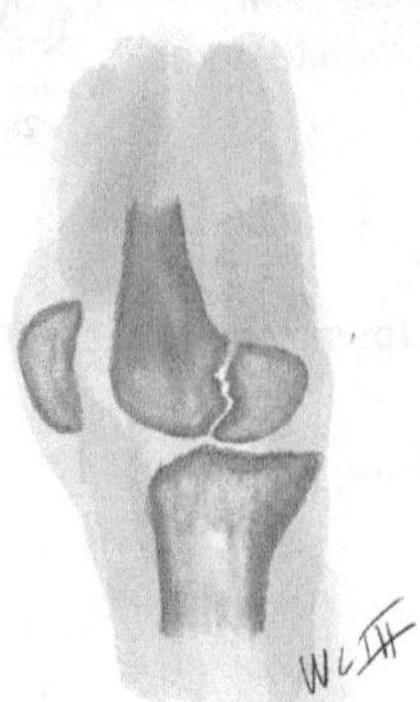

**Figure 1.28: Lateral of the knee showing a coronal plane fracture, often missed on plain films.**

**What are some of the general principles in the tx of intra-articular distal femur fractures?**

- Articular reduction + stable fixation of articular block to shaft

**What type of deformity is seen with non-locked plating tx for distal femur fractures?**

- Varus deformity

**What type of plating is preferred in patients w/ distal femur fx w/ metaphyseal comminution?**

- Fixed angle plating (95 degree platings/ locked plates)

**Should you use 95 degree plating for an intra-articular distal femur fx w/ an associated hoffa fragment?**

- No, it is a contraindication. Locked plating offers the advantage of multiple points of fixation in different planes
- Locked plating is also 5x more expensive than blade plating

**What is hybrid locked plating in the context of distal femur fractures?**

- Using locked (fixed angle fixation) + non-locked (plate used as a reduction tool) screw
- Plates w/ a longer working length allow stable and flexible fixation

**Does increased or decreased plate stiffness lead to healing with comminuted distal femur fx?**

- Decreased stiffness leads to healing

**What xray view do you use to assess screw length in distal femur?**

- 25-30 degrees internal rotation. Distal femur is trapezoidal in shape

**What are some pitfalls with plate position for distal femur fractures?**

- Too anterior- unicortical screws
- Too posterior- screw into intercondylar notch
- Too posterior- golf club deformity (medialization of condylar segment)
- Too distal- intra-articular screw placement + golf club deformity (convex part of plate pushes condyles medial)
- Too flexed/extended- unicortical screws/ posterior thrust

**What are some risk factors for failure of locked plating for distal femur fx?**

- Open fx, diabetes, smoking, increased BMI, and short plate length

**Ricci, 2014**

**In what cases is intramedullary nailing for distal femur fractures used?**

- Extra articular fractures, + some intra-articular fx after articular segment reduction and screw fixation

## Knee dislocations

**What is the most common direction and vascular injury for a knee dislocation?**

- Anterior/ popliteal

**Trauma 16: 1:50**

**What are some hard signs of vascular injury?**

- Pulsatile bleeding, expanding hematoma, absent pulses

**What are some soft signs of vascular injury?**

- Nonexpansile or nonpulsatile hematoma, abnormal ABI, or asymmetric pulses

**What is the next step when a patient is in the ED with a knee dislocation w/ no pulses?**

- Reduce knee, re- assess pulses and obtain ABI

**What to do if knee dislocation was reduced and w/ ABI> .9 and pulses are present?**

- Admit + observe. Serial exams

**What to do if knee dislocation was reduced and w/ ABI < .9 w/ pulses present or diminished?**

- Arteriogram

**What to do if knee dislocation was reduced and w/ absent pulses + noticeable bleeding/expanding hematoma or signs of limb ischemia?**

- Emergent revascularization. No need for CT. Ideally within 8 hours

**What is the surgical tx of a knee dislocation?**

- Vascular repair +/- ex fix
- Eventual cruciate ligament reconstruction (controversy in acute v subacute reconstruction)
  - Stiffness* is the most common complication

## Patella fractures

**What patella fractures are amenable to non-operative treatment?**

- Non displaced/ minimally displaced (<2mm) w/ intact extensor mechanism
- WBAT in hinged knee brace/knee immobilizer /cylinder cast

**Why do you try to preserve the patella if at all possible in patients with a patella fx?**

- Lever arm for quads function

**What are some tx options for ORIF of patella fx?**

- K-wire, cannulated screws, plate, tension band

**Is ORIF or partial patellectomy associated w/ better outcomes in comminuted displaced inferior pole patella fx?**

- ORIF when possible is associated w/ better outcomes

**If performing a partial patellectomy, where on the patella should the patellar tendon be reattached?**

- Anteriorly to prevent patellar tilt

**What is the most common complication after ORIF of the patella?**

- Symptomatic hardware

# Tibia plateau fractures

Ep: 24
w/ Dr. Githens

Trauma 16:
20:07

**What are the anatomical differences between the medial/lateral tibia plateau?**
- Medial plateau- larger and more concave
- The medial femoral condyle is stronger than lateral femoral condyle (lateral plateau fx are more common)

**What is the force mechanism that usually produces lateral tibia plateau fractures?**
- Valgus + axial compression

**What is the force mechanism that usually produces medial tibia plateau fractures?**
- Varus force + axial load

**What is the force mechanism that usually produces posterior column tibia plateau fractures?**
- Varus + flexion. ACL avulsion + lateral meniscus injuries common

**What is the Schatzker classification for tibia plateau fractures?**
- I- lateral split, II- split + depression, III- depression, IV- medial split, V- bicondylar w/ intact metaphysis, VI- metadiaphyseal dissociation

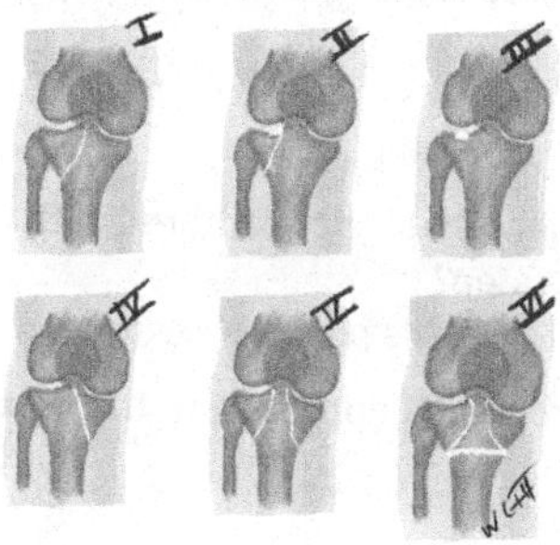


**Figure 1.28: Schatzker classification of tibia plateau fractures I-VI.**

**What are the common associated injuries seen with each classification type?**
- Lateral meniscus tears - type II (anterolateral approach)
- Medial meniscus tear + knee dislocation - type IV
- Compartment syndrome + ligamentous injuries are associated w/ higher energy mechanism injuries

**Which types are associated with a higher rate of complications?**
- Type IV-VI

**Which type is the most common?**
- Type II

**What is the AO classification for tibia plateau fractures?**
- 41 (4- tibia, 1- proximal)
- 41A, 41B, 41C (A- non-articular, B- partial articular, C- complete articular)

**What will you see on xray in patients w/ a medial tibia plateau fx dislocation?**

- Intact lateral column, centrolateral articular impaction, shortening + condylar widening

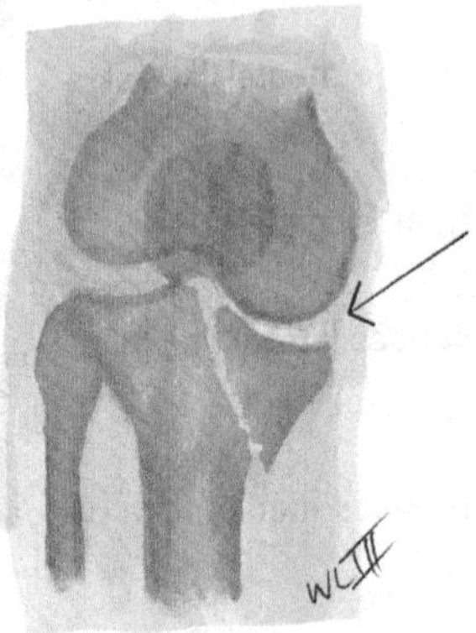


**Figure 1.29: AP of a knee showing a medial tibia plateau fracture dislocation. Notice how the femoral condyle is following the displaced tibia plateau fragment.**

**What are the operative indications for tibia plateau fractures?**

- Displaced articular fractures, fracture dislocations, medial tibia plateau fractures, bicondylar fractures, articular depression causing knee instability

**What are some situations where you may use a buttress plate in tibia plateau fractures?**

- Unicondylar (partial articular) fractures
- Split depression fractures w/ use of subchondral rafting screws to hold articular surface +/- bone void fillers

**What are some situations where you may use a locked plate for tibia plateau fractures?**

- Bicondylar fractures w/ poor bone quality, Some depression fractures
- Superficial peroneal nerve (SPN) is at risk w/ long plates

**If there is a separate posterior medial fragment that is not captured with a single laterally locked plate, what is the next step?**

- A separate posterior medial approach + buttress plate

**What is the interval between for the posteromedial approach to the tibia plateau?**

- Pes anserine and medial head of gastroc

**What are some items used to fill the void in tibia plateau fractures?**

- Autograft
- Calcium phosphate (highest compressive strength + lower rate of subsidence than autograft)

**What are some indications for temporary external fixation of tibia plateau fractures?**

- Severe soft tissue damage, polytrauma (damage control), joint subluxation/dislocation, bicondylar fractures

**How far away from the knee joint should pins be placed in tibia plateau fractures?**

- At least 15mm distal to avoid septic knee arthritis

**What are some complications seen with tibia plateau fractures?**

- Post-traumatic arthritis, malunion, ligament instability

**What correlates most with a satisfactory outcome in tibia plateau fractures?**
- Maintenance of the mechanical axis

**What is a treatment option for patients who fail to obtain 90 degrees of flexion at 12 weeks s/p ORIF tibia plateau?**
- Arthroscopic lysis of adhesions w/ gentle MUA

## Tibia shaft fractures

Ep 27
w/ Dr. Githens

**What is the acceptable alignment to treat tibia shaft fractures nonoperatively?**
- Varus/valgus <5deg
- Sagittal plane alignment <10deg
- Cortical apposition >50%
- Shortening <1cm
- Rotational alignment w/i 10 deg
- Stress fx & incomplete fx may also undergo non-op tx

Trauma 17:
18:30

**What should you be on the lookout for in patients with spiral distal ⅓ tibia shaft fractures?**
- Fracture of posterior malleolus

**What is the tx of choice for high energy unstable tibia shaft fractures?**
- Reamed, statically locked, intramedullary nailing

**What are some advantages to reaming in closed tibia shaft fractures?**
- Better healing rates w/ fewer complications
- Reaming allows use of a larger and stronger nails that improve stability

**When is the endosteal circulation destroyed by reaming the canal re-established by?**
- 8-12 weeks

**What is the most common complication w/ tibia nailing?**
- Anterior knee pain (no increased rates w/ suprapatellar approach) 50-75%

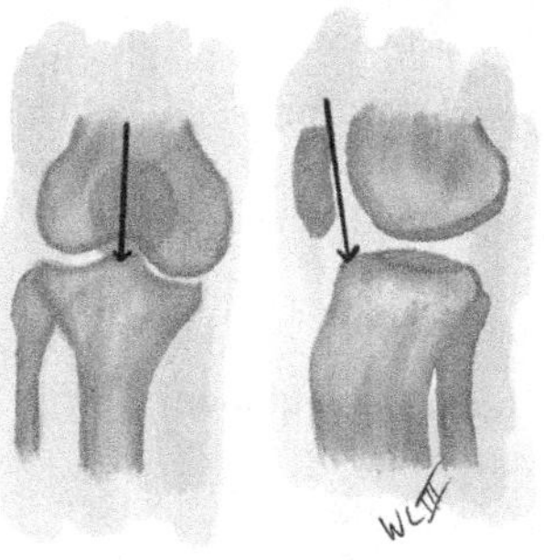

**What is the ideal start point for tibial nailing?**
- Medial to lateral tibial spine, anterior to intra-articular knee structures but proximal to tibial tubercle

**Figure 1.30: AP and lateral of the knee showing the ideal starting point for tibial nailing. A proper AP of the knee must be obtained to ensure accuracy.**

**What is a common deformity seen in proximal ⅓ tibia shaft fractures?**

- Valgus + procurvatum
- Patellar tendon + gastroc > procurvatum
- Anterior tibialis + pes tendon > valgus

**What are some ways to combat this deformity when using IMN for proximal tibia fx?**

- Correct starting point (too medial- valgus, too distal- procurvatum)
- Use of poller/blocking screws (placed posterior + lateral)
- Use of small LCP plate w/ unicortical locking screws
- Use of semi-extended leg position
- Use of multiple locking screws help stability

**What is the most important step to prevent infection in the open tibia shaft fx?**

- IV antibiotics

**What is the most important aspect of irrigation and debridement?**

- Urgent & thorough sharp debridement of devitalized tissue
- Improved results w/ early soft tissue coverage

(Sprint, 2008)

**Is there any difference in reamed vs unreamed nailing in open tibia shaft fractures?**

- No difference in outcomes
- In CLOSED fx there is a benefit for reaming

**What is the role of BMP-2 in open tibia shaft fractures?**

- When used w/ IM fixation, leads to fewer re-operations in acute open tibia shaft fx

**When would you consider ORIF vs IMN in tibia shaft fractures?**

- Too proximal or distal for nail fixation
- Adjacent hardware already in place (ie TKA)
- Revision with bone graft

**What are some of the difficulties with ORIF compared to IMN?**

- Larger incisions with more dissection
- Greater radiation exposure intraoperatively
- Risk of damage to superficial peroneal nerve at holes 11, 12, 13 with percutaneous screw placement (long proximal plate)

**What are some differences between plating and IMN for distal ⅓ tibia shaft fx?**

- Similar bony union, superficial/deep infections and wound complications
- Less chance of malalignment w/ plate fixation

**What is the most important predictor for eventual LE amputation?**

- Ipsilateral extremity soft tissue injury severity
- Timely admission to definitive trauma center- predictor of infection
- No diff in outcomes between limb salvage + amputations

- Worse outcomes w/ limb salvage if soft tissue flap required

**What is the difference between delayed union and nonunion for tibia shaft fractures?**

- Delayed union, 6-9 mo, Nonunion >9mo

**Trauma 18: 20:20**

**Delaying re-operation for nonunion until how many months may decrease the need for re-operation?**

- 6 months

**What are some of the treatment options for tibia shaft nonunions?**

- Dynamization - if axially stable
- Reamed exchange nailing- preferred for mid diaphyseal nonunions- not stable
- +/- bone grafts for defects

**Does tibial malrotation have significant effects on outcomes after IMN of tibia shaft fx?**

- No, try not to malrotate though
- (malrotation can be common in distal ⅓ tibia shaft fx)

**What are some prognostic factors for worse outcomes (nonunion, revision surgery, implant fracture) after IMN tibia?**

- High energy mechanism, use of stainless steel nail (compared w/ titanium), persistent fracture gap, full weight bearing

**(Schemitsch, 2012)**

# Pilon fractures

**What's the pathophysiology of tibial plafond fractures?**

- Talus is driven into distal tibia articular surface after high axial load

**What information can you get from looking at the fibula fx in pilon fx?**

- MOA
- Compression failure of fibula (valgus deformity)
- Tension failure (varus deformity)
- Fibula intact (axial load)- typically with multiple small articular fragments w/ poorer prognosis

**What are the 3 typical fragments of the distal tibia?**

- Chaput - AITFL
- Volkmann - PITFL
- Medial - deltoid

**Trauma 19: 4:45**

**What are some associated injuries?**

- 70% have fibula fracture
- 30% have ipsilateral lower extremity injury
- 20% are open
- Up to 10% are bilateral pilons

**Is there a classification for pilon fractures?**

- Ruedi-Allgower

- Type 1 - simple intraarticular, nondisplaced
- Type 2 - simple intraarticular, displaced/incongruous joint
- Type 3 - comminued, displaced/incongruous joint

**What's important to look for on presentation?**

- Open wounds
- Palpate pulses vs doppler – fracture fragments can impinge on neurovasculature
- Neuro exam
- Compartment syndrome

**What is the typical treatment algorithm for pilon fractures?**

- Staged treatment with initial external fixation +/- fibula fixation then definitive ORIF 2 weeks later

**What approaches are used to access the distal tibia?**

- Many useful approaches that are used dependent on fracture characteristics
- Unlikely to be tested on which approach to use, but may get tested on complications of a single approach
- Direct anterior
- Anterolateral - probably most widely used approach
  - Dangers include SPN with superficial dissection and DPN with deep dissection
- Anteromedial
- Direct medial
- Posteromedial
- Posterolateral
- Direct lateral

**What are some ways to manage open pilon fracture w/ metaphyseal bone loss?**

- Early debridement, fracture stabilization, soft tissue reconstruction
- Bone loss management- antibiotic beads or cement spacer > follow by grafting

**What is the most common complication seen w/ pilon fx?**

- Post-traumatic arthritis
- Patients socioeconomic factors are predictive of clinical outcome

**What cytokines are increased in post-traumatic arthritis?**

- IL-6, IL-8, MMP 1, 2, and 3

**What are predictors of poor outcome in pilon fractures?**

- Workers comp — will be tested
- Males
- Lower socioeconomic status
- Increased medical comorbidities
- Outcomes correlate with initial severity and quality of reduction
  - Studies have found that patients with pilon fractures scored lower

on SF-36 PRO on quality of life that those with AIDS, pelvic fractures, and coronary artery disease

**What are some treatment options for extra-articular varus malunion s/p ORIF pilon fx?**

- Osteotomy + revision fixation

**What is the treatment algorithm for post-traumatic arthritis?**

- Initially conservative with bracing, orthoses, injections
- Then consider arthrodesis vs arthroplasty (pros and cons will be covered in foot and ankle section)

## Podcast Episodes for a Deeper Dive into Trauma

- Episode 4 w/ Dr. Bernstein- Intro to Diaphyseal Femur Fractures www.naileditortho.com/femurbasics
- Episode 6: Intro to Pilon Fractures w/ Dr. Dixon www.naileditortho.com/pilonintro
- Episode 24 w/ Dr. Githens- Tibia Plateau Fractures https://naileditortho.com/tibiaplateau/
- Episode 27 w/ Dr. Githens- Tibia Shaft Fractures https://naileditortho.com/tibiashaft/
- Episode 30 w/ Dr. Spitler- Distal Femur Fractures https://naileditortho.com/30-distal-femur-fractures-w-dr-spitler/
- Episode 35 w/ Dr. Mauricio- Terrible Triad Injuries https://naileditortho.com/35-terrible-triad-injuries-w-dr-mauricio/
- Episode 46 w/ Dr. Harrison- Intro to Femoral Neck fractures https://naileditortho.com/femoralneck/
- Episode 54 w/ Dr. Sanders- Intro to Intertrochanteric Femur fractures w/ Dr. Sanders https://naileditortho.com/intertroch/
- Episode 62 w/ Dr. Vemulapalli & Dr. Hawkins- Intro to Pelvis Fractures https://naileditortho.com/pelvis/
  Video: https://youtu.be/Uyie6JQeNcg
- Episode 63 w/ Dr. Routt & Dr. Hawkins- Treatment of Pelvic fractures https://naileditortho.com/treatingpelvisfractures/
  Video: https://youtu.be/W2C1O1g4gNQ
- Episode 70 w/ Dr. Strelzow- Proximal Humerus fractures https://naileditortho.com/proximalhumerus/
- Episode 74 w/ Dr. Grandizio- Distal Humerus fractures https://naileditortho.com/distalhumerusfractures/
  Video: https://youtu.be/zwnKi5bAl-s
- Episode 83 w/ Dr. Sears- Intramedullary Nailing of Proximal Humerus Fractures https://naileditortho.com/sears/
  Video: https://youtu.be/4PdhAxmYxBY

## Specific Articles Mentioned in the Podcast

Vallier, H. A., Wang, X., Moore, T. A., Wilber, J. H., & Como, J. J. (2013). Timing of orthopaedic surgery in multiple trauma patients: development of a protocol for early appropriate care. *Journal of orthopaedic trauma*, 27(10), 543-551.

Richardson, M. (2012). Negative pressure wound therapy reduces deep infection rate in open tibial fractures.

Stannard, J. P., Volgas, D. A., McGwin III, G., Stewart, R. L., Obremskey, W., Moore, T., & Anglen, J. O. (2012). Incisional negative pressure wound therapy after high-risk lower extremity fractures. *Journal of orthopaedic trauma*, 26(1), 37-42.

Wilkerson, J., Paryavi, E., Kim, H., Murthi, A., & Pensy, R. A. (2017). Biomechanical comparison of superior versus anterior plate position for fixation of distal clavicular fractures: a new model. *Journal of orthopaedic trauma*, 31(1), e13-e17.

Petri, M., Warth, R. J., Greenspoon, J. A., Horan, M. P., Abrams, R. F., Kokmeyer, D., & Millett, P. J. (2016). Clinical results after conservative management for grade III acromioclavicular joint injuries: does eventual surgery affect overall outcomes?. *Arthroscopy: The Journal of Arthroscopic & Related Surgery*, 32(5), 740-746

Society, C. O. T. (2015). Multicenter randomized clinical trial of nonoperative versus operative treatment of acute acromio-clavicular joint dislocation. *Journal of orthopaedic trauma*, 29(11), 479-487

Schroder, L. K., Gauger, E. M., Gilbertson, J. A., & Cole, P. A. (2016). Functional outcomes after operative management of extra-articular glenoid neck and scapular body fractures. *JBJS*, 98(19), 1623-1630.

Hertel, R., Hempfing, A., Stiehler, M., & Leunig, M. (2004). Predictors of humeral head ischemia after intracapsular fracture of the proximal humerus. *Journal of shoulder and elbow surgery*, 13(4), 427-433

Rämö, L., Sumrein, B. O., Lepola, V., Lähdeoja, T., Ranstam, J., Paavola, M., ... & FISH Investigators. (2020). Effect of surgery vs functional bracing on functional outcome among patients with closed displaced humeral shaft fractures: the FISH randomized clinical trial. *JAMA*, 323(18), 1792-1801.

Bhandari, M., Devereaux, P. J., D Mckee, M., & H Schemitsch, E. (2006). Compression plating versus intramedullary nailing of humeral shaft fractures—a meta-analysis. *Acta orthopaedica*, 77(2), 279-284.

Kurup, H., Hossain, M., & Andrew, J. G. (2011). Dynamic compression plating versus locked intramedullary nailing for humeral shaft fractures in adults. *Cochrane Database of Systematic Reviews*, (6).

McKee, M. D., Veillette, C. J., Hall, J. A., Schemitsch, E. H., Wild, L. M., McCormack, R., ... & Leung, I. (2009). A multicenter, prospective, randomized, controlled trial of open reduction—internal fixation versus total elbow arthroplasty for displaced intra-articular distal humeral fractures in elderly patients. *Journal of shoulder and elbow surgery*, 18(1), 3-12

Duckworth, A. D., Bugler, K. E., Clement, N. D., & McQueen, M. M. (2014). Nonoperative management of displaced olecranon fractures in low-demand elderly patients. *JBJS*, 96(1), 67-72.

Duckworth, A. D., Wickramasinghe, N. R., Clement, N. D., & McQueen, M. M. (2014). Long-term outcomes of isolated stable radial head fractures. *JBJS*, 96(20), 1716-1723.

Firoozabadi, R., Spitler, C., Schlepp, C., Hamilton, B., Agel, J., & Tornetta, P. (2015). Determining stability in posterior wall acetabular fractures. *Journal of orthopaedic trauma*, 29(10), 465-469.

Foulk, D. M., & Mullis, B. H. (2010). Hip dislocation: evaluation and management. *JAAOS-Journal of the American Academy of Orthopaedic Surgeons*, 18(4), 199-209.

Nauth, A., Creek, A. T., Zellar, A., Lawendy, A. R., Dowrick, A., Gupta, A., ... & de Nies, F. (2017). Fracture fixation in the operative management of hip fractures (FAITH): an international, multicentre, randomised controlled trial. *The Lancet*, 389(10078), 1519-1527

Healy, W. L., & Iorio, R. (2004). Total hip arthroplasty: optimal treatment for displaced femoral neck fractures in elderly patients. *Clinical Orthopaedics and Related Research®*, 429, 43-48.

Ricci, W. M., Gallagher, B., & Haidukewych, G. J. (2009). Intramedullary nailing of femoral shaft fractures: current concepts. *JAAOS-Journal of the American Academy of Orthopaedic Surgeons*, 17(5), 296-305.

Ricci, W. M., Streubel, P. N., Morshed, S., Collinge, C. A., Nork, S. E., & Gardner, M. J. (2014). Risk factors for failure of locked plate fixation of distal femur fractures: an analysis of 335 cases. *Journal of orthopaedic trauma*, 28(2), 83-89.

Study to Prospectively Evaluate Reamed Intramedullary Nails in Patients with Tibial Fractures (SPRINT) Investigators. (2008). Randomized trial of reamed and unreamed intramedullary nailing of tibial shaft fractures. *The Journal of Bone and Joint Surgery. American volume.*, 90(12), 2567.

Schemitsch, E. H., Bhandari, M., Guyatt, G., Sanders, D. W., Swiontkowski, M., Tornetta III, P., ... & Study to Prospectively Evaluate Reamed Intramedullary Nails in Patients with Tibial Fractures (SPRINT) Investigators. (2012). Prognostic factors for predicting outcomes after intramedullary nailing of the tibia. *The Journal of bone and joint surgery. American volume*, 94(19), 1786.

# NOTES

# NOTES

# NOTES

# NOTES

# SPORTS CHAPTER 2

## General Sports

**What is a concussion and some of the symptoms?**

- Brain injury due to impulsive force transmitted to the head
- Sxs are highly variable: headache, emotional lability, cognitive impairment, behavioral changes, sleep disturbances
- LOC does not happen in majority of concussions

**Should a player return to play (RTP) after a concussion?**

- No same day RTP
- Gradual RTP after no symptoms
    - No activity > light aerobic exercise > sport specific exercise > non contact drills > full contact practice > RTP
    - Each stage at least 24hrs

**What can occur if the player returns to play and gets hit before their initial symptoms have resolved?**

- Second impact syndrome—can lead to loss of autoregulation of the brain's blood supply
- Mortality rate of 50%

**What is chronic traumatic encephalopathy?**

- Neurological degenerative disease due to repeated head trauma
- Early signs are cognitive difficulty

**What is a stinger/burner?**

**Sports 1: 8:20**

- Transient/unilateral neuropraxia brachial plexus injury (C5-C6 roots common)
- Burning pain + paresthesias to the neck > UE. Painless cervical ROM
- Resolution within 15 min- full ROM w/ no weakness/numbness

**What is a spear tackler's spine?**

- Acquired C-spine stenosis w/ pavlov ratio <.8
- Loss of cervical lordosis
- Hx of spear tackling
- Contraindication to RTP

**What is the female athlete triad?**

**Ep 61: w/ Dr Mulcahey**

- Low energy availability (+/- eating disorder), menstrual dysfunction, altered bone mineral density
- Stress fractures are common, DEXA scan is the study of choice for evaluating BMD

**What bones are commonly involved with stress fractures in athletes?**

- Femoral neck, pubic ring, tibia shaft

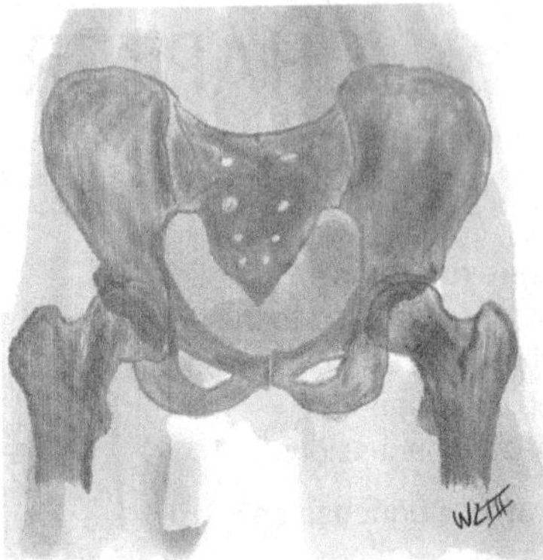

Figure 2.1: AP of the pelvis showing a femoral neck stress fracture of the left hip.

**In a young female athlete with a stress fracture, what should be a part of the history in talking with the patient?**

- Training frequency
- Diet
- Menstrual history

**What area of the tibia is involved with stress fractures?**

- Anterior cortex - it is the tension side
- Known as the "dreaded black line" on radiographs, but if radiographs are normal, consider MRI if there is point tenderness over anterior tibial cortex

**What's the treatment for tibia shaft stress fractures?**

- Nonoperative w/ restricted weight bearing, diet modifications
- If "dreaded black line" is present, reamed prophylactic nailing is preferred due to high rate of tibial nonunion after stress fracture completes

**What should you pay attention to with femoral neck stress fractures?**

- Side of fx
- Tension side fx (superior)- more serious and may need CRPP v DHS
- Compression side fx (inferior)- more common, tx w/ rest + PWB

**Sports 1: 20:30**

**What is the most common site of infection in athletes?**

- Skin from person-person contact
- HSV and staph a are most common pathogens

**What is the treatment for simple abscesses?**

- Moist heat + topical mupirocin for 10 days
  - Incision & drainage if no improvement
- Severe infections may need I&D and oral empiric antibiotic therapy

**What is the likely diagnosis if a cluster of vesicles on an erythematous base is seen on the lip of a wrestler?**

- HSV. Tx w/ oral systemic antivirals- i.e acyclovir & RTP in 120 hrs
- No RTP if: lesions within 48 hrs, less than 72hrs abx + moist lesions

**If a wrestler arrives w/ honey crusted lesions around their mouth, what is the likely dx and RTP protocol?**

- Impetigo from Beta-hemolytic strep or staph
- RTP once crusting is gone + on antiviral meds for 72 hrs and no new lesions for 48 hrs

**What should be on the differential for an athlete w/ a high fever, sore throat and lymphadenopathy?**

- EBV. Athlete complications:
  - Splenic rupture- usually within 3 weeks
  - Tonsillar enlargement- URT blockage
  - Chronic fatigue
- Limit contact sports for 3-5 weeks, splenomegaly must resolve

**What is hyphema?**

- Blood in the eye, associated w/ a vitreous or retinal injury in >50% of cases
- Protective eyewear reduces injuries

**How should an auricular hematoma (cauliflower ear) be treated?**

- Aspiration + wrapping + Rx

**When should a patient w/ epistaxis return to play?**

- Once bleeding stops. R/o CSF fluid

**What is the most common maxillofacial injury in ice hockey?**

- Crown fracture
- Tooth injuries can be placed in the buccal fold or milk
- Mouth guards can reduce injury

**What should you be on the lookout for in a football player w/ tachycardia, tachypnea, hypotension, anhidrosis and neurologic deficits?**

- Heat stroke. Rapidly cool the body core temp + hydrate

**What should you be on the lookout for in pts w/ dizziness, nausea, headache, and possible collapse while running a long distance race and drinking a lot of water?**

- Exercise associated hyponatremia (Na <135)

**What does creatine do and what are some of the side effects?**

- Increases muscle mass, increases water retention in cells
- Side effects: cramping, dehydration, renal issues (rare)

**How does steroids increase muscle mass and what are some of the side effects?**

- Increases muscle mass by increasing mRNA
- Dec HDL, LV hypertrophy, HTN, acne, inc aggression, testicular atrophy, hypercoagulability, alopecia

**What are the two most common causes of sudden cardiac death in athletes?**

**Sports 2: 9:00**

- Hypertrophic cardiomyopathy- autosomal dominant- murmurs > need further w/u
- Commotio cordis- chest wall trauma > Vfib
- Tx w/ immediate cardioversion + cardiopulmonary resuscitation

**What type of muscle does aerobic (endurance training) build?**

- Hypertrophy slow twitch (type 1) fibers, increases capillary density & mitochondria in muscle
- Decreased tension + increased reps

**What type of muscle does anaerobic (strength/resistance training) build?**

- Hypertrophy of fast twitch (type II- anaerobic) fibers
- Sprinting, interval training, weight lifting

**What is the difference between isotonic, isokinetic exercises?**

- Isotonic- constant resistance
  - Concentric- shortens
- Closed chain exercise- foot fixed
- Open chain exercises- foot free
  - Eccentric- lengthens
- Isokinetic- constant speed

**What are the energy sources for muscle?**

- 1st 10 seconds
  - ATP + creatine phosphate
  - Oxygen w/o lactate. Uses stored carbs
- 1-4 minutes- glycogen + lactic acid (aerobic + anaerobic)
- 4+ minutes-Glycogen + fatty acids

**What is the mode of energy utilization from IIa to IIb muscle?**

- IIa- anaerobic + aerobic
- IIb- primarily anaerobic

# Hip

**What is the acute treatment for a quadriceps contusion "dead leg"?**

- Cold compression + immobilization in 120 degrees of flexion
- Hemorrhage + late myositis ossificans expected

**What is the treatment for most hamstring strains?**

- Supportive, stretching and strengthening. Common tear at musculo-tendinous junction during sprinting

**What is the common mechanism for proximal hamstring avulsion?**

- Hip flexion + knee extension - water skiing injury
- MRI useful- early repair advocated

**What are common avulsion fractures seen in adolescents and treatment?**

- ASIS- sartorius avulsion
- AIIS- rectus
- Ischial Tuberosity- Hamstrings
- Tx- non-displaced fx- NWB x4 weeks followed by PT
- High level athletes w/ >2cm displacement- OR

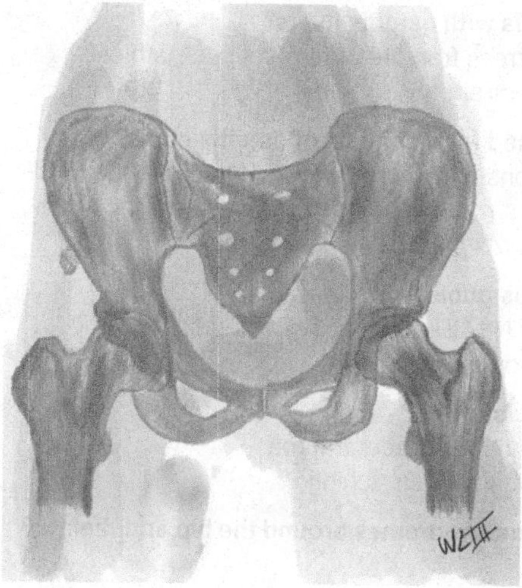


**Figure 2.2: AP of a pelvis in a skeletally mature individual (17M) showing an avulsion fracture of the ASIS.**

**What is the mechanism of injury for ASIS avulsion?**
- Forceful contraction of sartorius and tensor fascia lata (TFL) when the hip is in extension

**What nerves innervate the two muscles that attach to the ASIS?**
- Sartorius = Femoral nerve, TFL = Superior Gluteal nerve

**What imaging modalities are used to diagnose ASIS avulsion?**
- Usually only radiographs are needed, but CT and MRI can be useful for nondisplaced fractures

**What are the imaging differences between sartorius vs TFL avulsions?**
- Sartorius most commonly happens with sprinting and fragment is smaller and displaced anteriorly
- TFL most commonly occurs with twisting, is a larger fragment, and is pulled lateral

**What is the usual treatment for ASIS avulsion?**
- Nonoperative management, usually a post injury course of crutches and progressive WBAT over several weeks with return to activity when pain resolves

**When would ASIS avulsions require surgical intervention?**
- ORIF with displacement over 3 cm and symptomatic nonunions

**What structure is fractured with a forceful contraction of the rectus femoris?**
- AIIS avulsion

**What portion of the rectus femoris attaches to AIIS?**
- Direct head
- (Reflected head attaches to superior acetabulum + joint capsule)

**What's the treatment for AIIS avulsion?**
- Nonoperative management, crutches, progressive weight bearing

**What is the most likely diagnosis in a young, active soccer player that has pain when striking the ball and tenderness over the anterior pelvic ring?**
- Osteitis pubis, or an inflammation of the pubic symphysis

**What is the differential diagnosis with osteitis pubis?**

- Stress fracture of pelvis, stress fracture of femoral neck, athletic pubalgia/adductor muscle strain

**What imaging modalities are used for diagnosis of osteitis pubis?**

- AP pelvis may show erosions at symphysis if condition is long standing, MRI is useful to rule out more concerning diagnoses if those are a concern like stress fractures or oncologic processes

**What is the treatment for osteitis pubis?**

- Non-op management with NSAIDs, rest, activity modification
- May take several months to resolve

**What is a 'hip pointer' and what is the tx?**

- Iliac crest contusion secondary to direct trauma
- Tx: ice, compression, pain control, stretching

**What are some nerve entrapment syndromes around the hip and their tx?**

- Ilioinguinal nerve
  - Hypertrophy of abdominal muscles- worse w/ hip hyperextension
  - Release may be needed
- Obturator nerve
  - Medial thigh pain in athletes w/ well developed adductors, tx usually supportive
- Lateral femoral cutaneous nerve (LFCN)
  - Hip pain- worse w/ tight belts + prolonged hip flexion- can lead to meralgia paresthetica- tx- release compressive devices, NSAIDS, postural exercises
- Sciatic nerve
  - MC sites at level of ischial tuberosity + piriformis muscle
  - Tested by placing the leg in FADIR (flexion, adduction, internal rotation) which puts piriformis on stretch and can reproduce symptoms. Can get confused with FAI as there is pain with impingement with the same test

**What is the most specific test for detecting a hip stress fx?**

- MRI

**What should you pay attention to with femoral neck stress fractures (yes we asked this twice)?**

- Side of fx
- Tension side fx (superior)- more serious and may need CRPP v DHS
- Compression side fx (inferior)- more common, tx w/ rest + PWB

**What are the two types of snapping hip (coxa saltans)?**

- Internal / external
- Intra articular cases are there as well (loose bodies, etc)

**What is the external snapping hip and the tx?**

- Iliotibial (IT) band catches on greater trochanter (GT)

- Snapping is seen w/ hip adduction + knee extension, + ober test
- Tx: stretching/strengthening. IT band lengthening if needed

**What is internal snapping hip and its tx?**

- Iliopsoas tendon catches on bony prominences
- Dx- extension + IR of hip from flexed & ER position
- Dynamic ultrasound or bursogram
- Tx: conservative > lengthening

**What is a 'sports hernia (athletic pubalgia)?**

- Groin pain w/ heavy training + valsalva secondary to injury of abdominal wall muscles or adductor longus
- Combination of abdominal hyperextension + thigh hyperabduction
- Tx: 6-8 weeks rest + therapy > repair/reinforcement of anterior abdominal wall if non-op ineffective

**What is ischiofemoral impingement?**

- Pain w/ passive extension + adduction due to contact of LT and lateral border of ischium
- Affects quadratus femoris muscle
- Local injection is diagnostic

**What are some indications for hip arthroscopy?**

- FAI, labral tear, loose bodies, iliopsoas disorders, synovitis

**In what situations may hip arthroscopy lead to inferior results?**

- Pts w/ arthritis, severe pincer lesions, moderate - severe developmental dysplasia of the hip (DDH), instability s/p extensive capsulectomy

**What is a risk with prolonged traction during hip arthroscopy?**

- Pudendal nerve palsy secondary to perineal post

**What portals are commonly used during hip arthroscopy and what structures are at risk?**

Sports 4: 6:50

- Anterolateral (to greater trochanter)- superior gluteal nerve
- Posterolateral (to greater trochanter)- sciatic nerve- esp w/ ER
- Anterior- LFCN > femoral

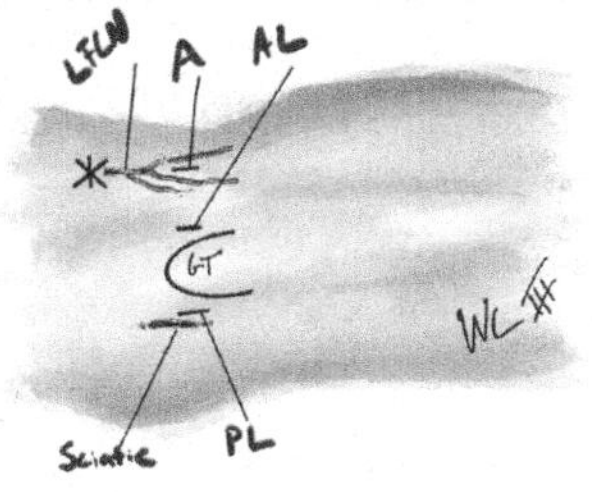


**Figure 2.3: A view of the right hip from the side showing portals that are commonly used in hip arthroscopy. GT marks the greater trochanter, AL is the anterolateral portal and PL is the posterolateral portal. A is the anterior portal. LFCN- lateral femoral cutaneous nerve**

**What are the compartments used for hip arthroscopy?**

- Central- intra articular portion between cartilaginous portions of prox femur/acetabulum
  - Labral repair/chondroplasty + acetabuloplasty

- Peripheral- intra articular portion of hip along neck of femur and edge of acetab
  - Femoroplasty
- Lateral- extra articular portion in peritrochanteric region + troch bursa
  - Gluteus medius repair, IT band release

Ep 17: w/ Dr. Okoroha

**What is FAI?**

- Abnormal contact between proximal femur + acetabulum > leads to chondral damage and sxs

**What do you look for on AP pelvis when evaluating for FAI?**

- Acetabulum morphology
- Lateral CEA- (vertical line along longitudinal axis of pelvis to a line towards edge of sourcil) Normal 25-40°, Hip dysplasia- CEA <20°
- Crossover sign- seen with acetabular retroversion causing pincer impingement. Anterior wall crosses lateral to the posterior wall. Ischial spines visible on AP pelvis
- Pistol grip deformity- nonspherical femoral head

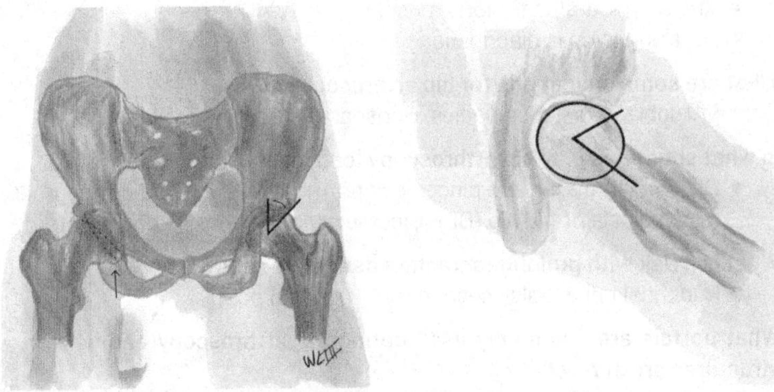

**Figure(s) 2.4 and 2.5: AP of the pelvis (2.4) showing the crossover sign on the right acetabulum and showing the lateral center edge angle of the left hip. A lateral of the hip (2.5) shows the alpha angle. A lateral CEA <20° is indicative of hip dysplasia. An alpha angle >55° is indicative of a cam deformity.**

**What do you look for on lateral xrays when evaluating for FAI?**

- Alpha angle- angle between line down middle of neck to center of femoral head & the point at which the femoral neck exits the circle
  - Normal <50°
  - >55° = cam morphology

**What are the types of FAI?**

- Cam + pincer lesion. Combined is most common

**What is cam impingement?**

- Common in young males
- Nonspherical femoral head + decreased head-neck offset
- Located anterolateral on femoral neck

- In hip flexion: aspherical head creates shearing force along acetabulum cartilage > leading to delamination/ cartilage flaps
- Labral tearing later in process
- Femoroplasty- normalizes offset

**What is pincer impingement?**

- MC in middle age females
- Acetabular overcoverage- results in abnormal contact between acetabular rim + femoral head-neck junction
- Results in intrasubstance tears of labrum- anterosuperior quadrant common
- Chondral injury is usually posterior inferior (contrecoup)
- Tx acetabuloplasty + labral repair

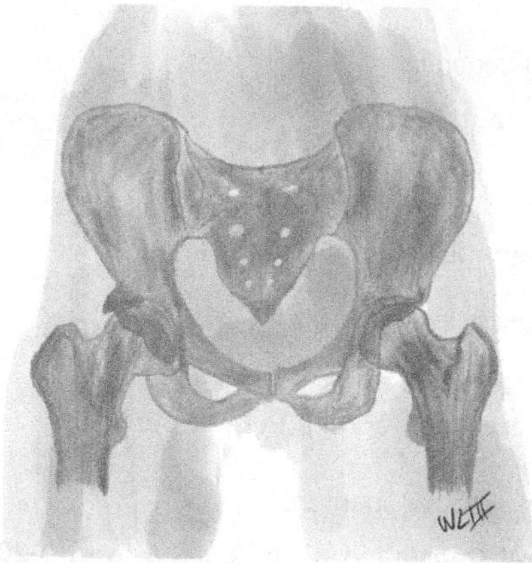

**Figure 2.6: AP of the pelvis showing a pincer lesion of the left acetabulum.**

**What is the most common reason for revision surgery in FAI?**

- Persistent FAI
- Also, poorer results w/ arthritis

**What are the symptoms of a labral tear of the hip and how is it diagnosed?**

- Anterior groin pain +/- mechanical sxs
- Pain w/ FADIR
    - MR arthrogram is most sensitive and specific test- anterior superior tears MC
- Tx: underlying hip disease + repair labrum
    - Inferior results w/ debridement

# Knee

**What nerve innervates the knee joint?**

- Posterior articular branch of PT

**Where in relation to the PCL does the nutrient artery to the tibia insert?**

- Below the PCL insertion

**What type of collagen makes up the articular cartilage of the knee?**

- Type II collagen
- Inc water + decreased PG's seen in OA

**Where is the origin and attachment site of the ACL?**

- Lateral femoral condyle > anterior tibia

**What artery supplies the ACL?**

- Middle geniculate artery

**What are the two bundles of the ACL and their functions?**

- Anteromedial bundle- tight in flexion and limits translation
- Posterolateral bundle- tight in extension and controls rotation

**What is the name of the structure that runs vertically with the knee in 90 flexion and divides the ACL bundles?**

- Lateral bifurcate ridge

**Sports 5: 4:08**

**Where does the PCL originate and attach?**

- Medial femoral condyle > posterior tibial sulcus

**What are the two bundles of the PCL and their functions?**

- Anterolateral - tight in flexion
- Posteromedial bundle- tight in extension

**What are the meniscofemoral ligaments?**

- Humphry- anterior to PCL
- Wrisberg- posterior to PCL

**What structures make up the posteromedial corner of the knee?**

- Sartorius (superficial)
- Superficial MCL, posterior oblique ligament, semimembranosus
- Deep MCL (deep)

**What structures make up the posterolateral corner (PLC) of the knee?**

- Biceps + iliotibial band
- LCL, popliteus (IR tibia), popliteofibular ligament

**What is the key restraint to lateral translation of the patella from 0-20 degrees of knee flexion?**

- MPFL

**The meniscus is primarily made up of what type of collagen?**

- Type I collagen
- Longitudinal + radial fibers

**What are some differences between the lateral and medial meniscus?**

- Lateral - semicircular shaped, more mobile, inserts near ACL

**What is a key feature w/ the history and pertinent PE for ACL injuries?**

- A hx of Pop + swelling. Or a non-contact twisting injury
- + lachman
- + pivot shift- lateral tibial plateau is subluxed anterior in extension, reduces with flexion due to IT band

**What is a key feature w/ the history and pertinent PE for PCL injuries?**

- Fall onto plantarflexed foot, ashboard injury
- + posterior drawer test + posterior sag noted w/ knee in 90 deg flexion

**What is the difference between opening to varus/valgus stress at only 30° of flexion vs in full extension?**

- Opening at only 30 degrees- isolated collateral injury
- Opening in full extension- combined cruciate + collateral injury

**What is a positive dial test indicative of?**

- Inc ER at 30 degrees of flexion- isolated PLC injury
- Inc ER at 90 degrees of knee flexion- Combined PLC + PCL injury

**What other physical exam maneuvers may be positive in LCL/PLC + PCL injury?**

- +Posterolateral drawer test, increased varus + tibial ER

**What is a positive J sign?**

- Patella takes an inverted J sign as knee goes from full extension into knee flexion
- Seen with PF instability

**What are some common radiographic findings in knee injuries and their significance?**

- Patella alta- patellar instability
- Segond fx- lateral capsule avulsion/ACL injury
- Fleck sign- small avulsion of MPFL from patella
- Square lateral condyle- discoid meniscus
- Pellegrini stieda fx- MCL avulsion

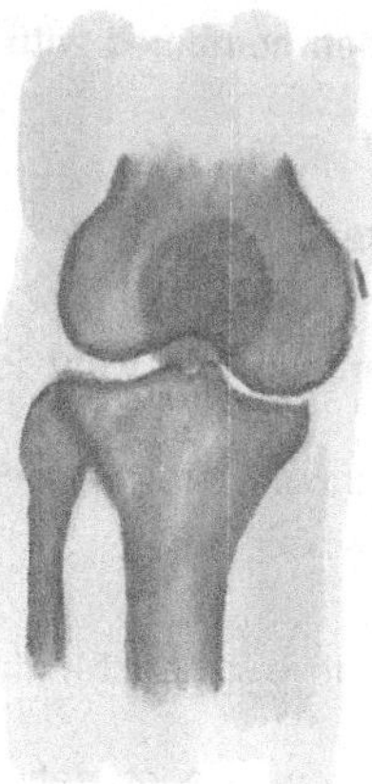

**Figure 2.7: AP of a knee showing a pellegrini stieda fracture, an avulsion of the medial collateral ligament (can be chronic).**

**What can you evaluate with weightbearing PA knee films (rosenberg)?**

- OA, OCD's, notch evaluation

**What can you evaluate w/ stress knee radiographs?**

- MCL/LCL injuries - varus/valgus
- PCL injuries

**What are some ways you can determine patellar height on lateral knee xray films?**

- Blumensaat's line
- Caton-deschamps ratio, insall-salvati, blackburne-peel

**What is the tibial tubercle to trochlear groove (TT-TG) distance?**

- Can be measured on CT or MRI. Distance between TG to TT apex on axial cut
- TT-TG>20 - some suggest TT anteromedialization osteotomy (fulkerson)

**What is the characteristic bone bruising seen on MRI w/ ACL injuries?**

- Mid ⅓ LFC + posterior ⅓ LTP bruising
- Kissing lesions

**What is a sign of a bucket handle meniscus tear seen on MRI?**

- Double PCL sign

**In an ACL deficient knee, injury to which meniscus is more common?**

- Medial meniscus (secondary stabilizer)

Sports 6: 6:45

**What type of meniscus tear is most common with acute ACL injuries?**

- Lateral meniscus

**What is a risk with partial meniscectomy if too much meniscus is removed?**

- DJD (arthritis)

**Which meniscus tears are amenable for repair?**

- Tears in the peripheral red-red zone
- Root tears, vertical tears, tears between 1-4cm, age <40

**What is the difference between outside in and inside out meniscus repair?**

- Inside out allows for better suture orientation than outside in for posterior horn tears

Ep 3 w/ Dr. Strauss Ep 60 w/ Dr. Saltzman

**What is the current gold standard for meniscus repair?**

- Inside out technique w/ vertical mattress sutures

**Is there improved healing of meniscal repair when combined with ACL reconstruction?**

- Yes

**What is the treatment of an acute meniscus root tear?**

- Repair, except when grade III or IV cartilage loss is present

**In what types of tears are meniscal cysts common and what is the treatment?**

- Common in middle ⅓ horizontal cleavage tears of lateral meniscus
- Tx: partial menisectomy + decompression through tear

**How do you diagnose a discoid meniscus?**

- Contiguous lateral meniscus on three consecutive sagittal MRI images
- Tx: observe if asymptomatic, partial meniscectomy (saucerization) for tears, repair for peripheral detachments

**When is a meniscus transplant indicated?**

- Controversial. Exhaust all non op management
- Prior total / near total meniscectomy, BMI <30, Age <50, no advanced arthrosis, normal alignment

**What is the most common complication after meniscus transplant?**

- Allograft tear

**Where is the most common location for an osteochondritis dissecans lesion?**

- Lateral aspect of medial femoral condyle
- Subchondral bone + overlying cartilage separation

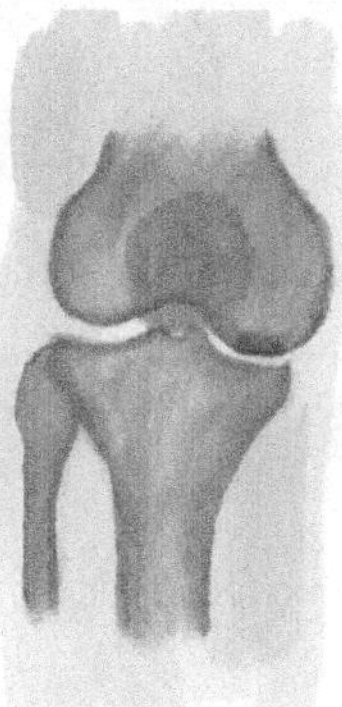

**Figure 2.8: AP of a knee showing an osteochondritis dissecans lesion. The most common location is on the lateral aspect of the medial femoral condyle.**

**What is the initial management of osteochondritis dissecans in an adolescent (open physes)?**

- Conservative w/ NWB 6-12 weeks, best prognosis
- Op tx for loose bodies, persistently symptomatic, and adult forms - arthroscopic drilling

**What are some tx options for articular cartilage lesions?**

Ep 40: w/ Dr. Nuelle

- Micro fracture- perforate subchondral bone- replaced by fibrocartilage -type I collagen will be replaced
- Autograft transfer <2.5cm
- Autologous chondrocytes- 2 stage
- Allograft - used for larger lesions

**What is the tx for spontaneous osteonecrosis of the knee?**

- Symptomatic tx, typically self limiting and seen after knee ATS in middle aged women

**Is arthroscopic synovectomy as effective as traditional open procedures for synovial lesions?**

- Yes, useful for PVNS, synovial chondromatosis, RA, etc

**What is a plicae?**

- Synovial folds that are embryologic remnants
- They can be pathologic, medial plicae is most common which can cause abrasion to the medial femoral condyle
- Tx- resect

## Knee Ligament Injuries

**What are some common history + PE findings with ACL tears?**

Ep 13 w/ Dr. Bonnaig

- Non-contact twisting injury, pop + knee effusion, quad avoidance gait (dec stride length and mid stance knee flexion is avoided)
- \+ Lachman, + Pivot shift

**What patients with ACL tears is non-op tx indicated?**

- Low demand patients, asymptomatic partial tears
- Operative tx: higher demand and active patients- reduces cartilage and meniscus injuries

Sports 7: 7:37

**What are different autograft choices ?**

- Bone tendon bone (BTB)- anterior knee pain, increased OA/DJD
- Quadriceps- 1.8x thick as patellar tendon
- Hamstrings: highest strength and stiffness

**What is a risk of graft harvest with a bone block?**

- Patella fracture

**Grafts less than what size are associated w/ increased failure rates?**

Ep 21: w/ Dr. Cooke

- <8.5mm

**Are allografts for ACL reconstructions associated w/ increased or decreased failure rate in young pts?**

- Increased rates
- Chemical processed or irradiated allografts have inc failure rates compared to fresh-frozen allograft

**What are key aspects of ACL rehab?**

- Early ROM- focus on extension
- Avoid isokinetic quad strengthening
- Eccentric strengthening inc quad + hamstring muscle mass
- No outcome difference in accelerated v nonaccelerated rehab

**What positions should the graft be placed on the femoral condyle?**

- 10 or 2 o'clock
- More horizontal placement- improved results, may reduce rotational instability

**What occurs when the femoral tunnel is too anterior / posterior?**

- Too anterior- tight in flexion
- Too posterior- tight in extension

**What occurs when the tibial tunnel is malpositioned?**

- Too anterior- roof impingement- tight in flexion

**What are some complications following ACL recon?**

- Tunnel malposition (ex: too vertical- rotationally unstable)
- Arthrofibrosis (begins in suprapatellar pouch)- ensure full ROM prior to surgery to ensure

**What are some complications seen with ACL hamstring harvest?**

- Graft amputation, saphenous nerve injury, possible loss of knee flexion strength

**What are some ways to prevent patella fracture?**

- Drill holes at corners, less rectangular graft, bone graft the defects, cutting undersurface, smaller saw blade

**What is a cyclops lesion?**
- A fibroproliferative tissue that blocks knee extension
- Sometimes a 'click' is heard/felt at terminal extension

**What is the most common organism seen w/ ACL infections?**
- Staph epi > aureus

**What are ways to prevent ACL tears in the female athlete?**
- Neuromuscular training/ plyometrics

**Sports 7: 25:50**

**What is the origin and attachment of the PCL?**
- Anterolateral aspect of medial femoral condyle + attaches to posterior tibia plateau

**What is the mechanism of injury for a PCL ligament injury?**
- Dashboard injury
- Fall onto a plantarflexed foot

**What is the PE finding in patients w/ a PCL injury?**
- Posterior drawer test
- Quadriceps active test
    - Knee flexed 90 deg. Quads are activated and look for anterior tibia translation/tibia reduction. Positive test = PCL injury
- Dial test

**What are the different grades of PCL injury?**
- Grade I- Isolated PCL injury- tibia is anterior to condyles
- Grade II- isolated complete PCL injury- anterior tibia is flush w/ condyles
- Grade III- possible ACL/PCL injury tibia is posterior to condyles

**What can be seen on xray w/ PCL injuries?**
- Avulsion injuries
- Subluxation on stress radiographs (>12mm difference indicative of PCL/PLC injury)
- PF compartment and medial compartment arthritis w/ chronic injuries (varus thrust)

**What is the treatment of PCL injuries?**
- Grade I/II- non-op w/ extension bracing and rehab to strengthen quads
- Grade III- Reconstruction
- Avulsion fx- ORIF

**What are some key techniques with PCL reconstruction?**
- Tibial inlay v transtibial
- Single bundle v double bundle

**What are some differences between tibial inlay and transtibial technique?**
- Tibial inlay- biomechanical advantages- avoidance of the killer turn/ acute graft bending leading to graft laxity

**What are some differences in PCL fixation between single and double bundle techniques?**

- Single bundle- fix graft at 90 flexion
- Double bundle- fix anterolateral at 90 of flexion (most important for posterior stability)
- PM bundle tighten in extension

**What is the mechanism and tx of most MCL injuries?**

- Valgus force to knee
- Non-op

**What is the mechanism and tx of most LCL injuries?**

- Varus force to knee
- Non-op
- Tx if combined injury (ex: PLC)

Ep 11: w/ Dr. Jorge Chahla

**What is the type of instability seen with posterolateral corner injuries?**

- Posterolateral rotatory instability- lateral tibial plateau moves posteriorly compared w/ lateral femoral condyle (increased ER)

**What are some PE findings in patients w/ a PLC injury?**

- Positive dial test
- Possible positive reverse pivot shift test - not sensitive/specific though
    - Subluxed tibia in flexion that reduces w/ knee extension

**What is the treatment of an acute PLC injury?**

- Repair

**In patients undergoing ligament reconstruction w/ multiligamentous knee injuries, what should you be on the lookout for when performing arthroscopy?**

- Fluid extravasation due to injured tissues
- Esp w/ pump use. Monitor compartments

**What is the optimal timing for ligament reconstruction after knee dislocation?**

- Controversial, but some studies show early tx is associated with superior clinical outcomes

Sports 8: 29:45

**What is a common complication after multiligamentous knee reconstruction + a way to avoid it?**

- Knee stiffness, early ROM

**What radiographs can you obtain to evaluate the extent of tibiofemoral arthrosis?**

- 45 degrees PA flexion WB radiographs (roseberg)

**What is the mechanical axis of the limb?**

- Center of hip through knee through ankle

**What is the normal knee joint line orientation in relation to the mechanical axis of the limb?**

- 3 degrees of varus

**Which patients are knee osteotomy indicated in?**

- Young patients (<50) w/ single compartment arthritis

**What are the goals of knee osteotomy?**

- Maintain joint line perpendicular to leg mechanical axis
- (mechanical axis is transferred to unaffected compartment)

**What is the typical treatment for varus knee deformity?**

- High tibial osteotomy
- Varus is usually due to proximal tibia varus

**What does increasing the tibial slope do to the tibia?**

- Increases anterior tibial translation- stress on ACL

**What does decreasing the tibial slope do to the tibia?**

- Increases posterior tibial translation- stress on PCL

**What is the typical treatment for valgus knee deformity?**

- Varus producing supracondylar femoral osteotomy
- Valgus is usually due to lateral femoral condyle hypoplasia

**What are some complications following HTO?**

- Loss of correction (most common), lateral cortex fx, delayed union/ nonunion, compartment syndrome, hardware prominence

## Patello-femoral joint

**What is jumper's knee and the treatment?**

- Patellar tendonisis (mucoid degeneration)
- Pain at inferior border of patella
- Tx: rehab- stretching, eccentric exercises

Sports 9: 16:54

**What is housemaids knee and the treatment?**

- Prepatellar bursitis. Assoc w/ prolonged kneeling
- Tx: supportive, aspirate in wrestlers to r/o infection

**What is IT band syndrome and its tx?**

- Lateral knee pain worse w/ knee flexed 90 degrees (hill runners/ cyclists common)
- Tx: rehab. Excision/Z- lengthening if necessary

**What are some different etiologies for patella-femoral instability?**

- MPFL rupture (traumatic)
- Patellar/trochlear dysplasia
- Patella alta
- VMO weakness
- Ligamentous laxity

Ep 31: w/ Dr. Yanke

**What are some PE findings in patients w/ patellar instability?**

- J sign- lateral movement of patella w/ knee extension
- Patellar glide- translation of patella w/ knee extension. Divided into quadrants
- Patellar apprehension- feeling of subluxation/dislocation episode w/ lateral patella translation
- Patellar tilt- abnormal laxity allowing increased tilt
- Craig's test- patient is prone, knee flexed + IR of leg. Increased IR – femoral anteversion

**What are some things to look for on xray to evaluate patients w/ patellar instability?**

- Lateral knee Xray
  - Trochlear dysplasia- crossing sign- lateral + medial trochlear facet + trochlear groove intersects. Indicates they are all same height and trochlea is flat
  - Patellar height-caton-deschamps ratio –based on articular surface– normal <1.2
- Merchant view
  - Sulcus angle >145 suggests dysplasia
  - Standing LE films
- Assess alignment- Q angle

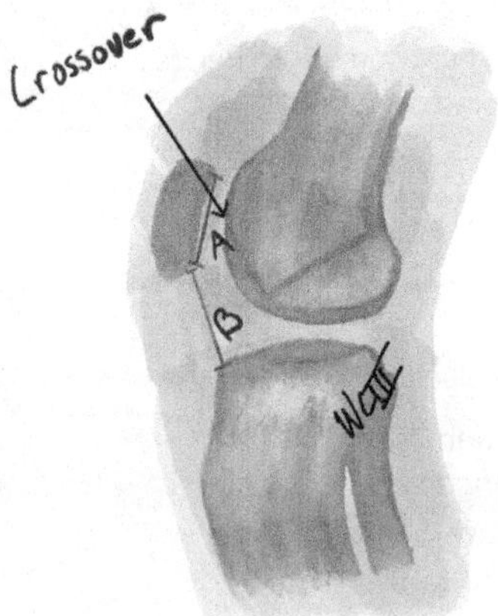


**Figure 2.9: A lateral view of the knee showing a crossover sign. This is seen when the lateral, medial trochlear facet and the trochlear groove intersect, indicating that trochlear dysplasia may be present. The Caton- Deschamps ratio is seen here (A/B) which can be used to assess patellar height.**

**What are some things to look for on CT scan to evaluate patients w/ patellar instability?**

- TT-TG distance
  - Superimpose axial image of TG and tibial tuberosity. Distance between lines. >15-20 are assoc w/ patellar instability
- Rotational alignment of limb
  - Assess cuts at hip, knee, ankle. Assess for anteversion
- Evaluate for trochlear dysplasia
- (Yes I know many of these are repeat questions... repetition is key!)

**What are some things to look out for on MRI to evaluate patients w/ patellar instability?**

- TT-TG distance
- MPFL ruptures

- Osteochondral fragments
- Articular cartilage defects (medial patellar facet / lateral femoral condyle)

**What is the initial management for patients w/ patellar instability?**
- Non-op: rehab, VMO strengthening, orthoses

**What is the treatment for a first time dislocator without a loose body / cartilage injury?**
- Non op tx. Some undergo operative tx if a loose body is present

**What are some common surgical options for patients w/ recurrent patellar instability w/ no improvement from non-op tx?**
- MPFL reconstruction - Anatomic recon at Schottles point
- Anteromedialization tibial tubercle osteotomy (Fulkerson)- TT-TG>20 + patellar tilt
- Lateral retinaculum release
- Trochleoplasty- controversial w/ mixed results
- Distalization/ distal femur osteotomy/ femoral rotational osteotomy

**Should an isolated lateral retinaculum release be performed for recurrent patellar instability?**
- No (most surgeons would say)

**Sports 10: 16:35**

**What is patellofemoral pain syndrome and its treatment?**
- Anterior knee pain worse w/ PF compressive maneuvers. Multifactorial etiology
- Tx: prolonged rehab

**What is lateral patellar facet compression syndrome?**
- Knee pain assoc w/ excessive patellar tilt + tight retinaculum
- Tx: conservative, rehab. Retinaculum release rarely indicated

**What is a bipartite patella?**
- Failure of an ossification center to fuse
- Characterized by smooth borders
- Tx of a symptomatic bipartite patella is conservative

**Are quadriceps tendon or patellar tendon ruptures more common in older patients?**
- Quad tendon rupture more common in pts >40 y/o

## Foot/Sports Injuries

**What is the most common ligament injured in ankle sprains + a common associated PE finding?**
- ATFL, + anterior drawer test. Plantarflexion injury

**What are some other commonly injured ligaments in ankle sprains?**
- CFL: +lateral tilt test
- Syndesmosis: + squeeze + ER test

**What is the treatment for an ankle sprain?**

- RICE, followed by PT + peroneal strengthening
  - Decreases recurrence

**What are some operative treatment options for patients w/ recurrent ankle instability w/ no improvement w/ PT?**

- Modified Brostrom—Anatomic ATFL reconstruction w/ extensor retinaculum augmentation
- Non-anatomic procedures—Chrisman Snook, Evans (peroneal tendon procedures)

**What is the most common complication following ankle arthroscopy?**

- Nerve injury (SPN) during anterolateral portal placement

**What are the sxs of chronic exertional compartment syndrome?**

- Pain + swelling with activity, quickly relieved by rest
- Common in runners/cyclists

(Roscoe, 2015)

**How do you diagnose exertional compartment syndrome?**

- Continuous pressure measuring at the following intervals:
  - At rest >15mmHg, after 1 minute >30mmHg, after 5 min >20mmHg
- Although, some studies suggest continuous monitoring until pain is too much and patients has to stop - higher sensitivity/ specificity

**What is the most common compartment affected w/ chronic exertional compartment syndrome?**

- Anterior compartment. Fasciotomy may be needed. Watchout SPN

# SHOULDER

**What artery contributes most to the blood supply to the humeral head?**

- Posterior circumflex artery

**What is an os acromiale?**

- An unfused secondary ossification center, most commonly at junction of mesoacromion and meta-acromion

**What are the static restraints of the shoulder?**

- Structures that provide unidirectional limitation to translation
- Glenoid labrum (increases depth), GH ligaments, humeral head retroversion, intra articular pressure, articular conformity

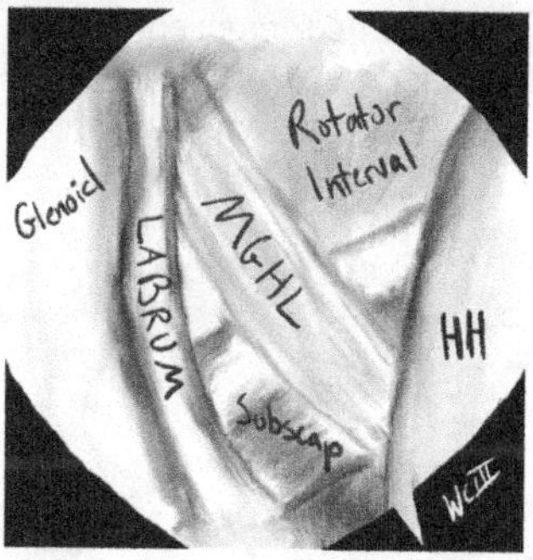


**Figure 2.10: Arthroscopic view of a right shoulder in beach chair position. Viewing from the standard posterior portal. MGHL- Middle glenohumeral ligament, HH- Humeral head, Subscap- Subscapularis tendon.**

**What are the different glenohumeral ligaments and their function?**

- Capsular thickenings that limit excessive HH rotation
- SGHL- Resists inferior translation w/ arm adducted
- MGHL- Resists anterior translation w/ 45 deg arm abduction
- IGHL
  - Anterior band- resists anterior translation @ 90 degrees abduction + ER
  - Posterior band- resists posterior inferior translation at 45-90 deg abd. Important in IR

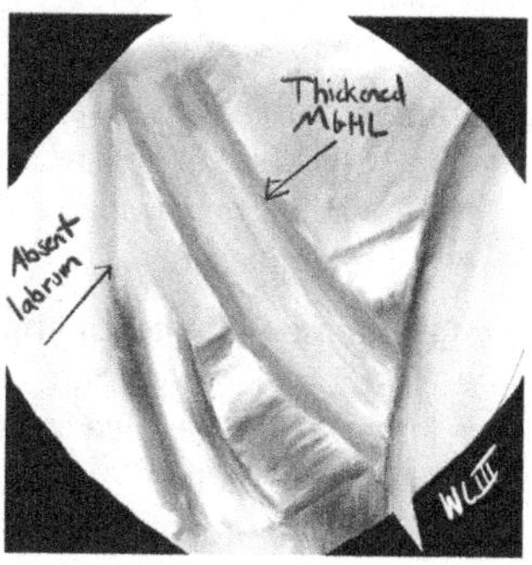


**Figure 2.11: An arthroscopic view of the right shoulder in the beach chair position, showing a buford complex.**

**What is a buford complex?**

- An absent anterosuperior labrum with a thickened cordlike MGHL

**What is a sublabral foramen?**

- Labrum not attached to glenoid anterior superior firmly. A variant

**What is the rotator interval and its borders?**

- Space between supraspinatus and subscap

- Medial border- lateral coracoid base
- Transverse humeral ligament forms apex laterally

Sports 12: 10:06

**What are the contents of the rotator interval?**

- Coracohumeral ligament, SGHL, biceps tendon, glenohumeral capsule

**What are some of the dynamic restraints of the shoulder?**

- Rotator cuff, scapular stabilizers, proprioception

**What is the rotator cable?**

- Thickening of the CH ligament located at medial aspect of rotator crescent formed by fibers perpendicular to the SS and IS
- Functions to transmit forces across rotator cuff complex

**What is the rotator crescent?**

- The thick crescent shaped sheet of RTC compromising the distal IS and SS insertions
- Relatively avascular area

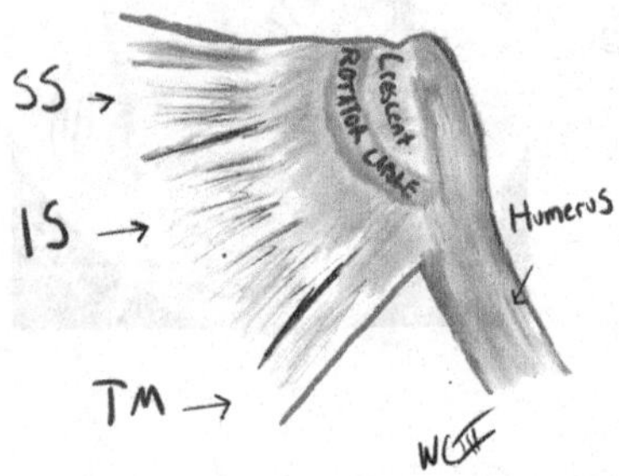


**Figure 2.12: A view of the rotator cuff muscles, the rotator cable, and the crescent. SS- Supraspinatus, IS- Infraspinatus, TM-Teres minor.**

## Shoulder Physical Exam

**What are some important parts when taking a shoulder history?**

- Patient age + chief complaint
- Young pts- shoulder instability, AC injuries, distal clavicle osteolysis
- Older pts- RTC tears, arthritis, fractures
- Night pain- RTC tear
- Contact w/ arm in Abduction/External rotation-instability

**What are some things to pay attention to on inspection PE for shoulder injuries?**

- Atrophy of SS/IS fossa/ obvious deformities
- Prominent medial scapula border
- Prior surgical scars

**What are some PE tests for impingement & how are they performed?**

- Neer Impingement sign- pain w/ FF in scapular plane > 90 degrees
- Impingement test- decrease in pain & ROM >90 degrees after subacromial injection
- Hawkins test- Pain w/ IR of the arm at 90 degrees of FF

**What are some PE tests for supraspinatus tears?**

- Jobe test- Pain/weakness w/ resisted FF at 90 degrees in scapular plane

- Drop arm test- patient is unable to maintain FF in plane of scapula- can indicated massive tear
- Whipple test- pain/weakness w/ resisted arm flexion while arm in FF and adduction

**What are some PE tests for infraspinatus tears?**

- ER lag sign- unable to hold an ER with the arm adducted
- Also weakness w/ resisted ER w/ arm adducted

**What are some PE tests for teres minor tears?**

- Hornblower sign- pain/weakness with resisted ER with the arm abducted to 90deg (can be pos with other lesions)

**What are some PE tests for subscapularis tears?**

- Lift off test- inability to elevate arm off back (lower>upper subscap)
- Bear hug- weakness with resisted ER while the hand is on the opposite shoulder and elbow is anterior to the body (upper subscap)
- Belly press test- inability to hold elbow forward while pressing on belly (lower subscap)

**What are some PE tests for anterior shoulder instability?**

- Apprehension test- apprehension when patient is supine, arm is abducted to 90 deg w/ ER and an anterior force is applied to humerus
- Relocation test- apprehension/ feeling of instability is relieved when a posterior force on the shoulder is placed in the same position
- Load & Shift - scapula is stabilized and the humerus is loaded to place HH in center of glenoid, then an anterior or posterior force is applied to the shoulder (ant/post instability)
    - 1+- translates to glenoid rim
    - 2+ translates over the glenoid rim and self reduces
    - 3+ translates over the rim but doesn't self reduce

**What are some PE tests for posterior shoulder instability?**

- Pain- block to ER may be seen w/ a fixed posterior dislocation
- Load & Shift- posterior translation
- Jerk test- posterior subluxation or a clunk heard when a posterior force is applied to humerus when arm is adduced and forward flexed
- Kim test- posterior shoulder pain when the arm is being elevated diagonally 45 degrees (above 90) with a downward and inferior pressure when the arm started abducted at 90 degrees- posterior inferior labrum test

**What are some PE tests for inferior shoulder laxity?**

- Sulcus sign- increased acromiohumeral interval w/ an inferior force when arm is hanging at side

**What are some PE tests for the superior labrum/ biceps?**

- No GREAT test
- O" Brien- pain w/ resisted FF with the arm in 10deg of adduction, pronated, and forward flexed that is reduced when the arm is supinated

at brought to neutral from an adducted position- SLAP- not very specific but is a little more sensitive
- Speed test- pain w/ resisted FF in scapular plane- biceps
- Yergason- pain w/ resisted supination- biceps

**What are some PE tests for AC joint pathology?**
- Pain w/ arm cross body adduction

**What are some PE tests for systemic hyperlaxity?**
- Beighton score- out of 9
  - 1 point for performing one on each side
- Little finger to touch arm (or bends >90 deg)
- Thumb to forearm
- Elbow hyperextension
- Knee hyperextension
- Palms to floor w/ knee straight (one point)

**What is a good xray view to evaluate for a shoulder dislocation?**
- Axillary lateral view

**Sports 13: 18:20**

**What can CT scan be useful for in the setting of shoulder pathology?**
- Visualize hill sachs/ bony bankart lesions
- Eval glenoid morphology- version/ bone loss

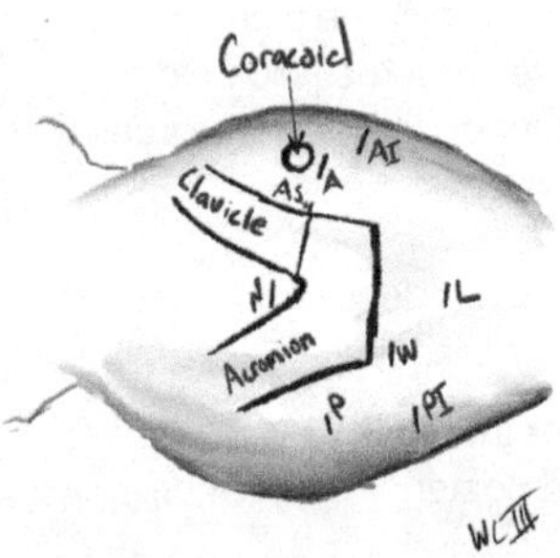


**Figure 2.13: A view of the shoulder showing some common portals used in shoulder arthroscopy. A-Anterior, AI- Anterior inferior, AS- Anterior superior, L- Lateral, W- Wilmington, P- Posterior, PI- Posterior Inferior, N- Nevaiser.**

**What are the standard portals for shoulder arthroscopy?**
- Posterior - 2cm distal/medial to PL acromion (viewing)
- Anterior - lateral to coracoid
- Lateral - 1-2cm distal to lateral acromial edge (RCR, SAD)

**What are some additional portals used in shoulder arthroscopy?**
- Wilmington (anterior to PL corner of acromion) SLAP
- Neviaser (through supraspinatus fossa)- SLAP + RC repair
- Anteroinferior (5pm)- bankart repair
- Posteroinferior (7pm)- stabilization procedures

**What nerve is 12mm distal to 6pm position?**
- Axillary nerve

# Shoulder pathology

**What is the spectrum seen in shoulder instability?**

- TUBS- traumatic unilateral dislocations w/ bankart lesions- may need surgery to prevent recurrence
  - TUBS- traumatic unidirectional bankart surgery
  - Anterior shoulder dislocation assoc w/ RTC tear in older pts
- Vs
- AMBRI- atraumatic multidirectional bilateral shoulder dislocation/ subluxation - rehab 1st
  - Atraumatic multidirectional bilateral rehabilitation inferior capsular shift

**What is the typical arm position for anterior shoulder instability / dislocation events?**

- Arm abduction to 90° and ER
- Anterior inferior GH ligament is the primary restraint to anterior dislocation
- Football, MMA

**What is a bankart lesion?**

- An anterior inferior labral tear - 'essential lesion of anterior shoulder instability'
- Bony bankart- a lesion to the glenoid as well

**What is a hill sachs lesion?**

- Posterolateral impaction of the humeral head

**What is an engaging hill sachs lesion?**

- When arm is placed into abduction + ER, HH subluxes or dislocates secondary to loss of glenoid contact

**What are some associated injuries seen with an anterior shoulder dislocation?**

- RTC tear in pts >40*
- GT fx, axillary nerve injury

**What is a HAGL lesion and the tx?**

- Humeral avulsion of the glenohumeral ligaments
- A coronal MRI image is shown w/ a lot of fluid
- Tx: Repair- open v arthroscopic

**What is an ALPSA lesion?**

- Anterior labrum periosteal sleeve avulsion- stripping of medial scapular neck periosteum
- Labrum is medialized + deficient. Seen w/ recurrent instability

**What is a GLAD?**

- Superficial anterior inferior labrum tear w/ a cartilage defect- causes a painful shoulder- not instability though

- Tx: Mobilize labrum into defect?

## Shoulder Instability

**Which patients may benefit from surgical stabilization after an acute, first time traumatic anterior shoulder dislocation?**

- Young active patients <23y/o- reduces recurrence

Ep 25: w/ Dr. Momaya

**Should you recognize any glenoid bone loss prior to surgery?**

- Yes... significant bone loss has been associated w/ instability recurrence w/ bankart repair
- 20-25% missing bone is considered significant bone loss and can require coracoid transfer vs distal tibia allograft

(Bottoni, 2002)

**In an arthroscopic bankart repair, how many anchors should be placed?**

- At least 3. (3-4)

**What are some factors that predict increased risk of recurrence after arthroscopic bankart repair?**

- Younger age, contact athlete, hyperlaxity, male gender, hill sachs lesion, glenoid bone loss

**What are some different techniques for open bankart repair?**

- Neer (subscap tenotomy)- longitudinal tenotomy w/ labral repair- humeral based capsular shift- shifting capsule superior and lateral-
- Jobe (subscap split)- horizontal capsulotomy w/ labral repair-glenoid based shift

**Is there any difference between open vs arthroscopic stabilization procedures?**

- Debated, possibly higher dislocation rates in arthroscopic group, equivalent QOL scores

(Mohtadi, 2014)

**What are some options for patients with an engaging hill sachs lesion?**

- Remplissage (soft tissue)
- Bone grafting / latarjet

**What is a latarjet procedure and its mechanism of stabilization?**

- Coracoid process transfer (consider in cases w/ glenoid bone loss)
- Sling effect from subscap + conjoined tendon, bone block effect from transferred coracoid, capsular repair effect of suturing CA ligament to capsule

**What are some complications associated w/ the latarjet procedure?**

- Nerve injury (MC), non-union/failure

**What is remplissage + complications?**

- Fills humeral defect w/ soft tissue (posterior capsule + infraspinatus)
- Used in conjunction w/ a labral repair
- Complications: decreased ROM

**What is the typical arm position for posterior instability?**
- FF, IR/neutral w/ a posterior force; may complain during bench press
- Lineman, seizures/ lightning strike (posterior shoulder dislocation)

**What is the light bulb sign?**
- Seen in posterior dislocation, HH appears like a light bulb
- Loss of ER- get axillary xray view!

**What is the tx for the 1st time posterior instability episode?**
- Rehab

**What are some other treatment options for posterior instability w/ no improvement w/ non-op tx?**
- Arthroscopic posterior labral repair
- Open stabilization procedures

**What is the presentation and treatment for patients w/ multidirectional instability?**
- Laxity in all planes, + beighton criteria, collagen disorders, + sulcus sign
- Tx: prolonged rehab
- If no improvement: capsular shift of plication +/- rotator interval closure

## Shoulder Impingement

**What is the treatment of a paralabral cyst w/ sxs of suprascapular nerve compression?**
- Shoulder arthroscopy w/ cyst decompression and labral repair (likely)

**What is the etiology of shoulder subacromial impingement syndrome?**
- Controversial
- Extrinsic- AL edge of acromion + CA ligament impinges
- Intrinsic- degeneration/tendinopathy in supraspinatus w/ SA space narrowing + abutment of RTC against acromion
  - Likely both

**What are the symptoms and PE findings of shoulder impingement syndrome?**
- Shoulder pain worse at night and w/ overhead activity
- +neer, + Hawkins, + impingement lidocaine test, strength normal

**What are the different types of acromion morphology?**
- Type 1- flat, Type II- curved, Type III- hooked
- Type II and III acromions are more common w/ RTC tears

**What is the initial treatment for shoulder impingement syndrome?**
- NSAIDs, activity modification, PT, Injections

**What is the treatment for shoulder impingement syndrome that does not improve w/ 6mo of PT?**
- Subacromian decompression (SAD), acromioplasty

**Which patients would you not want to do a SAD/acromioplasty on?**

- Overhead athletes or patients w/ massive irreparable RTC tears- limit acromial smoothing and perform a bursectomy
- Preserve CA arch- try to prevent anterior superior humeral migration

## Rotator cuff tears

(Mall, 2010 Keener, 2015)

**What percentage of asymptomatic full thickness RTC tears will become symptomatic or enlarge in ~3 years (2.8)?**

- 50%

**What is the function of the supraspinatus muscle?**

- Stabilizes the humeral head during early elevation and abduction

**What is the function of the infraspinatus?**

- External rotation of the humerus

**What are some areas of possible compression of the suprascapular nerve?**

- In suprascapular notch under ligament (both SS + IS)
- In spinoglenoid notch (IS)

Sports 14: 16:40

**What is the function of the subscapularis?**

- IR humerus (w/ PM, TM, ant deltoid, and lats)

**What symptoms do patients with a rotator cuff tear complain of?**

- Lateral shoulder pain, night pain, shoulder weakness, differences in AROM & PROM

**What are some things on xray you can assess in patients with a RTC tear?**

- AcromioHumeral Interval shortening - (8-10 normal), GH arthritis, AC joint arthritis

**What is the critical shoulder angle?**

- Measures the acromial overhand and glenoid inclination.
- >35-38deg may be assoc w/ recurrent RTC tears post-op
- <30 may be associated w/ GH arthritis due to inc GH forces

**What are different classification systems for RTC tears?**

- DeOrio and Colfield- based on the AP dimensions of the tear- Small <1cm, Medium 1-3cm, Large 3-5cm, Massive >5cm
- Patte- medial to lateral dimensions + thickness
- Burkhart- when viewed from lateral portal- crescent, U, L, Massive

**What is the goutallier classification system?**

- Grade 0- no fatty infiltration
- Grade I- some fatty streaks
- Grade II- fatty infiltration- more muscle > fat
- Grade III- equal fat and muscle
- Grade IV- more fat than muscle

**What is the tangent sign?**
- Supraspinatus muscle belly does not cross a line from the superior border of the coracoid to superior border of scapular spine
- Correlates w/ muscle atrophy + fatty infiltration- likely an irreparable RTC tear

**What does non-op treatment of RTC tears consist of?**
- PT, NSAIDS/Injections
- Patient expectations regarding PT is important (75% of patients get better- multiple studies)

**What patients w/ RTC tears would non-op management be indicated?**
- Pts w/ tendinitis, partial thickness, and some small <1cm full thickness tears
- Chronic full thickness tears in older pts (>65y/o)
- Irreparable tears (size, retraction, muscle quality + HH migration)

(Tashjian, 2012)

**What patients should RTC repair be considered in?**
- All acute full thickness tears (except some small tears)
- Chronic full-thickness tears in a young group (<65)

**What are the differences in outcomes between open and arthroscopic RTC repair?**
- Equivalent outcomes, but less pain and better visualization when done arthroscopically

**Where is blood flow to the repaired rotator cuff from?**
- The peribursal tissue and bone anchor site

**What is PASTA?**
- Partial articular supraspinatus tendon avulsion
  - Debridement v repair remains controversial
  - Consider: tear depth, pattern, amount of uncovered footprint, + patient activity level

**Is there any difference in clinical outcomes or healing rates after RTC repair with early vs delayed motion rehab protocols?**
- No

**What is an option for an irreparable SS + IS tear in a patient younger than 65 w/ no GH arthritis?**
- Tendon transfer- lat dorsi transfer to GT
- Lower trapezius transfer
- SCR

Ep 48: Superior Capsular Reconstruction w/ Dr. Mitchell

**What is an option for a patient w/ a massive irreparable RCT tear w/ OA?**
- RSA

**What are subscapularis tears associated with?**
- Coracohumeral ligament tear, Biceps tendon subluxation - biceps

tenodesis is an option for these patients

**What is the comma sign?**

- A sign of a subscap tear seen in arthroscopy, formed by an avulsed SGHL and CHL (leads you towards subscap)

**What is an option for an irreparable subscap tear in a young patient?**

- Pec major transfer

**What is rotator cuff arthropathy?**

- Massive RTC tear w/ superior HH migration + glenohumeral arthritis
    - Tendon transfers for younger, active patients may be an option

## Throwing/ Overhead athletes

**Sports 15: 26:00**

**What are the phases of throwing and what diagnoses are associated with some of the phases?**

- Wind up - No diagnoses
- Early cocking - no disorders
- Late cocking (high torque on shoulder and maximal elbow valgus stress)
    - MCL strain/tear, may see decreased ball velocity
    - Internal impingement occurs at this stage
    - SLAP tears - via peel back mechanism
- Acceleration
- Follow through/deceleration
    - Recognized as most harmful phase of throwing and highest torque on shoulder
    - Eccentric contraction of all rotator cuff musculature
    - See aggravation of SLAP tears and associated biceps tendinopathy, teres minor tears and distal biceps/brachialis tendonitis

**What are some common diagnoses/issues to look for in throwing athletes?**

- GIRD
- SLAP lesion
- Little league shoulder
- Internal impingement

**What is the pathoanatomy behind the thrower's shoulder?**

- SLAP lesion (peel back- described by Burkhart)
- PASTA lesion
- Humeral retroversion (inc ER), total arc maintained (hopefully)
- Posterior capsule contracture
- Anterior capsule laxity
- Bennett lesion

**What is GIRD?**

- Glenohumeral internal rotation deficit defined as >25 deg internal rotation deficit compared to contralateral shoulder mostly due to posterior capsular tightness

- Can also be due to excess humeral retroversion from repetitive torsional forces on the humerus from throwing as a kid

**What is the treatment for GIRD?**

- Posterior capsular stretching exercises aka "sleepers stretches"
- Only resort to posterior capsular release in refractory cases that don't respond to extended PT (most do)

**What is a Bennett lesion & its treatment?**

- Mineralization of the posterior inferior glenoid
- Conservative at 1st then shoulder ATS + excise

**What is little leaguer's shoulder?**

- A condition common in young baseball players- a stress reaction or salter harris type 1 fx
- Overuse of shoulder seen w/ repetitive pitching

**What are some imaging findings in little league shoulder?**

- May see widened lateral proximal humeral physis on XR
- Edema centered on physis with MRI
- This diagnosis is made primarily clinically though and should not rely on imaging

**What is the treatment for little league shoulder?**

- Rest for approximately 3 months with initiation of physical therapy directed toward proper mechanics and rotator cuff strengthening
- Advocate participation in multiple sports as total number of pitches and pitching year round are primary causes of little league shoulder

**What is a SLAP lesion?**

- Superior labral anterior to posterior tear
- Primarily occurs in overuse and overhead throwing athletes as their posterior capsule is tight and this causes a posterosuperior shift of the humeral head, especially in late cocking phase that puts shear stress on superior labrum

**What is the classification system for SLAP tears?**

- Snyder classification
- Type I- degenerative/ fraying
- Type II- detached from origin/anchor
- Type III- bucket handle tear
- Type IV- torn labrum w/ extension into proximal biceps

**What physical exam maneuver is very specific for SLAP tears?**

- None

**What are some anatomical variants of the superior labrum?**

- Sublabral foramen, sublabral foramen w/ thickened MGHL, buford complex (absent anterosuperior labrum w/ thickened MGHL)

**(Tuoheti, 2005)**

**What is the most common pattern of biceps attachment to superior labrum?**

- Posterior to 12 o'clock position
- Tuoheti classification goes over this but the true value of that study from 2005, was the description of the anterior IGHL attachment inferior or superior to 4 o'clock position on the glenoid for bankart repairs.
  - Posterior position showed all IGHL attachment inferior to 4 o'clock and any other biceps attachment the IGHL attachment was superior to 4 o'clock

**What associated condition might you see on MRI with a confirmed SLAP lesion?**

- Paralabral cysts, most concerning of which is the spinoglenoid notch cyst which can compress the traversing suprascapular nerve and lead to external rotation weakness in overhead throwing athlete

**What is the initial treatment for SLAP tears?**

- Rest, rehab, addressing GIRD with posterior capsular stretching

**What are the surgical options for SLAP Lesions?**

- Arthroscopic debridement, then rehab/GIRD stretching
- Repair is controversial and reserved for Type 2 tears in overhead throwing athletes
  - Return to play rates is lower for pitchers than position players
- Labral repair with biceps tenodesis v tenotomy
  - Mainstay for anyone over 36 and failed nonoperative management

**Sports 15: 6:07**

**What are some differences when it comes to biceps tenodesis vs tenotomy?**

- Tenotomy- assoc w/ cramping + popeye deformity
- Tenotomy is not associated w/ weakness
- Tenodesis- may have groove pain if tendon still in intertubercular groove (hence why subpec is used)

**What is internal impingement?**

- Impingement of the undersurface of the posterosuperior rotator cuff and posterior glenoid during late cocking

**What is the treatment for internal impingement?**

- Conservative, posterior capsular stretching, rest, rehab
- Surgical debridement vs RTC repair if conservative management fails

## Other shoulder conditions

**What are some PE findings of patients with DJD of the AC joint and treatment options?**

- TTP over AC joint, pain with cross body adduction
- Imaging- joint space narrowing + osteophytes

- Tx: conservative: AC joint injection
- Tx: surgical: distal clavicle resection (<1cm to avoid instability- preserve PS capsule)

**In what population is distal clavicle osteolysis common?**

- Weightlifters (hyperemia + inflammation w/ later bone resorption)
- Radiographs reveal: osteopenia + osteolysis
- Tx: Activity modification, injection > distal clavicle resection

**What is a typical mechanism of injury for pec major ruptures, and what part of the tendon is most often ruptured?**

**(Brown, 2021)**

- Eccentric contraction. Common in weightlifters. Tendon avulsion most common
- Treatment: Partial tear- non-op. Complete tear- repair lateral to biceps

**What is the etiology of frozen shoulder?**

- Female, age 40-70
- Associated w/ diabetes and thyroid disease

**How does frozen shoulder typically present?**

- Pain then a loss of external rotation
- As disease progresses, a global loss of ROM can be seen (AROM + PROM)

**What is the essential lesion in frozen shoulder and common histological findings + MRI?**

- Coracohumeral ligament + rotator interval capsule tightening
- Type III collagen + myofibroblasts and fibroblast seen under histology
- You can also see: GH joint capsule thickening, loss of axillary pouch, (none pathognomonic)

**What are the stages of frozen shoulder?**

- Early phase- pain- insidious onset (r/o locked dislocation)
- Mild phase- frozen- global ROM loss
- Late phase- thawing- gradual ROM return

**What are some tx options for frozen shoulder?**

- Therapy therapy therapy
- Operative: MUA + LOA, rotator interval release + capsular release (danger axillary nerve)

**What is the typical presentation of a stinger/burner?**

- Unilateral brachial plexopathy
- Resolves within minutes, normal C spine exam. Ok to RTP once symptoms resolve
- Careful if b/l sxs or C spine/ LE sxs

**What is the difference between suprascapular notch and spinoglenoid notch entrapment?**

- Both affect suprascapular nerve

- Suprascapular notch- affects SS and IS- compression by transverse scapular ligament
- Spinoglenoid notch-effects IS only- seen w/ paralabral cysts (cyst decompression + possible labral repair)

**What is quadrilateral space syndrome, its symptoms and diagnosis?**

- Axillary nerve or PCA compression in quadrilateral space (common to find a fibrous band between the teres major and long head of triceps)
- Pain + paresthesias w/ overhead activity- weakness in deltoid/ teres minor
- Dx w/ an arteriogram showing PCA compression
- Tx: release and decompress

**What is thoracic outlet syndrome?**

- Compression of neurovascular structures as they pass through scalene muscles + first rib
- Assoc w/ cervical rib, ptosis/ scalene muscle abnormalities
- Arm pain w/ paresthesias + positive wright test
- Tx: 1st rib resection

**What can an injury to the long thoracic nerve lead to?**

- Medial scapular winging (serratus anterior dysfunction)- C5-C7
- Can be due to compression injury or traction injury (backpacking/ weight lifting)
- Tx: PT for serratus anterior strengthening (1 year +)
- Operative: split pec major transfer +/- strip of fascia lata (chronic palsies)

**Injury to what structure leads to lateral scapular winging?**

- Trapezius - spinal accessory nerve- C2-C5
- Tx: therapy for trap strengthening
- Operative: nerve exploration, Eden-Lange Procedure: transfer of levator scapulae + rhomboid muscles, ST fusion

**What is snapping scapula syndrome?**

- Scapulothoracic crepitus- snapping scapula syndrome
- Painful scapulothoracic crepitus w/ arm elevation, pain relieved w/ manual scapula stabilization
- r/o osteochondroma and elastofibroma dorsi
- Tx: PT, injections, NSAIDs (works in most cases)
- Surgical: open or arthroscopic bursectomy +/- resection of superomedial scapula border

## Shoulder arthritis

Sports 17: 7:12

**What are some possible causes of glenohumeral arthritis?**

- Primary OA, post-traumatic OA, cuff tear arthropathy, RA, AVN, capsulorrhaphy arthropathy
- Chondrolysis, neuropathic arthropathy

**What are some common H&P findings in patients w/ shoulder OA?**

- Pain, ROM loss (ER loss due to anterior+inferior capsular tightness)

**What are some things to be on the lookout for in patients w/ shoulder OA?**

- Glenoid wear, humeral head flattening, inferior humeral head goat beard osteophytes, central humeral head wear, posterior subluxation of humeral head, rotator cuff pathology

**What are some radiographic features of rheumatoid disease?**

- Central glenoid wear, osteopenia, medialization of the humeral head w/ offset loss, minimal osteophytes

**What are some radiographic features of cuff tear arthropathy?**

- Proximal humeral head migration, acetabularization of the CA arch, femoralization of the proximal humerus

**What is the Hamada classification?**

- A classification system for rotator cuff arthropathy
  - 1 AHI >=6mm
  - 2 AHI <=5mm
  - 3 AHI <= 5mm w/ acetabularization of the coracoacromial arch
  - 4 GH joint narrowing
    - 4a no acetabularization
    - 4b with acetabularization
  - 5 HH osteonecrosis and eventual HH collapse

**What is the walch classification for GH arthritis?**

- A- humeral head centered on glenoid fossa
  - A1- no or minimal central erosion
  - A2- major central erosion
- B- posterior subluxation of humeral head
  - B1- no posterior bone loss
  - B2- posterior bone loss resulting in a biconcave glenoid
  - B3- enlarged biconcavity
- C- glenoid retroversion >25deg

**What are some things you can note on CT scan in patients w/ GH arthritis?**

- Glenoid morphology + bone stock
- Central wear + medialization- RA
- Posterior glenoid wear can be seen w/ ER contracture- OA

**What are some operative treatment options for patients w/ advanced OA?**

- Shoulder arthroscopy w/ debridement
- Arthrodesis
- Hemiarthroplasty w/ biologic resurfacing
- TSA
- RSA
- Resection arthroplasty

**What are some risk factors for failure of shoulder arthroscopy for shoulder arthritis?**

- Joint space <2mm
- Large osteophyte presence
- Grade 4 bipolar disease

**What are some indications for shoulder arthrodesis?**

- Failed prosthetic reconstruction
- Combined RTC and deltoid deficiency
- Paralytic disorders, intractable instability and infection
- Fusion position: 20° abduction, 30° FF, 40 IR°

**What are some indications for shoulder hemiarthroplasty?**

- Young patient w/ HH osteonecrosis w/o glenoid degeneration
- Decreasing indication, TSA shown to have better results

**Sports 17: 26:20**

**What is total shoulder arthroplasty?**

- Glenoid resurfacing, + HH replacement
- Preferred for shoulder OA and inflammatory arthritis
- Superior pain relief compared w/ hemi

**What are some contraindications for total shoulder arthroplasty?**

- Lack of sufficient glenoid bone
- Irreparable RTC or RTC arthropathy
- Deltoid dysfunction
- Brachial plexus palsy

**What are some things to consider w/ TSA on the humerus?**

- Humeral stem in 25-45° of retroversion
- Excessive humeral bone removal during osteotomy risks injury to RTC

**What are some glenoid things to consider w/ TSA?**

- Glenoid is positioned in neutral
- Address bone loss
- Pegs have lower loosening / revision risk compared w/ keel
- Uncemented glenoid/minimal is assoc w/ lower loosening rates

**What are some options to address posterior glenoid bone loss?**

- Eccentric reaming w/ 0-15° of retroversion
- 15° +
  - Posterior bone graft
  - Posterior augmented component
  - Correction w/ reaming
  - Ream + run
  - RSA w/ bone graft

**What are some complications with TSA?**

- *Glenoid loosening*
- RTC failure- subscap failure (inc ER compared w/ contralateral)

- Stiffness w/ overstuffed joint
- Infection (young males- C acnes- hold cultures 3x weeks)
- Nerve injury
- Instability

**What is a reverse shoulder arthroplasty?**

- Glenoid baseplate (cementless) w/ glenosphere (ball) assembled to baseplate
- Humeral stem w/ polyethylene socket

**What are some indications for RSA?**

- Proximal humerus fx / fracture malunion/nonunion
- RTC tear arthropathy
- Irreparable cuff tear
- Failed TSA
- Glenoid/humeral bone loss

**What is needed for a RSA?**

- A functioning deltoid + adequate bone stock

**What are some important things to know about the biomechanics of a RSA?**

- Design attempts to maximize compressive forces and minimize shear forces
- Grammont changed glenoid component to a hemisphere w/
    - Medialized joint COR + stabilizing bone-implant surface

**What has the medialization of shoulder COR been associated with?**

- Scapular notching, reduced IR, loss of shoulder contour

**What are some things to know about the glenoid component w/ RTSA?**

- Inferior positioning- helps decrease notching + gives more clearance between GT and acromial arch
- Inferior tilt- decreases notching

**What do lateralized glenoid designs do in regards to RSA?**

- Dec notching, better ROM w/o impingement
- Improved deltoid/posterior cuff tensioning
- May inc risk of implant instability

**Sports 18: 10:25**

**What do you generally want to limit in the immediate post-op period s/p TSA/RSA?**

- External rotation, esp w/ a subscap repair

**What is a common mechanism for anterior shoulder dislocation s/p RSA?**

- Pushing up from the chair
    - Shoulder hyperextension and ER
    - HH socket levers posteriorly

## Some elbow conditions

**What are common elbow disorders seen in athletes?**

- Tennis elbow "lateral epicondylitis"
- Golfer elbow "medial epicondylitis"
- MCL strain/rupture
- Valgus extension overload "pitchers elbow"
- LUCL injury
- Distal biceps avulsion
- Triceps rupture

**Starting with the most discussed- MCL rupture, what are the components of the MCL aka ulnar collateral ligament?**

- Anterior band - strongest and most important valgus stabilizer from 30-120 deg flexion
  - Medial epicondyle to sublime tubercle (2.8 mm distal to coronoid tip for those rotating on ortho sports service) with a mean length of 54 mm
  - Has anterior and posterior bands
- Posterior band - undergoes most change in length with elbow motion, tighter in flexion
- Transverse band

**What common tests diagnose UCL injury?**

- Milking maneuver and moving valgus stress
- Both place elbow in throwing position and stress UCL by pulling thumb posteriorly and placing valgus stress

**What imaging studies are typically obtained for UCL injuries?**

- Radiographs may show widened medial ulnohumeral articulation or bony avulsion
- MRI arthrogram more sensitive and specific than traditional MRI

**Sports 18: 24:00**

**What is the treatment for a UCL injury?**

- Strains are non-op with rest/PT
- Ruptures treated surgically with UCL reconstruction "tommy john"
  - 90% return to level of play
  - Humeral docking shown to be superior than figure of 8, and humeral docking with interference screw in ulna shown to be 95% of original UCL strength
  - Palmaris longus autograft vs gracilis vs allograft
  - Flexor pronator split better than release of flexor mass

**What is the muscle involved with lateral epicondylitis and what are some clinical tests to help diagnose it?**

- ECRB, originates on lateral epicondyle and inserts on base of third metacarpal
- Pain with resisted wrist extension

- Pain at the lateral epicondyle
- Maximal wrist flexion in pronation causes pain

**What is the classic histologic finding associated with lateral epicondylitis?**
- Disorganized collagen with angiofibroblastic dysplasia

## Podcast Episodes for a Deeper Dive

- Episode 3 w/ Dr. Strauss: Intro to Meniscus Injuries https://naileditortho.com/meniscusintro/
- Episode 11 w/ Dr. Chahla: Posterolateral Corner Injuries https://naileditortho.com/plcinjuries/
- Episode 13 w/ Dr. Bonnaig: Intro to ACL injuries https://naileditortho.com/aclintro/
- Episode 17 w/ Dr. Okoroha: Intro to Hip Labral Tears https://naileditortho.com/hiplabrum/
- Episode 21 w/ Dr. Cooke: Operative treatment of ACL Injuries https://naileditortho.com/acltreatment/
- Episode 25 w/ Dr. Momaya: Anterior Shoulder Instability https://naileditortho.com/25-anterior-shoulder-instability-w-dr-momoya/
- Episode 31 w/ Dr. Yanke: Patellar Instability https://naileditortho.com/31-patellar-instability-w-dr-yanke/
- Episode 40 w/ Dr. Nuelle: Cartilage Restoration https://naileditortho.com/cartilage/
- Episode 60 w/ Dr. Saltzman: How to read a Knee MRI +Operative Treatment of Meniscus Injuries https://naileditortho.com/readmriandmeniscus/
  YouTube Video: https://www.youtube.com/watch?v=zunUoKI_zuY
- Episode 61 w/ Dr. Mulcahey: The Female Athlete https://naileditortho.com/thefemaleathlete/
- Episode 71 w/ Dr. Jazrawi- SLAP tears https://naileditortho.com/slaptears/
  Video: https://youtu.be/Yw6_1EULPNA
- Episode 75 w/ Dr. Sherman- Early knee arthritis, high tibial osteotomy, knee deformity https://naileditortho.com/earlykneeoa/
  Video: https://youtu.be/9QDhfibFwdM
- Episode 78 w/ Dr. Erickson- UCL tears https://naileditortho.com/ucltears/
  Video: https://www.youtube.com/watch?v=api9lUsD0go&t=1096s
- Episode 83 w/ Dr. Freehill- The Throwers Shoulder https://naileditortho.com/throwershoulder/
  Video: https://www.youtube.com/watch?v=vIJZQZQn4c4&t=2616s
- Episode 86 w/ Dr. Abboud- Massive rotator cuff tears- Overview + SCR vs Balloon https://naileditortho.com/balloon/
  Video: https://youtu.be/LV9f_82B8x0
- Episode 88 w/ Dr. Bishop- Knee OCD lesions https://naileditortho.com/kneeocd/

Video: https://youtu.be/3W6sLW1rwlM

- Episode 89 w/ Dr. Shea- Elbow OCD lesions
https://naileditortho.com/elbowocd/
Video: https://youtu.be/qfU1DDVgSt0
- Episode 91 w/ Dr. Denard- Rotator Cuff Repair
https://naileditortho.com/rcrrepair/
Video: https://youtu.be/cYtF-NLX7VY

## Specific Articles Mentioned in the Podcast

Roscoe, D., Roberts, A. J., & Hulse, D. (2015). Intramuscular compartment pressure measurement in chronic exertional compartment syndrome: new and improved diagnostic criteria. *The American journal of sports medicine, 43*(2), 392-398.

Bottoni, C. R., Wilckens, J. H., DeBerardino, T. M., D'Alleyrand, J. C. G., Rooney, R. C., Harpstrite, J. K., & Arciero, R. A. (2002). A prospective, randomized evaluation of arthroscopic stabilization versus nonoperative treatment in patients with acute, traumatic, first-time shoulder dislocations. *The American Journal of Sports Medicine, 30*(4), 576-580.

Mohtadi, N. G., Chan, D. S., Hollinshead, R. M., Boorman, R. S., Hiemstra, L. A., Lo, I. K., ... & Paolucci, E. O. (2014). A randomized clinical trial comparing open and arthroscopic stabilization for recurrent traumatic anterior shoulder instability: two-year follow-up with disease-specific quality-of-life outcomes. *JBJS, 96*(5), 353-360.

Mall, N. A., Kim, H. M., Keener, J. D., Steger-May, K., Teefey, S. A., Middleton, W. D., ... & Yamaguchi, K. (2010). Symptomatic progression of asymptomatic rotator cuff tears: a prospective study of clinical and sonographic variables. *The Journal of Bone and Joint Surgery. American volume., 92*(16), 2623.

Keener, J. D., Galatz, L. M., Teefey, S. A., Middleton, W. D., Steger-May, K., Stobbs-Cucchi, G., ... & Yamaguchi, K. (2015). A prospective evaluation of survivorship of asymptomatic degenerative rotator cuff tears. *The Journal of bone and joint surgery. American volume, 97*(2), 89.

Tashjian, R. Z. (2012). Epidemiology, natural history, and indications for treatment of rotator cuff tears. *Clinics in sports medicine, 31*(4), 589-604.

Tuoheti, Y., Itoi, E., Minagawa, H., Yamamoto, N., Saito, H., Seki, N., ... & Abe, H. (2005). Attachment types of the long head of the biceps tendon to the glenoid labrum and their relationships with the glenohumeral ligaments. *Arthroscopy: The Journal of Arthroscopic & Related Surgery, 21*(10), 1242-1249.

Brown, S. M., Cole III, W. W., Provencher, M. T., & Mulcahey, M. K. (2021). Pectoralis Major Injuries: Presentation, Diagnosis, and Management. *JBJS Reviews, 9*(5), e20.

# NOTES

# NOTES

# NOTES

# NOTES

# BASIC SCIENCE

# CHAPTER 3

**What are the two types of bone?**

- Normal bone/ Lamellar/ Mature- cortical or cancellous bone- stress oriented- less cellular
- Woven/Immature - Pathologic bone (malignancy, infection, etc) or fx callus- not stress oriented. Weaker + more cellular

**BS 1: 4:20**

**What are some characteristics of cortical bone?**

- Higher young's modulus, stiffer, slower turnover
- Consists of tightly packed osteons/ haversian (or volkman) systems

**What are some characteristics of cancellous bone?**

- Lower young's modulus, less dense, high turnover

**What are the main types of bone cells?**

- Osteoprogenitor cells, osteocytes, osteoblasts, osteoclasts

**What cells are osteo-chondro progenitor cells derived from and via what transcription factor?**

- Mesenchymal stem cells, RUNX2 (BMP may also have a role in this)

**What is the differentiation of osteoprogenitor cells based on?**

- Strain + $O_2$
- High strain > fibroblast lineage
- Medium strain + low $O_2$ > Chondroblast
- Low strains + high $O_2$ > Osteocyte/osteoblast

**What are the transcription factors for osteoblast development + how do they work?**

- β-catenin, Runx2, Osx
- Mechanical stress- osteoprogenitor cells release Wnt proteins > causes production of β-catenin
- β-catenin- controls RUNx2 production, RUNx2 controls Osx for terminal osteocyte differentiation

**What are the transcription factors for chondrogenesis?**

- Sox9

**What are the transcription factors for adipogenesis?**

- PPARy2

**What are the transcription factors for tendon and ligament formation?**

- Scleraxis

**What does the osteoblast produce?**

- Bone
- A non mineralized matrix of type I collagen and alkaline phosphatase

**BS 1: 16:10**

- Matrix specific proteins, ex: osteocalcin
- Receptor activator of nuclear factor (NF)- kβ ligand (RANKL)
- Osteoprotegerin- binds RANKL- limits activity

**What are some receptors on the osteoblasts and their effect?**

- PTH- uses adenylyl cyclase as a mediator for cellular signaling
  - Pulsatile PTH stimulates osteoblast activity
  - Continuous PTH has opposite effect
- 1,25 (OH)2 vitamin D- stim alkaline phosphatase synthesis + production of bone specific proteins ex: osteocalcin
- Glucocorticoids- inhibit osteoblast protein synthesis
- Estrogen- prevents bone resorption + Inc mRNA levels for alkaline phosphatase, inhibits adenylyl cyclase
- Prostaglandins- activates adenylyl cyclase + stimulates bone resorption

**What is alkaline phosphatase required for?**

- Synthesis of inorganic phosphate and is important to bone matrix formation

**What are osteocytes?**

- Old osteoblasts trapped in the matrix

**Can osteocytes inhibit osteoblasts?**

- YES, via sclerostin

BS 1: 24:05

**What does sclerostin do, and how?**

- Limits bone formation
- Via Wnt-pathway antagonism
- Sclerostin (SOST) and dickkopf (dkk) are inhibitors of Wnt/b-catenin pathway
- Normal wnt/b-catenin pathway is as follows: (in absence of sclerostin)
  - Wnt binds to LRP5/6 and PREVENTS phosphorylation of β-catenin
  - Unphosphorylated β-catenin CAN pass into nucleus and upregulate osteoblastic differentiation, thus increasing bone formation
- With sclerostin and dkk present:
  - Sclerostin binds to wnt which causes phosphorylation of β-catenin because wnt cannot bind to LRP5/6
  - LRP5/6 then phosphorylates β-catenin and now it CANNOT pass into nucleus and increase osteoblastic upregulation, thus decreasing bone formation

**What are some things that increase or decrease sclerostin?**

- PTH increases sclerostin - which decreases bone formation.. Which makes sense from above (remember continuous PTH decreases bone formation)
- Calcitonin- decreases sclerostin- which increases bone formation

**If you are trying to increase bone production, do you want low or high blood levels of sclerostin?**

- Low... less osteoblast inhibition

**What are some things that stimulate osteoblast activity?**

- Wnt proteins
- Estrogen
- Intermittent PTH

**What are some things that inhibit osteoblast activity?**

- Sclerostin
- Glucocorticoids
- Continuous PTH

**What do osteoclasts do?**

- Take away bone (mineralized matrix only- they cant resorb unmineralized osteoid)
- They are multinucleated giant cells

BS 2: 1:30

**Where are osteoclasts derived from?**

- Hematopoietic cells in macrophage lineage

**What molecule activates osteoclasts?**

- RANKL

**What can stimulate RANKL to cause bone resorption?**

- PTH
- IL-1 and PTHrP- via metastatic pathways

**What molecule prevents osteoclast activation by inactivating RANKL?**

- Osteoprotegerin, the decoy receptor

**What molecule decreases osteoclast activity by directly binding to the osteoclast?**

- Calcitonin (from parafollicular cells of thyroid)
  - Opposite effect of PTH

**What is the effect of calcitonin?**

- Slows bone resorption, decreases serum calcium

**What cell makes osteoprotegerin?**

- Osteocytes

**Where does bone resorption occur on the osteoclast?**

- At the ruffled border (plasma membrane enfoldings that inc SA for resorption) > forms howship's lacunae

**How does the osteoclast actually bind to the bone?**

- Integrins (αvβ) on osteoclast mate w/ vitronectin on bone & seals space below osteoclast (like an alien spaceship)

**What is the amino acid sequence that is found on the bone for vitronectin where the integrins can bind?**

- Arg-Gly-Asp (RGD) sequence

**How does the osteoclast actually resorb the bone?**

- TRAP (tartrate resistant acid phosphate) lowers the pH using carbonic anhydrase
- This makes the hydroxyapatite crystals more soluble
- The matrix is removed by proteolytic digestion (cathepsin K- is a big one of these proteolytic enzymes)

**What happens when there is a mutation in carbonic anhydrase?**

- Osteopetrosis

**What is it called when there is a mutation in cathepsin K (autosomal recessive)?**

- Pyknodysostosis

BS 2: 16:00

**What type of collagen makes up the majority of organic bone matrix?**

- Type I collagen (tensile strength)

**What are some of the other components of organic bone matrix?**

- Proteoglycans- compressive strength of bone
- Osteocalcin- prod by osteoblasts- most abundant non collagenous matrix protein
    - Osteonectin produced too
- Hydroxyapatite- compressive strength of bone

**What is Wolff's law?**

- Bone remodeling occurs in response to mechanical stress

**What is Hueter-Volkmann law?**

- Compressive forces inhibit growth, tension stimulates growth

**Where do long bones get most of their blood supply from?**

- Nutrient artery- supply inner ⅔ of mature cortex via haversian system
- The rest come from the metaphyseal-epiphyseal system + periosteum

**What is the typical blood flow to bones and how does it change with fracture?**

- Centrifugal- inside to outside (from high to low pressure)
- When fx disrupts nutrient artery > centripetal (outside>in)

**Does blood flow play any part of how well a fracture heals?**

- Yes

**What are the three types of bone formation?**

- Intramembranous- no cartilage (distraction osteogenesis)
- Endochondral- cartilage replaced by bone (fracture callus)
- Appositional- on top of old bone (inc bone width)

**What is the process for endochondral bone formation?**

- Undifferentiated cells make cartilaginous matrix > chondrocytes
- Matrix mineralizes > vascular bud invasion which brings osteoprogenitor cells
- Osteoclasts absorb cartilage produced by chondrocytes
- Osteoblast makes bone on cartilaginous framework

**How are long bones formed?**

- Bones formed from mesenchymal anlage at 6 weeks gestation
- Vascular buds bring osteoprogenitor cells > osteoblasts > 1 ossification centers
- WNT protein to LRP5 or LRP6 stimulates differentiation
- Secondary ossification center develop at ends > forms epiphyseal centers > longitudinal growth

**BS 3: 1:30**

**How many growth plates exist in immature long bones?**

- Horizontal (physis)
- Spherical (epiphysis)

**What are the physeal cartilage zones + function?**

- Reserve zone- stores lipids, glycogen + proteoglycan aggregates
- Proliferative zone- chondrocytes stack, cellular proliferation, inc proteoglycans
- Hypertrophic zone- chondrocytes inc size, chondrocytes mature regulated by hormones + local growth factors, osteoblasts migrate
  - Maturation, degeneration, provisional calcification

**What are some common conditions that affect each of these zones?**

- Reserve zone- lysosomal storage diseases (ex: Gaucher)
- Proliferative zone- achondroplasia, growth hormone (gigantism)
- Hypertrophic zone- Widens in rickets, origin of enchondromas, mucopolysaccharidosis (Morquio / Hurler syndrome), physeal fractures, and slipped capital femoral epiphysis

**What does Indian hedgehog (Ihh) released by chondrocytes do?**

- Causes release of PTH-rP which...
  - In reserve zone- stimulates chondrocyte proliferation
  - In proliferative zone- inhibits
- Indian hedgehog is also responsible for osteophyte formation in arthritis

**What supplies chondrocytes to the periphery to help with lateral growth?**

- Groove of ranvier (a wedge shaped zone of cells at the periphery of epiphysis)
- Responsible for inc growth width (appositional)

**What is the perichondrial fibrous ring of La Croix?**

- Fibrous tissue that supports + anchors the periphery of the physis

**What are the two types of fracture healing and what determines the type of healing that will occur?**

- Primary + secondary
- Degree of stability determines strain which determines type
- <2% strain - primary, 2-10% strain- secondary

BS 3: 12:15

**When will there be primary bone healing and how does it occur?**

- Absolute stability constructs / < 2% strain
- Haversian remodeling- cutting cones (osteoclasts followed by osteoblast)
- Intramembranous healing

**What are the stages of secondary bone healing?**

- Inflammation:
  - Hematoma formation, osteoblast + fibroblast proliferation (due to BMP signaling), granulation tissue around fx ends
- Repair:
  - The mechanical environment drives differentiation
    - Low strain > osteoblastic
    - Higher strain > chondrocytic
  - Primary callus w/i 2 weeks- soft callus later replaced by hard callus (woven bone)
- Remodeling:
  - Wolff's law- allows bone to assume normal configuration

**What are some medications/ substances that can affect fracture healing?**

- Nicotine- increases nonunion risk
- NSAIDs- dec healing in lumbar spinal fusions (COX-2 needed in inflammatory stage)
- Diet- protein malnutrition- negative effects in fx healing

**What are some devices that can affect fracture healing?**

- Ultrasound- low intensity pulsed ultrasound- inc mechanical strength of callus
- Electrical bone stimulator- inc osteoblast activity by dec $O_2$ concentration + inc tissue pH

BS 3: 26:15

**What does osteoconductive / osteoinductive/ osteogenic mean?**

- Osteoconductive- acts as scaffold / framework for bone growth
- Osteoinductive- growth factors (BMP), that stimulate bone formation
- Osteogenic- primitive mesenchymal cells, osteoblasts + osteocytes

**What is creeping substitution?**

- Seen w/ cancellous bone graft w/ nonunions/cavitary defects- lays down new bone on old trabeculae

**When are cortical bone grafts used?**

- Structural defects, slow turnover + incorporation

**Do fresh allografts have more or less immunogenicity?**

- More (freeze dried is less immunogenic and is purely osteoconductive)

**What are the grafting properties of demineralized bone matrix (acidic bone matrix extracted from allograft)?**

- Osteoconductive w/o structural support, minimal osteoinductive

**What are the grafting properties of calcium phosphate?**

- Osteoconductive + highest compressive strength of any graft material

**Which synthetic bone graft is the fastest to resorb?**

- Calcium sulfate

**What is the dietary requirement of calcium?**

- 1300mg/day for adolescents/ young adults (10-25yo)
- 1200-1500 age >50yo
- 1500 mg/day for postmenopausal women + pts w/ healing fx of long bone

**BS 4: 1:00**

**What cells synthesize PTH and what is the synthetic form of PTH called?**

- Chief cells of parathyroid glands, Increases serum calcium & dec phosphate
- Teriparatide

**What cells synthesize calcitonin and what does it do?**

- Parafollicular cells of thyroid gland
- Decreases serum $Ca_2$+ (inhibits osteoclast bone resorption by decreasing osteoclast # and activity)

**What is the active form of Vitamin D3?**

- $1,25(OH)_2$ (works at kidneys, intestines, and bones)
- $24,25(OH)_2$ is inactive form

**What is the preferred laboratory study to examine vitamin D deficiency?**

- 25 Vitamin D

**What are the labs seen in primary hyperparathyroidism?**

- Inc: PTH, serum Ca2+, urinary phosphate
- Dec: serum phosphate

**What bony change is seen in primary hyperparathyroidism?**

- Osteitis fibrosa cystica (marrow replaced by fibrous tissue)
- Brown tumors- giant cells, hemosiderin staining, fibrous tissue hemosiderin
- Chondrocalcinosis

**What does the impaired renal function in renal osteodystrophy cause?**

- Less phosphate excretion & 1,25 vitamin D production
- This leads to:
    - High turnover bone disease- Inc PTH & secondary hyperparathyroidism

- Low turnover bone disease- Normal PTH

**What is the difference between rickets & osteomalacia?**

- Both are disorders of impaired mineralization
- Rickets- cartilage matrix is affected- *Zone of provisional calcification*
- Osteomalacia- bone matrix is affected (adults)

**What are some changes seen in rickets?**

- Increased physeal width and disorientation
- Bone bowing and cortical thinning

**What are some different causes of rickets?**

- Vitamin D deficiency (nutritional- malabsorption, chronic parenteral nutrition)
- Calcium deficiency rickets
- Phosphate deficiency rickets
- Hereditary vitamin D dependent rickets
- Familial hypophosphatemic rickets (Vit D resistant rickets or phosphate diabetes)

**What is the physiology and lab/xray findings with vitamin D deficient rickets?**

- Deficiency in vitamin D> dec calcium > Increased PTH + resultant dec phosphate
  - Inc osteoclast activity > increased alkaline phosphatase
- Xray- physeal cupping

**What is familial hypophosphatemic rickets?**

- Inability to absorb phosphate due to X linked dominant -inherited mutation of PHEX gene
- Labs will have normal calcium
- Tx: 1-3g phosphate daily + vitamin D3

**What is hereditary vitamin D dependent rickets?**

- Similar to nutritional rickets with worse sxs- may be bald
- Type 1- no renal 25 (OH)- vitamin D1 alpha-hydroxylase (no conversion to active vitamin D)
  - Autosomal recessive
- Type II - defect in intracellular receptor for 1,25 $(OH)_2$- vitamin D3

**What is osteoporosis?**

- Age-related decrease in bone mass, a quantitative not qualitative defect
- Diagnose via DEXA scan
  - L2-L4 density is 2.5 or more SD less than peak bone mass of a healthy 25 y/o-T score
- NOT Z score- thats for similar aged patients

**What are some labs to obtain to rule out secondary causes of osteoporosis?**

- 25 Vitamin D
- TSH + T4, albumin, creatine, CBC, serum calcium, 24 urine calcium + phosphorus, CMP, PTH

BS 5: 4:20

**What is osteopenia?**

- 1-2.5 SD less than the mean peak bone mass of a healthy 25 y/o

**What is osteomalacia?**

- A defect of mineralization leading to unmineralized osteoid (adult Rickets)

**What are the primary causes of osteomalacia?**

- Malabsorption and poor diet
- Renal osteodystrophy
- Chronic alcoholism

**What are some classic radiographic findings with osteomalacia?**

- Acetabular protrusion
- Biconcave vertebral bodies
- Looser's zones in insufficiency fractures
- Femoral neck fractures

**What is the treatment for osteomalacia?**

- Correct underlying cause (nutritional = high dose VitD until stores are normal then high dose maintenance)
- Give 25-VitD for hepatobiliary disease
- Give 1,25-VitD for renal disease due to enzymatic deficiencies

**What is oncogenic osteomalacia?**

- Overactivity of FGF 23
  - Decrease kidney phosphate reabsorption
  - + inhibition of 1 alpha hydroxylase (no conversion to 1,25 hydroxy vitamin D)

**Is a history of an osteoporotic vertebral compression fracture predictive of another vertebral fracture?**

- YES
- A vertebral compression fx increases risk of hip fx 5x

**What are some risk factors for developing osteoporosis?**

- White, female gender of northern European descent
- Thin, smoking, heavy drinking

**What are some indications to treat osteoporosis (in all postmenopausal women + men >50 y/o)?**

- Any hip/ vertebral fx
- Any prior fx + low bone mass (T-score)
- T score < -2.5 after secondary causes excluded
- Low bone mass and:

- FRAX 10 year probability of hip fx >/= 3%
- FRAX 10 year probability of any major osteoporosis related fx >/= 20%
- Secondary cause assoc w/ high fx risk (ex: immobilization)

**What are some ways to treat osteoporosis?**

- Exercise
- Calcium supplements- 1000-1500 daily + 400-800 Vit D daily
- Bisphosphonates
- Other medications

**What are the types of bisphosphonates?**

- Nitrogen and non nitrogen (etidronate, tiludronic acid, clodronate) containing

**BS 5: 21:10**

**How do bisphosphonates work?**

- Bind to mineralized bone surfaces and are taken up by osteoclasts during resorption
- Results in osteoclast apoptosis
- Because they bind to bone surfaces, they have lasting effects long after they are discontinued

**What is the difference in MOA of nitrogen and non-nitrogen bisphosphonates?**

- Nitrogen bisphosphonates- block farnesyl pyrophosphate synthase > leads to loss of GTPase formation
    - GTPase – is key for cell survival and ruffled border formation
    - Leads to cell apoptosis
- Non-nitrogen bisphosphonates- metabolized into a nonfunctional ATP analogue & induces apoptosis
    - Does not affect cell formation

**What type of side effects can be seen with bisphosphonates?**

- Atypical subtrochanteric femur fx (medial spike, lateral thickened cortex, transverse fx orientation)
- Jaw osteonecrosis

**What is teriparatide and risks associated with it?**

- Recombinant PTH, when used intermittently- anabolic effect on bone
- Risk of secondary osteosarcoma- contraindicated in pagets

**What is raloxifene?**

- SERM- reduces osteoclast activity

**BS 6: 1:35**

**What is denosumab?**

- A monoclonal antibody to RANKL (prevents RANK activation & inhibits formation, activation of osteoclast survival)

**What does calcitonin do to sclerostin?**

- Inhibits sclerostin formation

**How does bone metastasis play a role in bone resorption?**

- Cause an increase in RANKL- activates osteoclasts

**What is romosozumab?**

- A sclerostin antibody

**How is zoledronic acid administered?**

- Yearly infusion

**How is denosumab administered?**

- Q6 months subQ injections (danny the dinosaur does dos injections yearly)

**How is calcitonin administered?**

- Intranasal spray (sniffing that cocaine calcitonin.. Used when other therapies have failed, kind of similar to using cocaine after other drugs have failed- if you listened to the podcast you'd get this joke!)

**How is teriparatide administered?**

- Daily injection

## Orthopaedic Tissues

**What are the main types of cartilage found in the body?**

- Hyaline - articular surfaces
- Fibrocartilage - bone/tendon interface, menisci (fibroelastic cartilage)
- Elastic - found in trachea
- Epiphyseal - found in growth plates

**What transcription factor designates toward a cartilage lineage?**

- Sox-9
- Run-X2 is for bone
- Easy way to remember is "put on your SOX before you RUN" (as cartilage forms before bone)

**What are the zones of articular cartilage and how are they oriented in relation to the joint line?**

- Superficial/tangential zone - Type II collagen oriented in parallel to joint line, flat chondrocytes, high collagen to proteoglycan ratio, only zone where articular cartilage progenitor cells have been found
- Intermediate zone - collagen oriented in random/oblique orientation, largest zone with round chondrocytes and abundant proteoglycans
- Deep zone - collagen is perpendicular to joint line and crosses tidemark, highest concentration of proteoglycans, round chondrocytes oriented in columns
- Tide mark - divides the noncalcified articular cartilage to the calcified remnant of the epiphysis, this is found only in joints and not at other cartilage-bone interfaces
- Subchondral bone

**What is the most superficial layer of the articular surface called?**

- Lamina splendens- has densely packed collagen fibrils but no chondrocytes, these fibers resist the shear forces placed on the joint through the range of motion

**What makes up the extracellular matrix of articular cartilage?**

- Water makes up around 70%, more prominent at the surface and helps with lubrication, around 60% at the deeper levels
  - Deeper levels need high proteoglycan content (specifically aggrecan) to help pull in as much water as possible
  - Increased in arthritis and decreased in normal aging (water that is)
- Collagen with type II being most prominent at 90-95%
  - Makes up 20% of cartilage mass
- Proteoglycans make up 10%
  - Function to provide compressive strength and attract water, keratan sulfate, chondroitin sulfate, and aggrecan
  - Produced by chondrocytes

**What type of cartilage forms after full thickness articular injury?**

- Fibrocartilage

**Where does cartilage get its nourishment from?**

- It is avascular so it relies on the synovial fluid and subchondral bone for diffusion and exchange of nourishment and products of metabolism
- Because it is avascular, it relies on anaerobic metabolism (ie glycolysis) for ATP production

BS 6: 24:15

**What are forms of lubrication at the articular surface?**

- Elastohydrodynamic - elastic deformation of cartilage through dynamic joint function allows for slight differences in the shape of the cartilage where synovial fluid can form a boundary between the gliding surfaces
  - A truly fully congruent joint won't let a fluid boundary to form between the surfaces
- Boundary - aka slippery surfaces where non deformable joint surfaces have a fluid film only partially separating them and certain constituents of synovial fluid (such as lubricin, hyaluronic acid, and surface activated phospholipid) bound to the surface act as the boundary between the two allowing gliding
- Boosted - pools of lubricant form between areas that are in contact with each other
- Hydrodynamic - the gliding of joints creates negative pressure, pulling in synovial fluid between the surfaces
- Weeping - axial load on a joint pushes some of the entrapped water into the joint space and helps form a boundary layer

**What are some of the main differences between normal aging and osteoarthritis in articular cartilage?**

BS 7: 1:15

- Water is decreased in aging, but increased in arthritis
- Young's modulus - increased in aging, decreased in arthritis
- Glycosaminoglycan ratio is opposite of each other
  - Aging has high keratan sulfate: chondroitin 4 sulfate
  - Arthritis has high chondroitin 4: keratan sulfate

**What are the contractile units of muscle called?**

- Sarcomeres- the contractile units seen in myofibrils

**How are sarcomeres arranged?**

- Into bands and lines
- A sarcomere is from Z line to Z line

**What kind of filaments make up a sarcomere?**

- Thick + thin
- Thin filaments- actin (I band)
- Thick filaments- myosin (H band) (looking my so thick today)

**How does muscle contraction occur?**

BS 7: 11:30

- Acetylcholine diffuses across synaptic cleft > binds to muscle membrane receptor > depolarizes the sarcoplasmic reticulum
- This releases calcium > $Ca_2$+ binds w/ troponin > shifts tropomyosin molecules to expose myosin binding sites on actin > myosin cross bridges form > contraction/motion
- ATP needed to break the link + get ready for upcoming cycle

**What type of injection functions by blocking presynaptic acetylcholine release?**

- Botulinum A, used for spactic muscles
- There is a shortage of acetylcholine receptors in myasthenia gravis

**What type of muscle contraction is most efficient to build muscle strength?**

- Eccentric contraction (muscle lengthens while contracting)
- Also where many injuries occur commonly at myotendinous junction

**Does the number of muscle cells increase or the muscle fiber increase with muscle strength conditioning?**

- Muscle fiber Increases

**What are the different types of muscle fibers?**

- Type I- slow twitch- first lost w/o rehab- activated first- endurance
- Type II- fast twitch- short duration activities
  - IIA- fast oxidative glycolytic
  - IIB- fast glycolytic

**What is the primary energy source used for the first twenty seconds?**

- ATP-creatine phosphate system
- From 20-120 seconds- lactic anaerobic system

- Afterwards- aerobic metabolism- replenishing ATP through oxidative phosphorylation

**How does a strained muscle heal?**
- Initial inflammation phase w/ later TGF-b mediated fibrosis
- Satellite cells are most responsible for muscle healing
- Muscle mid belly lacerations recover about half the muscle strength

**How is a nerve organized (structure wise)?**
- Axon > myelin sheath > endoneurium > fascicles > perineurium > epineurium

**Does myelination make the nerve signal move faster or slower?**
- Faster- myelinated + thicker myelin is faster

**What is the loss of function order after nerve injury?**
- Motor, proprioception, touch, temperature, pain, sympathetic
- (return of function is opposite, motor is last)

**What is Wallerian degeneration?**
- Axon breakdown distal to level of nerve injury that is initiated 48-96 hrs after transection

**What is neurogenic shock?**
- Hypotension + bradycardia
- Occurs after C / Upper T spinal cord injury

**What type of tissue are tendons composed of?**
- Collagen - 75% dry weight
  - Of that 95% is type I, 5% is type III
- Proteoglycans- 5% dry weight

**What is decorin?**
- Most predominant proteoglycan in tendons
- Regulates tendon diameter, transfers loads, + forms cross links between fibers

**What is aggrecan?**
- A large proteoglycan that forms macromolecular aggregates w/ HA via interaction stabilized by link protein
- Has avidity to water up to 50x its weight- keeps scaffold of collagen and other matrix molecules inflated
- Allows cartilage capability to dispense contact forces evenly to underlying bone
- It is also present at tendon compression points

**What are keratin sulfate and chondroitin sulfate?**
- GAG rich domains, both which make up domains in aggregan
- They have high charge density- so a high degree of hydration for proteoglycan aggregate- leading to effect in cartilage and IV discs to resist compression under load

**What type of collagen do tenocytes produce in response to rupture?**
- Type III (inflammation phase)- greater proportion of type III collagen naturally in achilles tendon - predisposes to rupture
- Type I collagen is seen in the remodeling phase

**What are some different structures that can cover tendons?**
- Paratenon- high paratenon vascularity can lead to better healing results
- Synovium- ex: flexor tendons- allows for gliding motion.
  - Vincula carry blood supply to one tendon segment

**What are the four transitional tissues by which tendons attach to bone?**
- Tendon > fibrocartilage > mineralized fibrocartilage (Sharpey fibers connect w/ periosteum), bone

**When is tendon repair the weakest?**
- 7-10 days s/p repair
- Original strength regained around 21 days
- Max strength- 6 months

BS 8: 5:50

**What is the most prevalent glycosaminoglycan of cartilage?**
- Chondroitin sulfate

**Does keratin or chondroitin sulfate increase with age?**
- Keratin sulfate increases w/ age (provides compressive strength)
- Chondroitin 4 sulfate decreases w/ age

**What is the role of the negative charge sulfate ions at the end of the molecules?**
- Attract positive ions + trap & hold water

**What does a defect in the SO4- transporter protein (DTDST) cause?**
- Diastrophic dysplasia
- Dwarfism + short extremities, hitchhikers thumb

**What is synovial fluid?**
- An ultrafiltrate of plasma
- Hyaluronic acid- mucin- main molecule responsible for viscosity
- Viscosity decreases as shear rate increases- non newtonian fluid (thixotropic)
  - (Example of a Newtonian fluid is water- the viscosity does not change with mixing speed)

**What is a viscous fluid?**
- A "thicker fluid"
- A stronger molecule-molecule interaction causes the molecules to stick together- Ex: water vs honey

**What are the synovial fluid lab findings seen with septic arthritis (in a native joint)?**
- WBC cell count >50k
- High % PMNs (>85%)

BS 8: 16:40

- Appearance: cloudy/opaque
- Gram stain + cultures often positive
- Low glucose

## Arthritis

**What is osteoarthritis and key radiographic findings?**

- Degenerative joint disease- a progressive loss of cartilage structure and function
- The innate immune system stimulates degradative enzymes
- Joint space narrowing, osteophytes, subchondral cysts

**What are the tissue changes seen in osteoarthritis?**

- Cartilage degradation + loss of smooth lamina
- Cartilage fragmentation
- Increased matrix permeability
- Increased water content
- Dec modulus of elasticity

**What are the tissue changes seen with increased age (as opposed to osteoarthritis) ?**

- Dec water content
- Increase modulus of elasticity
- Inc decorin (more crosslinks)
- Increase in glycosylation end products
- Stiff

**What are some enzymes seen in osteoarthritis?**

- IL-1β (beta)- destroys cartilage- main proinflammatory cytokine
- MMP's (matrix metalloproteinases): 1,3, 13
- ADAMTS - Extracellular protease enzymes (aggrecanases, proteoglycans, etc)

**What is neuropathic arthropathy (charcot joint disease) and its presentation?**

- Arthritis caused by disturbed sensory innervation
- Swollen red joint, typically painless, pts may feel unstable
- Xrays- severe joint destruction, bone in fibrous tissue

**What are some causes of charcot joint disease?**

- Diabetes, syringomyelia (upper extremity), leprosy, tabes dorsalis

**BS 9: 4:48**

**What is syringomyelia?**

- Cyst in the cervical spinal cord
- Pts have early pain/temperature sensory deficits over shoulders/ arm/back
- Most common cause of UE neuropathic joint

**What condition is noted by OA, chondrocalcinosis, and black urine?**

- Alkaptonuria

- Autosomal recessive defect of homogentisic acid oxidase>> excess homogentisic acid deposited in joints
- Stiff cartilage > early arthritis + thin spinal discs

**What condition is noted by a caucasian with hand arthritis, skin hyperpigmentation, and diabetes?**

- Hemochromatosis, HFE gene C28Y mutation
- "Bronze diabetes"- triad- liver cirrhosis, DM + skin pigmentation
- Osteoarthritis of the hands common- hook like osteophytes on 2nd and 3rd metacarpal heads
- Screen: high serum ferritin (>200 µg/l), high transferrin saturation (>45%)

**What condition is noted in a 35 y/o F w/ polyarthralgia, fatigue, and skin rashes around her face?**

- Lupus, autoimmune disorder (fatigue, non-erosive arthritis, butterfly malar rash, + renal issues)
- + antinuclear antibodies (ANA) in 95% (screening)
- + anti-dsDNA, anti-Sm - specific tests for lupus
- + anti-histone abs- drug induced lupus

**What are some other types of autoimmune disorders and their distinguishing features?**

- Sjogren's syndrome- dry mouth, eyes, polyarthralgia- + SS-A, SS-B
- Scleroderma- calcinosis, indurated skin- Raynaud syndrome is common
  - Localized- CREST- anticentromere Ab
  - Diffuse- anti-DNA topoisomerase I Ab

**What condition is noted in a 35 M w/ back pain and morning stiffness?**

- Ankylosing spondylitis
- HLAB27 in 95%
- Sacroiliitis common, bamboo spine on xray, hip OA

**What condition is noted in a 55 caucasian female w/ b/l shoulder + pelvic AM pain that lasts 1hr, anorexia, fever & headaches with an elevated ESR?**

- Polymyalgia rheumatica- assoc w/ giant cell arteritis
- Temporal artery biopsy needed if temporal arteritis present (prevents blindness)

**What is a common presentation seen in rheumatoid arthritis?**

- Female w/ morning joint pain in multiple symmetric joints

**What is the pathophysiology behind rheumatoid arthritis?**

- Antigen triggers a genetically susceptible person (ex: HLA-DR4) > citrullinated proteins create auto antigens
- B cells make: anti CCP + RF
- CD4+ T Lymphocytes infiltrate around joint tissues + release inflammatory cytokines
  - IL-1- leads to inflammation + matrix destruction, main cartilage destroyer

- TNF-alpha- activates synovial fibroblasts, drives osteoclastogenesis
  - Fibroblasts (type B): release cadherin 11(mediates fibroblast migration to cartilage), MMP's, RANK-L
- IL-6- stimulates immunoglobulin from plasma cells
- Synovial cells invade cartilage pannus + release MMP's

**What are some bony changes seen in RA & why?**

- Periarticular erosions- RANKL released by fibroblasts, T/B cells + macrophages

**What are some treatment options for RA?**

- NSAIDs- helps early sxs
- Low dose steroids
- DMARDs

**How long do DMARDs take to work?**

- 2-6 months

(Krause, 2014)

**What are some of the DMARDs that can be continued throughout surgery?**

- Methotrexate (folate analog) - continue throughout surgery (hold pre op for renal insufficiency, alcohol abuse + severe diabetes)
- Hydroxychloroquine- continue
- Sulfasalazine- continue
- (can also continue aspirin- although not a DMARD)

**What are some DMARDs that should be stopped prior to surgery?**

- TNF alpha inhibitors- etanercept, infliximab, adalimumab
- IL-1 inhibitors- anakinra
- (at least one dose interval should elapse before surgery) ~2 weeks or so but this can vary. Inc risk of atypical infections
- Rituximab - stop ~6months in advance

**What are some cytokines commonly seen with inflammatory reactions?**

- IL-1
- IL-6 (causes liver ESR/CRP release)
- TNF-alpha
- Toll like receptors (TLR's)- are also upregulated in OA (TLRs turn on the innate immune system)

**What are some anti-cytokine drugs?**

- IL-1 blocker- anakinra receptor antagonist
- TNFalpha blocker
  - Etanercept- acts as a TNF receptor
  - Infliximab - chimeric IgG (molecule made up from a domain of another species)
  - Adalimumab- monoclonal antibody
- IL-6 blocker- Tocilizumab- IL-6 receptor antibody
- Side effects: increase risk of atypical infections

**What is the mechanism of action of etanercept?**

- TNF-alpha antagonist

**What is the mechanism of action for abatacept?**

- MHC receptor antagonist (blocks T cell activation)

**What is seen with wear particle osteolysis?**

- Macrophage phagocytose particles + release cytokines (IL-1, IL-6, RANKL)
- Osteoclast stimulation > bone dissolves

**What are some other types of arthritis and distinguishing features?**

- Psoriatic arthritis- skin lesions, nail lesions, sausage digit, DIP pain, pencil in cup deformity
- Reactive arthritis- conjunctivitis, urethritis, mono/oligoarthritis (cant see, pee, or bend a knee)
  - Can occur w/ recent extra-articular infections (i.e: chlamydia, shigella, salmonella, gonorrhea)
- Relapsing polychondritis- migratory arthritis + ENT involvement (saddle nose deformity, auricle thickening, trachea involvement). Parasternal pain, antibodies to type II collagen + matrilin-1
- Lyme arthritis- chronic episodic oligoarthritis, US northeast/ pacific northwest,erythema micgricans (early) neurologic sxs (late) - tx 3-6wks amoxicillin <8y/o, >8y/o doxycycline

**What are some conditions seen in young patients w/ arthritis?**

- Juvenile idiopathic arthritis- pt age <16 y/o, persistent (>6wk) joint swelling
  - Oligoarticular JIA- age<8 asymmetric, painless iridocyclitis/uveitis (eye exam), good prognosis
  - Seronegative polyarticular JIA, 8-12 y/o, large joint involvement, negative RF
  - Seropositive polyarticular- teenage girls, aggressive, + RF, + HLA-DR4 in some
  - Systemic onset JIA (Still disease)- any age, diurnal fevers,lymphadenopathy, hepatosplenomegaly, salmon macular rash. Macrophage activation system. Can be fatal
  - Psoriatic JIA- any age, asymmetric, spine involvement possible, DIP joints, nail involvement, dactylitis. Painful uveitis (eye exam)
  - Enthesitis- related JIA (juvenile ankylosing spondylitis)- boys >girls, age 8-12, hip + sprint involvement, + schober lumbar flexion test

**What is crystal deposition arthropathy?**

- Crystal deposition / formation in / around joints

**What are some different forms of crystal deposition arthropathy?**

- Gout- monosodium urate crystals- negatively birefringent under polarized light- tx: indomethacin, colchicine for recurrence

- Chondrocalcinosis- pseudogout- rhomboid shaped crystals- weakly positive birefringent. Tx: NSAIDs, cortisone. Colchicine for recurrence
- Calcium hydroxyapatite crystal deposition- destructive arthropathy in knee + shoulder (milwaukee shoulder- deposition w/ cuff tear arthropathy), turmeric calcinosis, - crystals too small for light microscopy. Purple aggregates on wright stain
- Calcium oxalate deposition- secondary oxalosis (more common), metabolic abnormalities w/ renal insufficiency, birefringent bipyramidal crystals

## Molecular Biology

**What are some autoimmune antibodies seen in orthopaedics and their function and associated condition?**

- ANA antibodies- antibodies to nuclear contents- screening tool for autoimmune disorders
- Anti-dsDNA Ab - Lupus
- Anti-histone Ab- protein for spooling DNA- drug induced lupus, RA, scleroderma
- Anti-topoisomerase (Scl-70) Ab- unwinds DNA- diffuse scleroderma
- Anti-Jo-1 Ab - tRNA synthetase ab- polymyositis + dermatomyositis
- Anti- Smith - transcription modification of introns/exons (splicing)- Lupus
- Anti-Ul-rnp Ab- post-transcription modification of introns/exons (splicing)-mixed connective tissue disease

**What is the difference between an exon and an intron?**

- Exon- DNA regions that code for mRNA
- Introns- regions of DNA that don't code for mRNA

**What are some important proteins that regulate progression through the cell cycle?**

- pRB-1 (retinoblastoma protein)- retinoblastoma + osteosarcoma
- p53- prevents entry to S phase- osteosarcoma, rhabdomyosarcoma + chondrosarcoma

BS 10: 7:50

**Using cytogenetic analysis, what are some chromosomal translocations seen in orthopaedic oncology?**

- t(11:22)- Ewing sarcoma
- t(X:18)- Synovial sarcoma
- t(2:13)- rhabdomyosarcoma
- t(12:16)- myxoid liposarcoma
- t(12:22)- clear cell sarcoma

**What's the difference between northern/southern/western blotting?**

- Southern blotting- detects DNA sequence
- Northern blotting- detects RNA sequence
- Western blotting- detects protein

**What are some common orthopaedic autosomal dominant conditions?**

- Syndactyly/polydactyly, Marfan syndrome, hereditary multiple exostoses (MHE), malignant hyperthermia, Ehlers-danlos syndrome, achondroplasia, osteogenesis imperfecta (OI) (type I & IV)
- Story to remember them: Autozone (autosomal) dominant basketball game:
  - 1st team, Tall lanky players with 9 fingers on each hand, with bright blue eyes (marfan/ehlers, syndactyly/polydactyly, OI)
  - 2nd team: Short guys with a short temper who cheat (achondroplasia, malignant hyperthermia)
  - Basketball rim isn't round and has a strange shape with multiple branches (MHE) –refer to podcast for more context

**What are some of the structural protein defects in the autosomal dominant disorders?**

- Marfans - fibrillin (also TGF-beta excess)
- Ehler's Danlos - COL5A
- OI - COL1
- Achondroplasia- FGF-R3

**What are some common orthopaedic autosomal recessive conditions?**

- Diastrophic dysplasia, hurler's syndrome, sanfilippo, morquio
- Story to remember them: Kids outside playing recess at autozone (autosomal recessive)
  - **Sam** is sitting against a pole **flipping** a quarter (Sanflippo), meanwhile a giant mosquito bites her, and she hurls up all her lunch (Morquio + Hurler), she becomes **diastropichally displeased** that she threw up because she had ice cream for lunch and it's her favorite (diastrophic dysplasia)

**What are the gene deficits in some common autosomal recessive disorders?**

- Diastrophic dysplasia- sulfate transport
- Hurlers syndrome- alpha-L-iduronidase
- Sanfilippo- heparan sulfamidase
- Morquio- galactose sulfatase

**What are some X-linked recessive disorders?**

- Hunters mucopolysaccharidosis, hemophilia A/B, Duchenne + Becker muscular dystrophy
- Story to remember: All male school recess
  - There's a kid in the bushes with a spear, he is **hunting** another kid (Hunters), he throws the spear at him and barely hits him in the arm. He starts **bleeding** everywhere (Hemophilia A/B). His friend tries to get up to go to his rescue but he's taking a long time because **he has to use his hands to try and stand up** (DMD/Becker)

**What are some X-linked dominant disorders?**

- Hypophosphatemic rickets- mutation of X-linked PHEX- inc FGF 23> renal PO4 wasting
  - Story to remember: At the father daughter dance, they are playing tennis using tennis **rackets** (rickets)

**What is the gene mutation seen with osteogenesis imperfecta (AD)?**

- COL1A1, COL1A2

**What is the gene mutation seen with Ehlers-Danlos syndrome?**

- COL5A1, COL5A2

**What is the gene mutation seen with Marfan syndrome?**

- FBN1, w/ superior lens dislocation

**What is the gene mutation seen with achondroplasia?**

- FGFR3

**What is the gene mutation seen with spinal muscular atrophy?**

- SMN1 (survival motor neuron-1)

**What is the gene mutation seen with spondyloepiphyseal dysplasia?**

- COL2A1

**BS 10: 27:20**

**What is the gene mutation with McCune Albright syndrome?**

- GNAS gene

**What are some distinguishing features of McCune Albright syndrome?**

- Fibrous dysplasia of bone, shepherd's crook deformity of hips, cafe au lait spots (irregular- coast of Maine), endocrinopathy

**What are some orthopaedic issues seen in patients with Trisomy 21?**

- Atlanto-axial instability (no contact sports), hip instability, patellar instability, pes plano-valgus. (non-ortho: heart problems, thyroid issues)
- COL6 on chromosome 21

**What orthopaedic condition is associated w/ a deletion of the long arm of chromosome 13?**

- Multiple myeloma (B cell proliferation, M spike, multiple lytic lesions cold on bone scan

## Genetics

**What is the most common form of dwarfism?**

- Achondroplasia - FGF-R3 receptor
- Affects proliferative zone

**Are the arms or legs short or maintained with achondroplasia?**

- Arms/legs are shorter
- Trunk and head are normal
- Varus knees

**BS 11: 1:40**

**What are some conditions where dwarfism is proportionate?**

- Constitutional dwarfism
- Mucopolysaccharidoses
- Endocrinopathies + familial

**What are other FGF-R3 dysplasias?**

- Achondroplasia
- Hypochondroplasia (milder than achondroplasia)
- Thanatophoric dysplasia (no proliferative zone, fatal by 2 years old)

**What's the difference between FGF-R3 and FGF-23?**

- FGF-R3- associated with the dysplasias
- FGF-23- decreases renal reabsorption of PO4 (produced by osteocytes+blasts)

**In what condition is a mutation of the FGF23 inhibitor called?**

- Genetic hypophosphatemic rickets - PHEX mutation, so no FGF23 inhibition

**What are some other conditions that increase FGF 23 (>hypophosphatemia)?**

- Fibrous dysplasia
- Tumoral- induced osteomalacia

**What are some conditions that decrease FGF 23 (>hyperphosphatemia)?**

- Familial tumoral calcinosis (dec FGF-23 activity)
- Tumoral calcinosis (kidney failure MC, can't excrete phosphate)

**What conditions are caused by a mutation in the cartilage oligomeric matrix protein (COMP) gene instead of FGF-R3?**

- Pseudoachondroplasia - COMP gene (thrombospondin 5)
  - Short limb dwarfism, normal face
  - Spine involvement (C1-C2 instability, lordosis)

**What condition is noted by a short stature w/ multiple abnormal epiphysis, early arthritis, but does NOT have spine involvement?**

- Multiple epiphyseal dysplasia
- COMP gene (most often), also MATN-3 (Matrillin) and COL9 (collagen type IX)

**What are some skeletal dysplasias where collagen is affected?**

- COL1- OI
- COL5- Ehlers-Danlos syndrome
- COL2- Spondyloepiphyseal dysplasia (spine involvement), Kniest dysplasia (dumbell bones), achondrogenesis (lethal at birth), stickler syndrome (pierre robin face)
- COL9- multiple epiphyseal dysplasia
- COL10A1- metaphyseal chondrodysplasia

**What condition is noted by joint hypermobility, dislocation, vascular problems (aneurysms) and cutis elastis?**

- Ehlers-danlos syndrome- COL 1,3,5
- Try not to operate

**What condition is noted by joint laxity, hip protrusio, aortic dissection, and ectopic lens (superior)?**

- Marfan's syndrome (fibrillin-1)

**What condition is noted by a marfanoid (tall & thin) appearance, ectopic lens (inferior), + DVT/PE?**

- Homocystinuria

**What does excess Sonic Hedgehog (Shh) expression lead to?**

- Post-axial polydactyly

**What does poor Shh expression cause?**

- Postaxial hypoplasia
- Fibular hemimelia - missing fibula, anteromedial tibia bowing, loss of lateral foot rays

**In what condition can antero-lateral tibial bowing be seen?**

- Neurofibromatosis

**What condition is noted in a patient with absent clavicles, proportional dwarfism, and skull deformities?**

- Cleidocranial dysplasia
- 1CBFA/1RUNx gene - Autosomal dominant
- Impaired intramembranous ossification

**What condition is noted with an aplastic/hypoplastic patella, iliac horns, and nail problems?**

- Nail-patella syndrome
- Gene involved: LMX1B

# Infections

**A lot of the information in these sections was covered in medical school and STEP 3. Also, you can check out Miller's review book or Orthobullets for a deeper dive into this.**

**What is the mechanism of action of penicillin?**

- Inhibits peptidoglycan bonds of bacterial cell walls

BS 12: 1:20

**What does MSSA stand for?**

- Methicillin- sensitive *S. aureus*
- Methicillin, nafcillin, dicloxacillin work against staph beta-lactamase (bla gene mutants create beta-lactamase)

**What gene helps make methicillin resistant staph?**

- mecA gene- codes for penicillin binding protein 2A (PBP2A)... which doesn't bind to penicillin well

- Staphylococcal chromosome cassette mobile element-carrying IV (SCCmecIV) carries the mecA gene

**What are some differences between hospital and community acquired MRSA?**

- Hospital- larger SCCmec- more drug resistant
- Community acquired- smaller SCCmec- less drug resistance- almost all have panton-Valentine leukocidin (PVL) cytotoxin that lyses PMN's

**What gene causes increased adhesion of S. aureus to titanium?**

- Fnb gene

**What does bacterial glycocalyx-biofilm-slime-polysaccharide capsule protect against?**

- Phagocytosis and antibiotics
- Can grow very slow (years)
- Biofilm can also start to form within hours of inoculation

**What condition is noted by a rapidly progressing subcutaneous tissue and fascia infection with foul-smelling dishwater pus seen in surgery?**

- Necrotizing fasciitis- polymicrobial
  - Monomicrobial (Type II)- strep pyogenes MC
  - Vibrio vulnificus w/ saltwater laceration,
- Aeromonas hydrophila- freshwater lac
- Pain out of proportion + outside erythema margin
- LRINEC score

**What is the treatment for necrotizing fasciitis?**

- Emergent wide debridement
- Increasing mortality w/ delay in treatment >24hrs
- IV abx

**What condition is noted in a patient s/p lawnmower wound closure in ED 2 days prior w/ soft tissue crepitus and air in the soft tissues on xray?**

- Gas gangrene (clostridium perfringens)
- (don't close war wounds/ tornado injuries/ lawnmower injuries)
- Tx: I&D, IV PCN, clinda

**What is the most common organism seen in orthopaedic infections?**

- *S aureus*

**What are some host factors for surgical site infections?**

- Inc BMI >30
- Malnutrition
- Active infections
- Heavy alcohol use
- Smoking**
- Diabetes
- Anemia

- Immunocompromised (ex: HIV, RA)
- Recent gingivectomy or tooth extraction (bacteremia w/ strep)
- Bacteriuria + urinary sxs - postpone surgery

**What is an organism seen with human bites?**

- *Eikenella corrodens*
- Treat fight bite w/ I&D
- Tx: amoxicillin/ Clavulanic Acid

**What is an organism seen in dog and cat bites?**

- *Pasteurella multocida*
- Tx: amoxicillin/ clavulanic acid or cefoxitin

**What is an organism seen in fish bites and marine injuries?**

- *Mycobacterium marinum*
- Slow culture at low temp (Lowenstein-Jensen medium at 30° celsius)
- Tx: 3 months minocycline or clarithromycin

BS 12: 22:06

**What condition is noted in a farmer with fish and swine who shows up with a wound with a painful, itchy ring shaped lesion with a purple border?**

- Fish handler's disease
- *Erysipelothrix rhusiopathiae*
- Tx: oral PCN

**What is the most common route of joint infections in kids and adults?**

- Kids- hematogenous spread
- Adults- direct inoculation

**What is the most sensitive lab finding in acute osteomyelitis?**

- Elevated CRP
- Dx w/ cultures
- Treat w/ abx

**What is sequestra?**

- Necrotic dead bone

**What is involucrum?**

- New periosteal bone

**Should antibiotics for chronic osteomyelitis be based on sinus tract biopsy or deep cultures?**

- Deep cultures... a sinus tract is diagnostic for infection though

**What type of malignancy can chronic osteomyelitis lead to?**

- Marjolin's ulcer > Squamous cell carcinoma (seen in sites of inflammation)

**What is the *most common* organism seen in sickle cell patients with osteomyelitis?**

- *S aureus*
- Salmonella is common, but S aureus is still most common

**What is the *most common* organism seen in a puncture wound through the shoe?**
- *S aureus*
- Should cover pseudomonas as well

**What is a common cause of septic arthritis in a young healthy sexually active individual?**
- Gonococcal arthritis
- Tx: ceftriaxone

**What is the most common organism in shoulder infections?**
- *Cutibacterium acnes* (gram + rod)
- **Slow culture growth** - hold cultures 2+ weeks
- Rx: PCN, tetracyclines, clinda

## Biomaterials

**What is force?**
- A push or pull on an object in a certain direction that causes external (acceleration) and internal (strain) effects

BS 13: 3:10

**What are some different types of force?**
- Linear + rotational

**What are some different types of linear forces?**
- Normal force- perpendicular to surface on which it acts
- Tensile force- elongates a body
- Compressive force- a force that squeezes something together
- Tangential force- parallel to the surface

**What are some types of rotational forces?**
- Moment- rotational effect of a force
- Torque- moment perpendicular to long axis causing rotation
- Bending moment- force parallel to long axis
- Mass moment of inertia- resistance to rotation

**What is stress?**
- Force/ area, the intensity of internal force

**What is shear stress?**
- Stress is parallel to the material surface (rather than perpendicular, i.e. normal stress)

**What is strain?**
- Change in length / original length... the relative measure of deformation from loading

**What is the difference between plastic and elastic deformation?**
- Elastic- temporary (returns to resting length)
- Plastic - permanent- (doesn't return to resting length after lengthened/shortened)

**What is Hooke's law?**

- Stress is directly proportional to strain up to a limit (the linear part in the stress/strain curve)

**What is the point called where the material changes from elastic to plastic behavior?**

- Yield point

**What is young's modulus of elasticity?**

- Measure of a materials stiffness
- Stress/strain

**In the first part of the stress/strain curve, what is the material experiencing?**

- Elastic deformation (like a rubber band)

**What does the slope in a stress/strain graph equate to?**

- How stiff the material is (it changes with different materials)
- The more vertical / higher the modulus is... the more force it can take

**What type of deformation is seen in the non-linear part of the stress/strain curve?**

- Plastic deformation (material doesn't go back to normal size)

**What is the ultimate strength?**

- The most stress a material can take before breaking (this isnt when the material breaks though)

**What is fatigue?**

- Progressive and localized structural damage that occurs when a material is cyclically loaded
- Failure of material below the ultimate strength (on the graph)

**What is necking?**

- A type of plastic deformation seen when there is a tensile stress and there is a reduction in the cross sectional area of the material (giving it a V or neck appearance)
- There is a large amount of local stress, but overall decreased stress
- This is what's going on in the area after ultimate strength

**What is the breaking point?**

- Failure of material
- Fracture, the end of the curve

**What is stiffness?**

- Resistance to a force causing a material to bend
- Young's modulus (depends on elastic deformation)
- Slope of linear portion of stress/strain curve

**What is strength?**

- Load required to break material (depends on plastic deformation)
- (ultimate tensile strength)

**What is ductility?**
- Amount deformation a material can undergo before fracture
- Distance between yield point and fracture point

**If a material is brittle, is it very ductile?**
- No, that's the opposite.
- I.e- glass
- There will be a small difference between the yield and fracture point

**What is toughness?**
- Ability of material to absorb energy
- (Area under the stress/strain curve)

**What is a viscous type of material?**

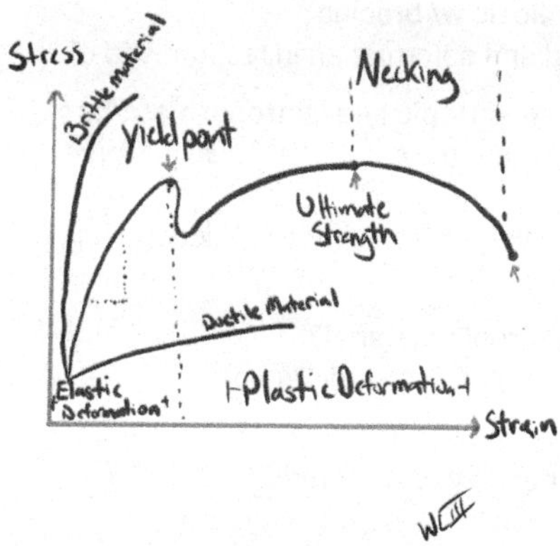


- A material that is sticky/ thick/ or adhesive
- Think- internal friction between the molecules
- Friction due to sliding (ex: liquids like honey)

**What is an elastic material?**
- Energy storage and return (ex: metal, rubber band)

**BS 13: 30:00**

**Figure 3.1: The labeled stress strain curve. Toughness is the area below the curve.**

**What is a viscoelastic material?**
- A material that exhibits both fluid (viscous) and solid (elastic) properties

**What are some properties seen with viscoelastic materials?**
- Stiffness is time/rate dependent
- Hysteresis
- Creep
- Load relaxation

**What property is characterized by a change in deformation as the load on a material is held constant (i.e. a constant stress)?**
- Creep
- The strain increases over time

**What happens when an increasing rate/load of magnitude is applied to a viscoelastic material?**
- When a quick load is applied over a short period of time- material is stiffer (higher youngs modulus)
- I.e: dropping playdo rolled into a ball on the ground (it will bounce back up)

**What is noticed when you apply a set change in length to a tendon and measure the change inforce overtime (strain held constant)?**
- Load drops off and force (stress) decreases over time

BS 14: 4:00

**What is hysteresis?**
- Energy lost as you load and unload a material (area between curves is lost)
- A characteristic of viscoelastic behavior

**What types of tissues in the body are viscoelastic?**
- Tendons, bone

**What type of property is seen when you stretch your calf muscle?**
- Load relaxation

**What property is noted when tx scoliosis w/ bracing?**
- Creep response (constant load and deformation in response to it)

**What is the difference between an anisotropic and isotropic material?**
- Isotropic- mechanical properties are the same regardless of force direction
- Anisotropic- mechanical properties behave differently depending on force direction

**Is cortical bone an anisotropic or isotropic material?**
- Anisotropic (bone is stronger w/ axial than radial load)
- Cartilage also is anisotropic

**What metal has the highest E (stiffness / young's modulus)?**
- $Al_2O_3$ - Ceramic

**What metal has the closest E to cortical bone?**
- Titanium
- PMMA is less stiffer than cortical bone, followed by polyethylene

**If ceramic has the highest E, and titanium has the closest E to bone, where do the other two metals lie as far as young's modulus?**
- Stainless steel is stiffer than titanium
- The alloy is stiffer than stainless steel (Co-Cr-Mo)

**What is the order of material stiffness from highest to lowest stiffness?**
- Ceramic ($Al_2O_3$)> Co-Cr-Mo Alloy > stainless steel > titanium
- CORTICAL BONE
- Matrix polymers>PMMA> polyethylene > cancellous bone > tendon/ ligament > cartilage

**What is an alloy?**

- Two or more metals
- Useful because pure metals can be weak/soft

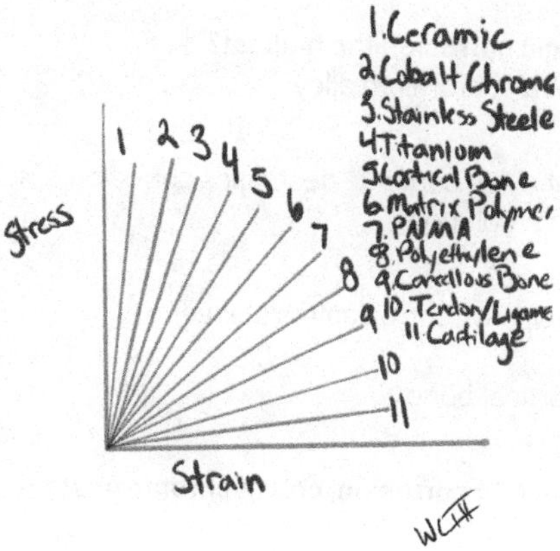


**Figure 3.2: Young's modulus for different elements. It is seen that titanium is the metal with the closest modulus of elasticity to cortical bone.**

**What are the three types of alloys commonly used in orthopaedics?**

- Steel (iron based), cobalt-based, titanium based

**What is 316 L stainless steel made from?**

- Iron-carbon, chromium, nickel, molybdenum, manganese
- Carbon- adds strength
- Chromium nickel- enhances corrosion resistance
- Susceptible to pitting and crevice corrosion

**What is the cobalt alloy made of?**

- Cobalt (~70%), chromium (~27%), molybdenum
- Very strong implant

**What is corrosion?**

- Chemical dissolving of metals (can occur in the body)

**What type of corrosion occurs when there is a depletion of oxygen inside a small crack or gap which eventually converts the metal inside the gap to a cathode?**

**BS 14: 26:50**

- Crevice corrosion
- The can occur between two metals or a metal and non metal
- 316L steel is most susceptible, titanium is the least

**What type of corrosion occurs when there is an electrochemical process where one metal corrodes in preference to another metal that it is in contact with through an electrolyte?**

- Galvanic corrosion (bimetallic corrosion)
- Galvanic = relating to electrical currents produced by chemical action
- Avoid by using similar metals

**What type of corrosion is seen when material deterioration occurs at the interface of two contacting surfaces due to small oscillatory movements?**

- Fretting corrosion
- Often seen in devices w/ tapered junctions (titanium is susceptible)

**What type of corrosion is the most severe form where there is damage to the metal (cavities or "holes" are produced in the material) and possible release of metal ions?**

- Pitting corrosion

**Between what metals is galvanic corrosion the highest?**

- 316L stainless steel + cobalt-chromium alloy

BS 15: 1:40

**What is self passivation?**

- Formation of an adherent oxide coating - decreases corrosion
- It separates the metal from solution

**What are some properties of titanium?**

- Excellent biocompatibility (helps w/ corrosion resistance)
- Self passivation
- Young's modulus close to cortical bone
- But poor wear resistance

**What metal has better resistance to corrosion, cobalt chrome or stainless steel?**

- Cobalt chrome alloy

BS 15: 5:19

**What is tantalum?**

- A transition metal
- Useful for bony ingrowth to prosthesis
- Can be used to augment cancellous defects

**What are ceramics and some characteristics of ceramics?**

- A brittle + corrosion-resistant material with elements linked together by covalent or ionic bonds
- Many are oxides of a metallic element (ex: zirconia $ZrO_3$)
- Brittle + stiff (high young's modulus), not tough, insoluble
- Best wear characteristics w/ polyethylene and a low oxidation rate
- Biocompatible

**What are some different types of ceramic?**

- Inert (alumina zirconia)
- Bioactive- degradable- (beta-tricalcium phosphate hydroxyapatite)

**What are some materials that can be useful as a coating to help with implant strength + bone healing?**

- Calcium phosphates (hydroxyapatite) - plasma sprayed

**What are some characteristics of bioactive ceramics?**

- Degradable
- Osteoconductive only - large pore size

**What is ultra-high-molecular-weight polyethylene (UHMWPE)?**

- A polymer of long carbon chains
- Structure of long chain affects properties
  - Longer + linear = stronger

BS 15: 16:50

- Cross linking = stronger + stiffer
- It is also ductile, tough, and has viscoelastic properties

**What effects does gamma irradiation in air do to polyethylene?**
- Increases free radical formation > oxidative polyethylene degradation
  - (Oxygen free irradiation helps prevent free radical formation)
  - Irradiation w/ nitrogen or argon helps minimize free-radical formation
- Increases polymer chain cross links > improved wear characteristics

**What is annealing and what are some effects seen w/ polyethylene annealing?**
- Heating to below melting point
- Decreases free radicals

**Are thinner or thicker polys associated with wear particles?**
- Thinner polys <6mm
- Wear debris are associated w/ a histiocytic osteolytic response

**What are many poly biodegradable implants made of?**
- Polylactic acid polymer
- Material undergoes hydrolysis > lactic acid > excreted from lungs as $CO_2$
- Other biodegradable polymers include polyglycolic acid, polydioxanone + polycaprolactone

**What does PMMA (bone cement) do?**
- Mechanically interlocks w/ bone & reaches ultimate strength w/i 24 hrs
- Mixing technique important- vacuum mixing, centrifugation (avoid inc porosity)

BS 15: 23:20

**What substance helps give bone its compressive strength?**
- Hydroxyapatite (helps w/ stiffness + strength of bone)

**What are some key points about the mechanical properties of bone?**
- Strongest in compression/ weakest in shear
- Aniostropic (properties change w/ force direction: ex: strong in compression)
- Viscoelastic (stronger / stiffer when loaded quickly)

**What does stress shielding do?**
- Induces osteoporosis in adjacent bone next to a load sharing implant

**A hole of what percent of the bone diameter reduces the bone strength up to 50%?**
- 20-30%, whether a screw is in hole or not
- Area returns to normal 9-12mo after screw removal

**What kind of a force results in what type of fracture (typically)?**
- Tension- transverse fx
- Compression- crush fx

- Bending- transverse/oblique (fx starts on tension side)
- Torsion- spiral fx

**What does the inner diameter, outer diameter, and pitch of a screw have to do with the pullout strength?**

- Smaller inner diameter, larger outer diameter, & a finer pitch increase pullout strength

**To what power is the bending stiffness proportional to the thickness of a plate?**

- To the third power - r3

**What side of a fracture is the plate most effective on?**

- On the tension side
- A plate is a load bearing device (vs load sharing would be a IMN)

**What are some functions that a plate can be used?**

- Dynamic compression, static compression, neutralization mode, buttress

**What is the difference between a locking and a nonlocking plate?**

- Locking- does not require compression to bone
- Absorb axial forces transmitted from screws

**What is a hybrid locking plate?**

- A plate where unlocked + locking screws are used

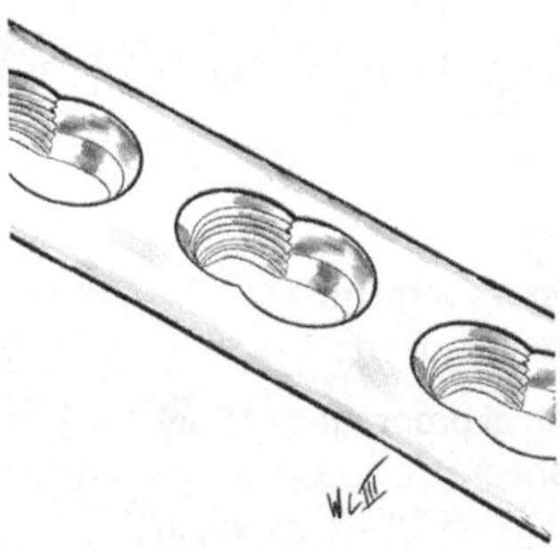

**Figure 3.3: A photo showing a hybrid locking/non locking plate. The locking portion of the plate allows the threads in the head of the screw to screw into the plate.**

**What are some things that improve locking plate stability?**

- Bicortical screws (better than unicortical screws for resisting torsion)
- Longer plate
- Increase screws

**What is the working length of a plate?**

- The screws in the plate closest to the fracture
- Decreasing working length increases stiffness

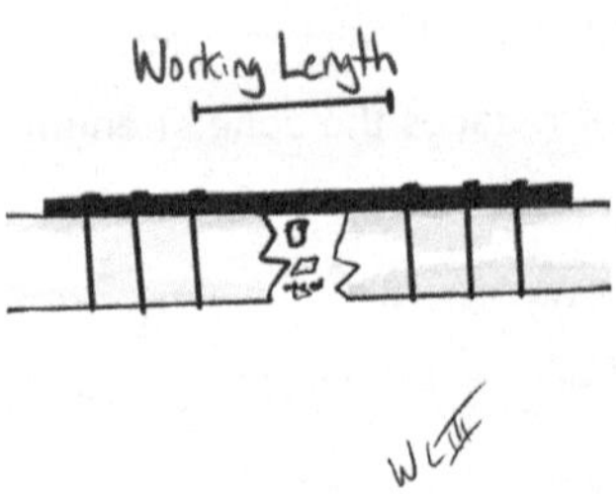


**Figure 3.4: A photo showing the working length of a plate. It is the distance between the two screws that are closest to the fracture.**

**What is the stiffness of an intramedullary nail proportional to?**

- The radius to the 4th power

**What is the most important factor for stability with external fixation?**
- Fracture ends in contact with each other

**What are some other ways to enhance stability when using an ex fix?**
- Inc pin diameter (2nd most important)
- Inc pin #, decreasing bone-rod distance, multiplanar, increasing rod #, increasing spacing between pins, pins closer to fracture site (central pins), peripheral pins further from fracture site

## Perioperative stuff

**What would you be worried about if a patient had a petechial rash on their chest, was tachypneic and was confused after a closed femoral shaft fracture?**

BS 16: 2:10

- Fat emboli syndrome
- Triad- petechial rash, mental status changes, ARDS (fluid leak into alveoli > right sided heart failure > death)
- Can be seen after an asymptomatic interval w/ long bone fx

**How can you try to prevent fat embolism syndrome?**
- Stabilize long bone fx early

**What is the treatment for ARDS (in general)?**
- Oxygen (100%)
- Address the fx
- PEEP (Positive end expiratory pressure) ventilation

**What is the difference between a thrombus and an embolism?**
- A thrombosis is a clot at an improper site while an embolism is a clot that has migrated

**What is a strong recommendation from the AAOS regarding VTE prophylaxis in patients undergoing THA/TKA?**
- No post-op duplex ultrasound
- Moderate recommendation - pharmacologic/mechanical compression for pts not w/ inc risk for DVT

**How does a sequential compression device work?**
- Decreases venous stasis by increasing peak venous flow

**Is recurrent deep venous thrombosis (DVT) more common after the first DVT?**
- Yes, 4-8x more common

**What is post- thrombotic syndrome?**
- A complication of chronic venous insufficiency- venous HTN, skin pigmentation + ulceration. Swelling & pain

**Does a proximal or distal DVT have a greater PE risk?**
- Proximal DVT (above knee)

**What are some risk factors for thromboembolic disease?**

- Prior TE disease
- Inc age (>40)
- Immobility
- Obesity

**What is Virchow's triad?**

- Endothelial damage (trauma > exposes collagen + triggers platelets)
- Venous stasis (clotting proteins + cells bond)
- Hypercoagulability (inc clotting factors >> insoluble fibrin)

**What is the final product of the clotting cascade?**

- Thrombin IIa (converts soluble fibrinogen to insoluble fibrin)

**What are some genetic clotting disorders?**

- Dec anti clotting factors: Protein C + S deficiency, antithrombin III deficiency
- Inc clotting factors: Factor V Leiden, (Homozygous > heterozygous) Inc Factor VIII, hyperhomocysteinemia

**Are most patients w/ DVT symptomatic?**

- No more are asymptomatic

**Should you screen everybody for a DVT w/ a duplex ultrasound?**

- No

**What are the initial tests you should obtain if a PE is suspected?**

- EKG, arterial blood gas, CXR

BS 16: 21:15

**What is the best test for a suspected PE?**

- Spiral CT angiography (no evidence that it decreases mortality)
- V/Q scan for dye sensitive patients

**What is a risk with DVT ppx?**

- Bleeding, causing hematoma formation & possibly requiring return to the OR

**What are some mechanical ways to prevent a DVT?**

- Early mobilization
- Ankle pumps
- Intermittent pneumatic compression- lowers bleeding risk
- IVC filter (in cases where anticoagulation may be contraindicated- thrombocytopenia/hemorrhage)
- Compression stockings + CPM- no value for DVT prevention

**What are some common anticoagulants used in orthopaedic surgery?**

- Aspirin, heparin, fondaparinux, rivaroxaban, dabigatran, coumadin

**What is the mechanism of action of aspirin?**

- Irreversible COX inhibitor- decreases TXA2 and prostaglandin production

**What is the mechanism of action of acetaminophen?**

- Inhibits prostaglandin E2 through IL-1

**What is the mechanism of action of heparin?**

- Enhances the ability of antithrombin III to inhibit factor IIa, IXa, XIa, XIIa (reversible)
- Also binds to platelet factor 4 which can lead to heparin induced thrombocytopenia
- IV and SubQ forms

BS 17: 3:20

**What is the reversal agent for heparin?**

- Protamine sulfate

**What's the difference between heparin and low molecular weight heparin?**

- Heparin has a long chain that binds to different proteins
- LMWH- short molecule that only inhibit Xa & thrombin

**What is the mechanism of action for LMWH and some advantages when compared to heparin?**

- Blocks Xa through ATIII and IIa (thrombin)
- Sub Q administration
- No need for monitoring
- Dec dose in renal insufficiency
- Reversible

**What is the mechanism of action of fondaparinux?**

- Irreversibly binds Xa through ATIII
- No antidote, Higher bleeding risk than LMWH

**What is the mechanism of action of rivaroxaban (and the other xabans- i.e. apixaban)?**

- Direct Xa inhibitor
- ORAL medication
- Higher risk of bleeding that LMWH

**What is the antidote for apixaban?**

- Andexanet - decoy recombinant factor Xa molecule

**What is the mechanism of action of hirudin (isolated from leech glands)?**

- Direct thrombin IIa inhibitor
- Cloned hirudin recombinant proteins
  - Dabagitran (pradaxa) PO & Desirudin (Revasc)

**What is the reversal agent for hirudins (dabigatran + desirudin)?**

- Idarucizumab

**What is the mechanism of action of warfarin (coumadin)?**

- Vitamin K epoxide reductase inhibitor
- Prevents vit-K gamma carboxylation
- Decreases production of II, VII, IX, and X

- Monitoring needed + dietary modifications to maintain therapeutic levels

**What is the reversal agent for coumadin?**

- Fresh frozen plasma

**Do flyers have an increased risk of a TE event compared to non- flyers?**

- Yes, 8x the risk
- No chemical DVT recommended

BS 17: 20:45

**What should you consider in a 25 M w/ RUE pain, swelling, dilated veins with a feeling of arm heaviness?**

- Effort thrombosis (Paget-Schroetter syndrome)
- An UE clot in an athlete
- Dx w/ Ultrasound. Tx: pt may need thoracic outlet decompression

**What is the mechanism of action for tranexamic acid?**

- Competitive inhibitor of plasminogen activation (plasmin dissolves fibrin clots)
- It is a synthetic lysine analogue

**How does a bone scan work?**

- Technetium-99m phosphate complex
- Absorbed on to hydroxyapatite crystals in bone
- Shows inc blood flow and activity (trauma, infection, neoplasia)

**What are some areas where a bone scan may be of use?**

- Osteomyelitis
- THA/TKA component loosening
- AVN

## Specific Resources Mentioned in this Episode

**Krause ML, Matteson EL. Perioperative management of the patient with rheumatoid arthritis. World J Orthop. 2014 Jul 18;5(3):283-91. doi: 10.5312/wjo.v5.i3.283. PMID: 25035831; PMCID: PMC4095021.**

**Osteoporos Int. 2014; 25(10): 2359–2381. Published online 2014 Aug 15. doi: 10.1007/s00198-014-2794-2 PMCID: PMC4176573 PMID: 25182228 Clinician's Guide to Prevention and Treatment of Osteoporosis**

# NOTES

# NOTES

# NOTES

# NOTES

# SPINE CHAPTER 4

**What is cervical spondylosis?**

- Chronic disk degeneration + associated facet arthropathy

**What is the difference between radiculopathy, myelopathy, discogenic back pain, and myeloradiculopathy?**

- Radiculopathy- nerve root disease (radiating pain)
- Myelopathy- spinal cord disease
- Discogenic - vertebral disc disease
- Myeloradiculopathy- spinal cord + nerve root dysfunction

**Do the cervical nerve roots exit above or below their corresponding vertebrae?**

- Above,a disc herniation at C4-C5 involves C5 nerve root
- At C7-T1- C8 nerve root

**Spine 1: 5:00**

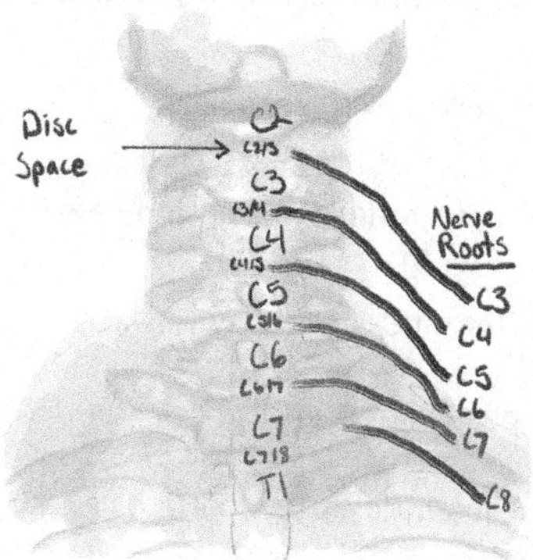


**What does a positive spurling test suggest?**

- Nerve root pain
- The neck is rotated w/ a lateral bend and axial compression of the head

**What does a positive Lhremitte test suggest?**

- Specific for cervical myelopathy (not specific or sensitive for radiculopathy)
- C-spine flexion/extension causes radiating pain to arms/legs (spinal cord stretching/compression)

**Figure 4.1: Imaging of the C-spine showing the exiting nerve roots in the cervical spine. The nerve roots exit above the disc.**

**What test is performed by "flicking" the long finger distal phalanx while looking for thumb IP flexion?**

- Hoffman test, sensitive for cervical myelopathy
- Tests the long tract neural pathway

**What does a positive babinski or positive clonus suggest?**

- Upper motor neuron pathology

**What cervical nerve root and C-spine level is affected in a patient w/ weakened wrist extension and numbness along the radial forearm and thumb, and an abnormal brachioradialis reflex?**

- C6 reflex- brachioradialis
- C5-C6

**What maneuver tests the C7 reflex arc?**

- Triceps reflex test
- C5- biceps, C6- brachioradialis, C8- none

**What cervical nerve root and spine level is affected in a patient with grip weakness and numbness over the small and ring finger?**

- C8 (no reflex)
- C7-T1

**What cervical nerve root and spine level is affected in a patient with shoulder abduction weakness, numbness over the lateral arm and an abnormal biceps reflex?**

- C5 reflex- biceps
- C4-C5

**What is a tandem gait and what is it indicative of?**

- Heel/toe walking (like walking in a straight line)
- Balance issues doing this may indicate possible cervical myelopathy

**What does heel and toe walking evaluate?**

- Strength of tibialis anterior (heel) and gastrocnemius- soleus complex (toe walking)

**What does recovery of the bulbocavernosus reflex typically indicate?**

- The end of spinal shock (~48 hrs after the start)

**Spine 1: 17:45**

**What are some things to look for on different C-spine xray views?**

- AP- uncovertebral joint pathology
- Lateral- sagittal alignment, disk space narrowing, listhesis, osteophytes
- Flexion/Extension lateral- C- spine instability, pseudoarthrosis
- Oblique- neuroforaminal stenosis
- Odontoid view- C1/C2 fx

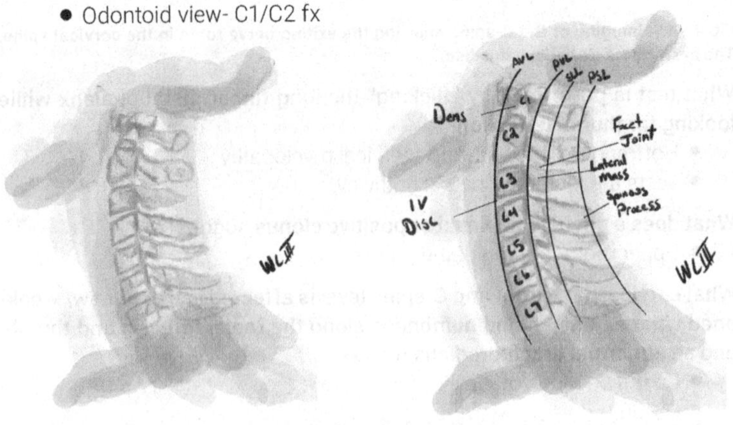


**Figure(s) 4.2 & 4.3: Lateral view of the C-spine shows structures marked out and the lines to use when evaluating cervical spine xrays. AVL- anterior vertebral line, PVL- posterior vertebral line, SLL- spinolaminar line, PSL- posterior spinous line**

### What are some causes of cervical radiculopathy (nerve root compromise)?

- Disc herniation, uncovertebral osteophyte, facet arthropathy, thickened ligamentum flavum, degenerative spondylosis (foraminal stenosis from chondro osseous spurs)

### What are some symptoms of cervical radiculopathy?

- Pain, numbness, + paresthesias in a dermatomal distribution

### What is a way to distinguish between C8-T1 radiculopathy and cubital tunnel syndrome?

- Ulnar forearm involvement (innervated by MABn, not ulnar nerve)
  - Ulnar n innervates small + ring finger

### If all intrinsic hand muscles are weak, what are some potential causes?

- Median + ulnar nerve compression or C8-T1 radiculopathy

### What are some things you may see on xray in patients with cervical radiculopathy?

- Uncovertebral joint arthritis, osteophytes > causing foraminal stenosis

### What are some things you may see on MRI in patients with cervical radiculopathy?

- Disc herniation
- CSF effacement (on sagittals)
- Disc/osteophyte complex w/ foraminal stenosis

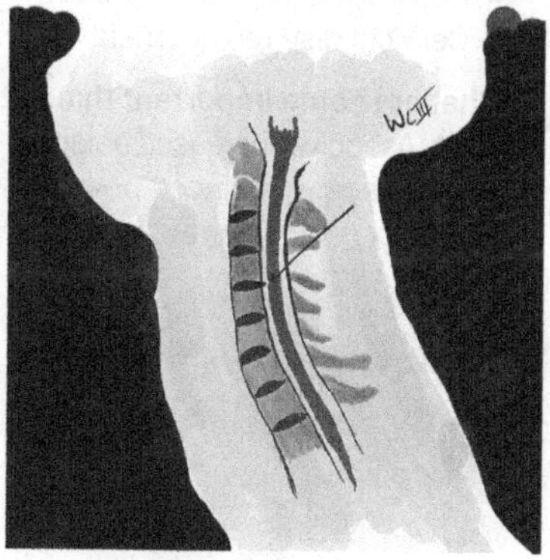

**Figure 4.4: Sagittal view of the cervical spine showing a disc herniation, pointed out by the arrow.**

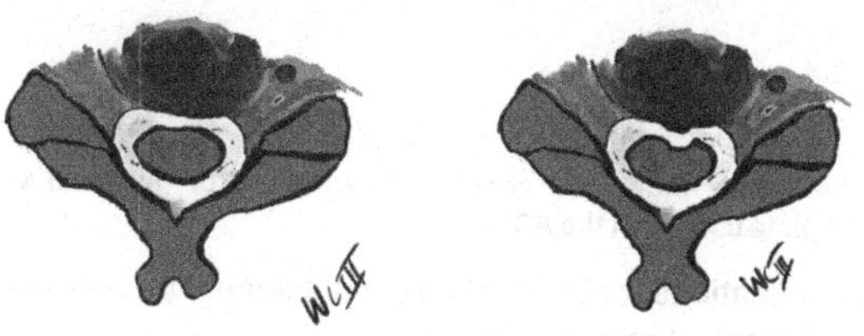

**Figure(s) 4.5 & 4.6: Axial cuts of the cervical spine in a normal person (left) and a cervical disc herniation.**

### What is the non-op treatment for cervical radiculopathy?

- NSAIDs, oral steroids, epidural injections (can be diagnostic + therapeutic), physical therapy
- 75% get better w/ non-op tx

**What are the surgical indications for patients w/ cervical radiculopathy?**

- Persistent sxs despite non-op tx (after 6-12 weeks)
- Worsening neurological sxs (ex: motor weakness)

**What is a corpectomy?**

- Vertebral body removal (ACCF = Anterior cervical corpectomy and fusion)
- w/ fusion - possible complications: pseudoartrosis, graft dislodgement

**What is an ACDF?**

- Anterior cervical discectomy and fusion
- (direct decompression of structures)

**What are some surgical options for patients with cervical radiculopathy?**

- ACDF- removal of herniated disc + osteophyte excision + strut graft fusion w/ or w/o instrumentation (can be one or multilevel)
- ACCF- if compression due to pathology behind vertebral body
- Posterior laminoforaminotomy- enlarges foramen
- Cervical disc replacement

Spine 2: 7:12

**What are some important things to note about ACDF?**

- Assoc w/ increased adjacent segment disease, also pseudoarthrosis
- Assoc w/ reduced post-op neck pain
- Poorer fusion rates w/ 3+ levels

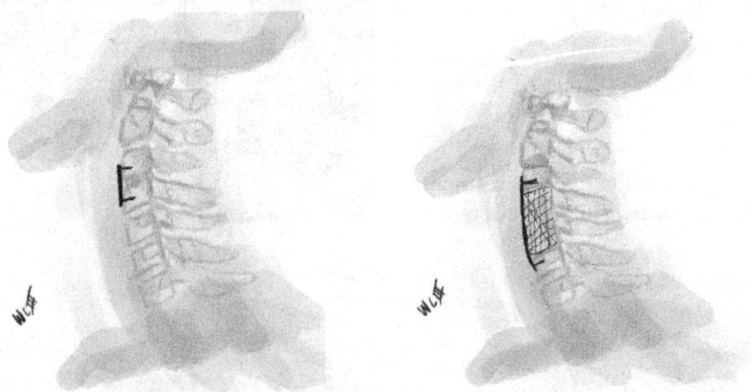

**Figure(s) 4.7 and 4.8 show films of the cervical spine after ACDF (left) and ACCF (right). Note the cage and plate used with the ACDF.**

**What are some indications for cervical disc replacement (maintains motion)?**

- Radiculopathy / myelopathy
- Single + two level disease
- Equivalent outcomes to ACDF, possible reduced reoperation rate when comparing w/ 1 level ACDF (for radiculopathy, but some recent studies show no difference)
  - Associated w/ HO formation

(Johansen, 2021)

(Nunley, 2018)

**What are some important things to note about posterior foraminotomy?**
- Assoc w/ increase same level radiculopathy recurrence
- Assoc w/ increased neck pain

**What are some soft tissue landmarks and their C-spine correlation w/ the anterior approach?**
- C2- Angle of mandible
  - C2/C3 herniation- superior laryngeal n a risk during approach (high phonation)
- C3- Hyoid bone
- C4-5 - Thyroid cartilage
- C5-C6- Cricoid membrane
- C6- Carotid tubercle

**What is the degenerative spinal cascade seen in cervical spondylosis?**
- Cervical disc collapse > loss of cervical lordosis > kyphosis > Anterior disc osteophyte spurs
- Facet + uncovertebral joint loading > spondylotic changes in foramina > nerve root compression

**What are some causes of cervical myelopathy?**
- Cervical spondylosis- MC- (bulging osteophytes, ossified discs, thickened ligamentum flavum, etc)
- Ossified posterior longitudinal ligament (OPLL)
- Rheumatoid arthritis
- Oncological tumor
- Epidural abscess

**Spine 2: 15:55**

**Ep 5 w/ Dr. Cyriac**

**What are some symptoms of cervical myelopathy?**
- Finger clumsiness, dropping items, trouble buttoning shirt, balance issues, tingling in hands

**What are some physical exam findings that can be seen with cervical myelopathy?**
- **Hoffmann sign**, clonus, hyperreflexia (indicate spinal cord compression)
- Finger escape sign (small finger abduction due to weak intrinsics) + balance issues

**What is the natural history of cervical myelopathy due to spondylosis (cervical spondylotic myelopathy)?**
- Progressive stepwise decline is most common
- Do well for a while then do worse
- Worse outcomes w/ symptom severity when being treated

**What are some things to note on C-spine xray when evaluating for cervical myelopathy?**
- Amount of kyphosis (C2-C7 alignment)
- Degenerative changes (joint space narrowing, anterior osteophytes, facet arthropathy)

- Congenital stenosis
- OPLL (ossified posterior longitudinal ligament) presence
- Flexion/Extension films- flexible vs rigid kyphosis

**What are some things to look for on MRI when evaluating cervical myelopathy?**

- Myelomalacia
- CSF effacement (thinning of the CSF fluid)
- Disc herniation

**What is another imaging modality that can be obtained if the patient cant get an MRI (i.e.- pacemaker)**

- CT myelogram - may show ossified PLL better

**What patients with cervical myelopathy can undergo non-op treatment?**

- Pts w/ no functional impairment (no myelopathy/radiculopathy- radiographic cord compression only)
- Frequent follow up required

**What patients w/ cervical myelopathy should undergo operative intervention?**

- Patients w/ any functional impairment
- The disease is progressive and will only get worse
- Surgery improves functional outcomes

**What are some operative treatment options for patients w/ cervical myelopathy?**

- Anterior: ACDF, corpectomy
- Posterior- laminectomy w/ or w/o fusion, laminoplasty
- Anterior + posterior procedure

**What is a way to decide which procedure should be performed?**

- Measure kyphosis
    - If >10 degrees, must go anterior (unable to decompress spinal cord if you go posterior)
- Measure levels of compression
    - 1 or 2 levels compression- ACDF/corpectomy
    - 3+ levels of compression
        - And >10° kyphosis- Anterior (to decompress/ correct kyphosis) + posterior
        - And <10° kyphosis - Posterior (laminoplasty v laminectomy & fusion)

**What is an important thing to consider in the surgical treatment of patients w/ kyphosis?**

- Rigid kyphosis doesn't allow spinal cord to float back w/ a posterior approach only

**What is the difference between laminectomy and laminoplasty?**

- Laminectomy- removal of the lamina

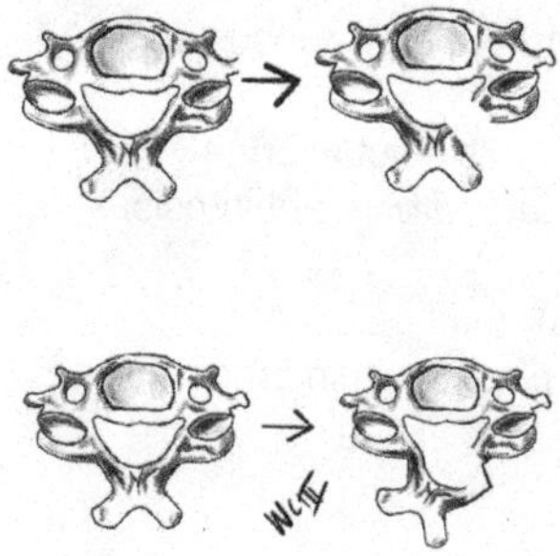

- Laminoplasty- lamina is cut and hinged open and held w/ some type of fixation (graft/sutures/ plate)
    - Preserves motion

**Figure 4.9: An example of a cervical laminectomy (top) and laminoplasty (bottom) is shown.**

**What is a complication that can be seen in a patient that had a laminectomy w/o fusion?**

- Post-laminectomy kyphosis
- (w/ fusion- avoids post-laminectomy kyphosis + may help w/ spondylotic neck pain)

**What is the difference between an open door and french door laminoplasty?**

- Open door- unilateral hinge at contralateral lateral mass + lamina junction
- French door- bilateral hinge created at midline

**What are some potential complications w/ laminoplasty?**

- Neck pain (no fusion), motion loss, segmental root level palsy

**Is there any difference between posterior and anterior approaches?**

- Anterior approach- dysphagia
- Posterior approach- infection

**When should both anterior and posterior approaches be considered?**

- Post-laminectomy kyphosis
- Kyphotic patients that need multilevel decompression

**Spine 3: 7:40**

**Is there any difference when placing screws in C3-6 vs C7 when you are aiming?**

- C3-C6 lateral mass screws are aimed 15° cranial and 30° lateral
- C7 pedicle screw is aimed 30° medial

**What is the likely diagnosis in a patient s/p 2 level ACDF w/ lateral arm numbness and abduction weakness?**

- C5 palsy, possibly due to stretching of C5 nerve root
- Tx: Observe

**What is on the differential diagnosis in a patient 6mo s/p 2 level ACDF w/ continued neck pain and incomplete fusion seen on xrays?**

- Pseudoarthrosis (rate inc as levels fused inc ~10% three levels)
- Smoking is a risk factor
- Tx:
    - Asymptomatic- observation
    - Symptomatic- revision ACDF or posterior cervical fusion

**What are some other complications seen w/ ACDF?**

- Dysphagia (higher risk at C3-4, decrease by: steroids at end of case,

limit retraction, low profile hardware)
- Recurrent laryngeal nerve injury (watch at first, ENT consult at 6 weeks)
- Hypoglossal nerve injury (tongue deviates to side of injury)
- Horner's syndrome (sympathetic chain injury- ptosis, anhidrosis, miosis, enophthalmos)
- Airway compromise (edema / hematoma)
- Adjacent segment disease (inc if plate is placed within 5mm of superior endplate)

## Rheumatoid

**What is the Ranawat classification for patients with RA w/ myelopathy?**

**Spine 4: 1:33**

- I- no neurological deficit
- II- subjective weakness, dysesthesias, + hyperreflexia
- III- objective weakness + UMN signs
  - IIIA- ambulatory
  - IIIB- non-ambulatory (surgery doesn't do as well)

**What are the C-spine conditions that should be on your mind in any patient with rheumatoid arthritis?**
- Atlantoaxial subluxation (first presentation of C- spine instability in rheumatoid pt)
- Basilar invagination
- Subaxial subluxation

**What is the cause of atlantoaxial subluxation?**
- Pannus formation between dens and C1 leading to destruction of the transverse ligament
- Leads to C1-C2 instability & subluxation

**What are some symptoms seen in atlantoaxial subluxation?**
- Neck pain, occipital headaches (occipital branch of C2 compression)
- Myelopathy/radiculopathy can also occur

**What is the atlanto-dens interval?**
- Distance between anterior arch of atlas and dens of axis
- >10 mm of motion on flex/extension films- assoc w/ inc risk of neurologic injury (operate)
- >3.5mm increase- instability (common in RA, may not indicate surgery)

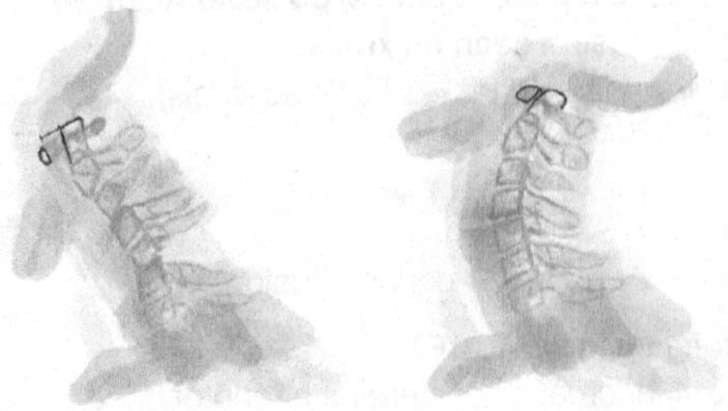

**Figure 4.10: Lateral flexion and extension films of the cervical spine, showing atlantoaxial subluxation. An increase in the ADI is noted with motion (black outlines).**

**What is the difference between the posterior ADI (PADI) and the space available for the cord (SAC)?**

- Nothing, they are the same
- PADI < 14 may require surgical tx

**What are the surgical indications for patients with atlantoaxial subluxation?**

Spine 4: 9:43

- Worsening sxs/ neurological instability
- PADI <14, ADI >10 motion

**What are some of the surgical options for patients w/ atlantoaxial subluxation?**

- C1-C2 transarticular screw (C1+C2 lateral mass fusion- vertebral artery +C2 nerve injury risk)
- C1 lateral mass- C2 pedicle/pars fixation (strongest C1-C2 fixation construct, doesn't require C1/C2 to be reduced)
- Odontoidectomy

**What is basilar invagination/ atlantoaxial invagination?**

- Tip of dens migrates above foramen magnum
- Due to bone loss + erosion between C1/C2 and occiput
- Can lead to brainstem compression + vascular compromise

**What can you use radiographically to clue you in to basilar invagination on lateral xray?**

- Ranawat index (detects vertical subluxation)
- Distance between a point on C2 and C1 measured (normal 15mm+ men, 13mm+ women)
- McGregor's line can also be used (odontoid shouldn't protrude >4.5mm above line)

**What is the surgical tx for basilar invagination (pts w/ intractable pain +/- neurologic compromise)?**

- Occiput to C-spine fusion
- Transoral/ anterior retropharyngeal odontoid resection (if brainstem is compromised)
- C1 arch removal may also be considered for decompression
- In severe cases- cervical traction may be used 1st to reduce dens

**What is subaxial subluxation?**

- Pannus formation in uncovertebral + facet joints > subluxation that can be at multiple levels
- Subluxation >4mm or >20% - there may be cord compression
- Tx: PSF w/ or w/o decompression

## Ankylosing Spondylitis

**What is ankylosing spondylitis?**

Spine 2: 2:15

- A seronegative inflammatory disease that affects axial skeleton
- Entheses are affected > leads to bony erosions > new bone formation > ankylosing
- Sacroiliitis common

**If a patient with ankylosing spondylitis (AS) falls and has neck pain, but a negative xray, should you do any further workup?**

- Yes, consider advanced imaging (CT/MRI)
- Must have high suspicion for occult fracture
- Fractures are unstable - they extend across all three columns > spinal instability
- Missed fracture can have bad consequences and neurological compromise

**What is a positive lab finding in a patient w/ ankylosing spondylitis?**

- HLA- B27, positive 95% of the time

**What are some things that you may note on xray in a patient with ankylosing spondylitis?**

- Kyphotic deformity, ossification of C-spine disc space, sacroiliitis (sometimes fusion), bamboo spine
- Marginal syndesmophytes

**What are some things you may note on xray in a patient w/ diffuse idiopathic skeletal hyperostosis (DISH)?**

- Large non-marginal syndesmophytes
- Flowing candle wax appearance, preservation of disc space
- No SI joint involvement

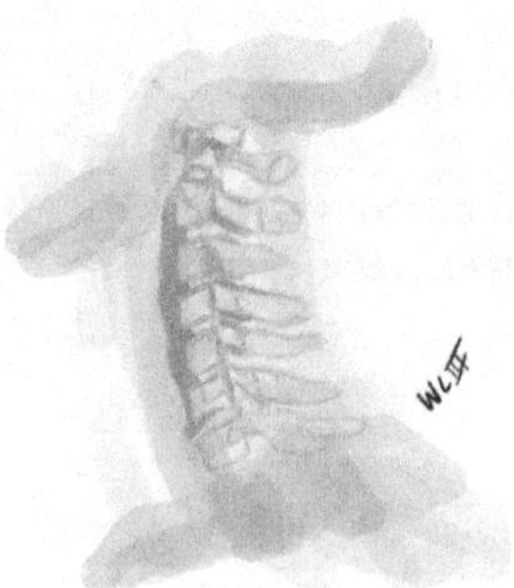

**Figure 4.11: Lateral C-spine films showing the classic appearance of DISH, with the flowing candle wax appearance and preservation of disc space.**

**Should you be concerned if there is a patient that has neck pain after a fall with DISH or AS?**

- Yes, the injury can be devastating!
- Higher rates of neurological injury

**What is the treatment for a patient w/ AS after a fall w/ neurological deficits?**

- Decompress + long stabilization

**What are some surgical options in patients with AS and a kyphotic deformity?**

- Anterior opening osteotomies or pedicle subtraction osteotomies (restore sagittal balance)

**What is a surgical option for a patient w/ a fixed C-spine flexion deformity (i.e.- chin on chest)**

- C- spine osteotomy (sometimes done at C7-T1, to avoid injury to vertebral a)
- C spine laminectomy + osteotomy + fusion

**What is an ossified posterior longitudinal ligament (OPLL) and the tx if symptomatic?**

- PLL ectopic ossification
- Posterior approach
  - Indirect spinal cord decompression, lordotic or neutral alignment needed
  - Laminectomy alone- not done due to post-laminectomy kyphosis
  - Laminectomy + fusion (w/ instrumentation most often)
  - Laminoplasty- don't do in kyphotic spine
- Anterior approach
  - ACDF/ACCF - higher incidence of dural leak (OPLL assoc w/ dural ossification)

**What is a burner/stinger? (yes this is the third + time we are mentioning this)**

- Transient neurapraxia commonly assoc w/ stretching of brachial plexus
- Typically unilateral burning/weakness- eval for C-spine pain, TTP, or neuro sxs

## C-Spine Trauma

**What is the difference between a complete and incomplete spinal cord injury?**

- Complete- no function below a level
  - Recovery can't be determined until end of spinal shock (return of bulbocavernosus reflex), or 48 hrs after injury
- Incomplete- some sparing of distal motor/sensory function

**What is the American Spinal Injury Association (ASIA) Classification?**

Spine 6: 2:34

- A- complete- no motor, sensory or sacral sparing
- B- incomplete- sensory only, no motor
- C- 50% muscles <grade 3- can't raise arms/ legs
- D- 50% muscles >grade 3- can raise arms/legs
- E- motor + sensory normal
  - E- strong as an elephant !

**Is there any indication for halo vest immobilization, and what is the safe zone for pin placement?**

- To control Occiput-C2 motion (less effective to control subaxial spine)
- Safe zone- anterior pin- above eyebrow in middle-lateral ⅓

- Avoids supraorbital nerve
- Kids- 8-10 pins w/ 2inch-lb pressure pin
- Adults 4 pins (6-8 inch-lb pressure pin)
- Not tolerated well in elderly

**What PE findings would you see in a patient w/ Brown- Sequard syndrome (cord hemitransection)?**

- Ipsilateral- motor weakness + loss of posterior column (vibration + sense)
- Contralateral- loss of spinothalamic function (pain + temperature)
- Best prognosis

**What PE findings would you see in a patient with anterior cord syndrome (anterior a injury)?**

- Paraplegia/ quadriplegia + a sensory deficit below level of injury
- Worst prognosis

**What PE findings would you see in a patient w/ central cord syndrome?**

- UE weakness > LE weakness +/- burning in UE
- Usually caused by hyperextension
- Good prognosis- full functional recovery rare though

**What is the treatment for most incomplete SCI?**

- Decompress w/i 12 hrs
- Treatment for most complete SCI- decompress + stabilize w/i 24hrs

**What SCI can be typically treated non-op?**

- Central cord syndrome + GSW
- Take to the OR if worsening neuro exam or fragment in CSF

**Is there a clear cut role for methylprednisolone for treating SCI?**

- No, it is controversial
- Historically used for non-penetrating trauma w/i 8 hrs of injury
- Mechanism by which it works: inhibits lipid peroxidation + cytokines, prevents calcium channel influx and accumulation + improves vascular perfusion

**What are some other things to note in the medical management of SCI?**

- Rigid backboards + patient repositioning every 2 hours- prevent ulcers
- Urinary retention- catheter placement- monitor for UTI / urosepsis
- DVT/PE ppx for up to 3 months

Spine 7: 1:00

**What is traumatic occipitocervical dissociation (OCD) and its treatment?**

- When the head is not connected to C1
- Often lethal & hard to detect on xrays
  - Use powers ratio to help in diagnosis with anterior OCD
- Tx: light traction can help reduce dislocation > occipitocervical fusion

**Can occipitocervical dissociation be acquired?**
- Yes, due to bony dysplasia/ ligament and soft tissue laxity
- Can be see in patients w/ down syndrome
- Tx: consider occipitocervical fusion if myelopathic

**What is the classification for atlas fractures?**
- Type I- isolated arch fx
- Type II- Jefferson fracture
- Type III- Isolated lateral mass fx

**What is a burst (Jefferson) fracture?**
- Bilateral fracture of anterior + posterior C1 arch
- Typically due to axial force
- Look for lateral mass displacement on xray
  - If sum of displacement >8.1mm assoc w/ transverse lig rupture = unstable

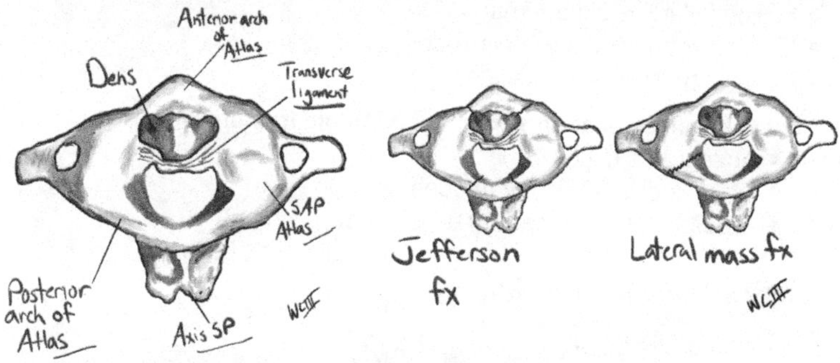


**Figure(s) 4.12 and 4.13: Axial view of the C-spine showing the atlas/axis with the corresponding structures marked (left), and fracture patterns of a C1 Jefferson and Lateral mass fracture (right).SAP- Superior articular process, SP- Spinous process.**

**Injury to what structures (ligaments) can result in an ADI >5mm?**
- Alar, apical, and transverse ligaments

**What does long term stability of burst fractures depend on?**
- Transverse ligament healing
- On MRI:
  - Type 1 lesion- midsubstance rupture of transverse ligament
  - Type 2 lesion- avulsion of ligament

**What are the stable atlas fractures and their treatment?**
- Isolated arch fx, transverse processes fx, + lateral mass fx- 6-12 weeks C-collar
- Jefferson fx w/ intact ligament (<8.1mm displacement) - Halo immobilization

**What are the unstable atlas fractures and their treatment?**
- Unstable fx (>8.1mm displacement)
  - ADI >3.5 indicates transverse ligament injury, ADI >5mm indicates

injury + transverse & alar ligaments

- Tx- bed rest w/ Halo conversion if reduction maintained, C1/C2 fusion, occipitocervical fusion

**What is the blood supply to the axis (C2)?**

- Internal carotid artery- apex
- Vertebral artery- base

**Where does most of the C-spine flexion and rotation come from?**

- Flexion- occiput - C1 (50%)
- Rotation- C1-C2
- Lateral bend- 60% from subaxial spine

**What is the dens?**

- Odontoid process (part of axis that articulates w/ C1)

**What is an os odontoideum due to?**

- Fusion failure vs old trauma
- Look for round fx edges on imaging
- Contact sports contraindicated

**Spine 8: 0:55**

**What is the classification system for odontoid fractures?**

- Anderson & D'Alonzo
- Type I- oblique fracture through tip
- Type II- fx through base of dens (most common)
    - Type IIa- comminuted fracture through base of dens
- Type III- fx through C2 body

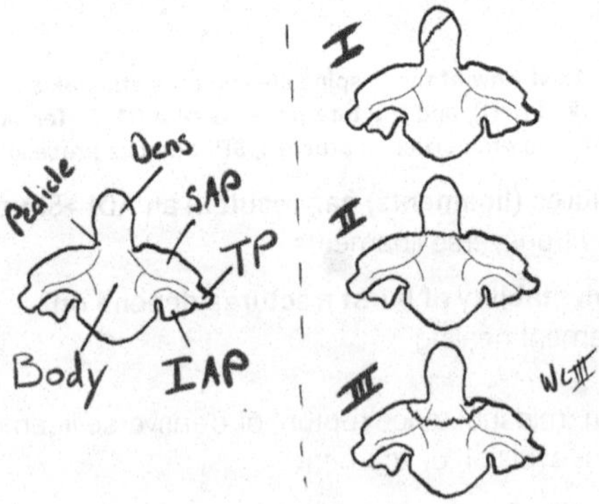


**Figure 4.14: Shows the axis labeled (left) and the different types of odontoid fractures according to the Anderson & D'Alonzo classification.**

**What is the imaging modality of choice for C2 fractures to further assess fracture?**

- CT scan
- MRI- get if cord injury suspicion- can tell if injury to transverse ligament

**What is the tx for type I & type III odontoid fractures?**

- C-collar

**What is the nonunion rate + risks for type II odontoid fracture?**

- 32%
- *>5mm displacement*, angulation >10°, 40 y/o+, posterior displacement assoc w/ inc nonunion rates w/ non-op treatment **(Koivikko, 2004)**

**What is the treatment of choice for type II odontoid fractures?**

- Controversial
- Nondisplaced fx w/o nonunion risk factors- halo vest
  - If elderly, consider C1-C2 fusion or orthosis (poorly tolerated)
    - Orthosis may allow fibrous union to develop
- Nondisplaced fx w/ nonunion risk factors- surgical stabilization
- Displaced fx- surgical stabilization

**What are some different surgical options for type II odontoid fractures?**

- Anterior odontoid screw (fracture must be reduced prior to screw placement)
- C1-C2 transarticular screw + wire (internal carotid @ risk w/ screw placement)
- C1 lateral mass - C2 pedicle screw placement w/ grafting

**Where does the vertebral artery course in relationship to the cervical spine?**

- In transverse foramen of C2 then onto superior aspect of C1
- Injury associated w/- facet dislocations, OC dissociation, displaced transverse foramen fx

**What is traumatic spondylolisthesis of the C-spine and its mechanism?**

- Bilateral fractures of the pars interarticularis (hangman)
- Mechanism- hyperextension, compression, + rebound flexion

**What is the Levine and Edward classification for Traumatic Spondylosthesis of the axis?**

- Type I- axial compression + hyperextension - <3mm displacement w/ no angulation
- Type II- hyperextension + axial load + rebound flexion- >3mm translation + angulation
- Type IIa- flexion/distraction - significant angulation w/o much translation
- Type III- flexion/distraction + hyperextension- Type I + bilateral C2/C3 facet dislocation

**What is the treatment for traumatic spondylolisthesis?**

- Type I- rigid orthosis
- Type II w/ severe angulation + type IIa
  - Reduce > halo immobilization
  - Consider surgery if unable to maintain reduction / displacement >5mm

- Type III- surgery
- Surgical options
  - Posterior C1-C3 fusion, anterior C2/C3 interbody fusion, b/l C2 pars a. screws

**What's the management for an awake patient w/ bilateral facet dislocations?**

- Close reduce w/ traction - monitor neurological deficits- stop if change in deficits
- Obtain MRI after reduction (eval for hematoma or remaining disk materials/cord compression)
  - Also ***obtain MRI in obtunded patients** + patients w/ a failed closed reduction

**Do you not do a closed reduction if they are awake with neurological deficits?**

- You still do a closed reduction w/ traction whether neurological deficits are present or not
- (AAOS Review book)

**What surgery should be considered if residual herniated disk is present after closed reduction of a cervical facet dislocation?**

- Anterior decompression 1st before posterior procedure

**What is the treatment for unilateral and bilateral facet dislocations (after reduction)?**

- Unilateral- immobilize w/ close follow up
- Bilateral- surgical stabilization. Both anterior + posterior procedures work
  - Sometimes posterior preferred due to biomechanical and anatomic advantages

## LUMBAR SPINE

**What nerve root does the patellar tendon reflex test?**

- L4

**What is the reflex that can be used to test the L5 nerve root?**

- None

**What is the reflex that can be used to test the S1 nerve root?**

- Achilles tendon reflex

**What nerve root may be affected in a patient with ankle dorsiflexion weakness and numbness about the medial foot?**

- L4 (also possible quadriceps loss)

**What nerve root may be affected in a patient with gastroc weakness and numbness about the posterior calf and plantar foot?**

- S1

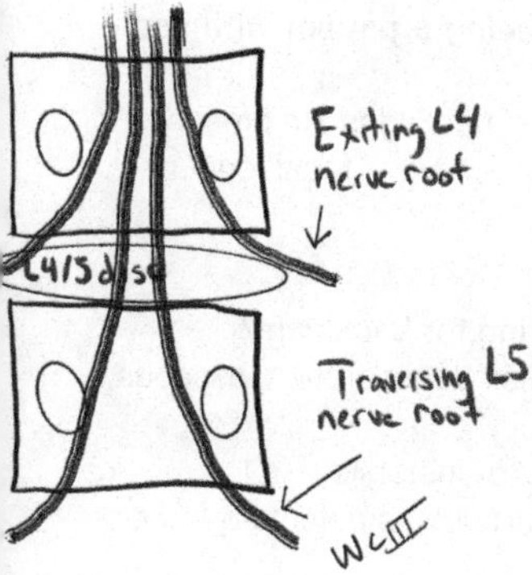


**What nerve root may be affected in a patient with big toe extension weakness and numbness about the lateral calf and dorsal foot?**
- L5

**Figure 4.15: Image showing the lumbar spine and the relation between the traversing and exiting nerve roots. The nerve roots exit below the corresponding vertebral pedicle. A central disc herniation at L4/5 would affect the traversing L5 nerve root.**

**What nerve root(s) may be affected in a patient with hip flexion weakness and sensory loss around the anterior thigh?**
- L2, L3

**What is the lasegue (straight leg raise) sign?**
- Hip flexion w/ knee extension to 90° leads to radiating pain down leg
- Sensitive for L4-5 or L5-S1 herniated disc

**Spine 9: 8:15**

**What is the crossed straight leg test?**
- Extension of contralateral leg produces symptoms down symptomatic leg
- Specific for contralaterally herniated disc

**What is the femoral stretch test?**
- Tenses upper lumbar roots
- Passive hip extension + knee flexion
- Sensitive for herniated discs at L1-2, L2-3, L3-4

**What is a physical exam test that tests for hip arthritis?**
- Pain w/ internal / external hip rotation

**What is a physical exam test used for sacroiliitis?**
- Patrick/FABER test (flexion- abduction- external rotation of hip)

**What do the Waddell signs indicate and what are they?**
- Non- organic pain, 3+ PE findings are suggestive
- Overreaction, simulation- back pain w/ pushing on head, superficial tenderness, regional disturbances (whole leg numbness/weakness that doesn't match a dermatome), distraction

**What is the leading cause of disability in patients under 50 y/o?**
- Low back pain (LBP)
- Can be due to: muscle sprain, discogenic tears/ annular tear, facet joint arthropathy, spondylolisthesis, & spinal stenosis

**Do you always need to get xrays when first seeing a patient with acute back pain?**

- No, you can wait up to 6-8 weeks unless red flag signs are present
  - Red flag: weight loss, altered mental status, fevers, focal tenderness, decline in physical abilities
  - Also if there is a traumatic event

**What are you looking for on xrays when evaluating for back pain?**

- AP+ lateral- coronal + sagittal alignment, disc degeneration, osseous abnormalities
- Dynamic flexion/extension views- evaluate for instability
- Oblique views- useful to rule out pars interarticularis defects & facet joint arthropathy

Spine 10: 2:50

**What are some indications to get an MRI in a patient w/ LBP?**

- No improvement w/ non op tx for 3 months, malignancy, infection, lumbar radiculopathy patients w/ no improvement w/ 6 weeks tx or worsening sxs, or patients w/ unbearable leg pain

**Are herniated discs common to find in patients >50 y/o?**

- Yes, 25-37% of asymptomatic patients have a herniated disc on MRI

**What is the best imaging study for recurrent herniated disc?**

- MRI w/ gadolinium contrast

**What is the most sensitive method for detecting isthmic spondylolisthesis?**

- SPECT (Single-photon Emission Computerized Tomography)

**What are the disc changes seen with intervertebral disc degeneration?**

- Decrease of proteoglycan>loss of hydration
- Increase in pentosidine (arginine and glycine) cross links + advanced glycosylation
- Relative increase in decorin

**Is there any correlation between degenerative disc disease and low back pain?**

- No, altered segmental biomechanics seen in DDD may play a role though

**What is the pathoanatomy seen in DDD?**

- IV disk collapse > loss of lordosis > chronic anterior cord compression > anterior disc osteophyte spurs > spondylotic foraminal changes > possible segmental instability

**What is a discography?**

- Dye injected into IV disks > should reproduce pain
- Controversial
- Correlates MRI findings w/ clinical pain generator

**What is the difference between acute and chronic back pain?**

- Acute 6 weeks - 3 months

- Chronic > 3 months

**What is the typical treatment for acute low back pain?**

- Non-op, usually self resolves
- Acetaminophen, NSAIDS, muscle relaxants, active physical therapy
- Avoid bedrest

**What are some possible reasons to operate for acute low back pain?**

- Infection, neoplasm, cauda equina syndrome, fractures
- Non op tx first unless: progressive neuro deficits, intractable pain, no improvement in neuro sxs

**What is the typical treatment for chronic back pain?**

- Non-op
- NSAIDs, PT, conditioning, behavioral modifications (smoking cessation, weight loss, etc)
- Tx can be anywhere from 1-6 months

**What are some surgical options for chronic low back pain w/ no improvement w/ non-op tx due to DDD?**

- Controversial whether or not to do surgery, try to avoid
- Fusion- open vs minimally invasive (no single fusion superior to another)
- Total disk arthroplasty- no difference in outcomes between fusion v TDA
  - May better restore disk height

**What is the most sensitive and specific finding with a lumbar disc herniation?**

- Sciatica

**What are some different types of lumbar disc herniation LDH?**

- Central- assoc w/ back pain (possible cauda equina sxs in certain situations)
- Posterolateral (paracentral)- more common- affects traversing nerve root (Ex: left L4-L5 affects L5 root)
- Foraminal (far lateral)- affects exiting nerve root (Ex: left L4-L5 affects L4 nerve root)

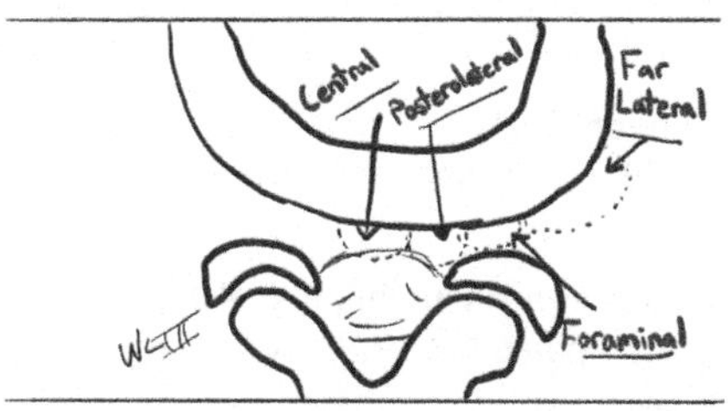


**Figure 4.16: A simplified example showing the difference in location between central vs foraminal and far lateral disc herniations.**

**What symptoms do people with a LDH present with?**

- Back pain, leg pain worse w/ sitting, relieved by standing
- Pain / numbness in a dermatomal fashion

Spine 11: 5:25

**What imaging should be obtained in patients w/ a possible LDH?**

- XRays- flex/extension- assess for instability
- MRI- false positives are common- clinical exam important
  - w/ gadolinium for recurrent disc herniations

**What is the treatment of an acute LDH?**

- Non-op, unless progressive neurological sxs/ intractable pain
- NSAIDs, PT, epidural steroid injections
- Other tx options: oral steroids, muscle relaxants

**What are some surgical indications for LDH?**

- Cauda equina / progressive neurological deficit (rare)
- No improvement w/ non-op tx

**What are common surgical options for patients w/ LDH?**

- Partial discectomy (open/ limited open/ microscope assisted - similar outcomes)
- Hemilaminectomy + discectomy - common
- Total laminectomy- possibly needed for large central herniations
- Para-medial / muscle splitting (Wiltse)- useful for far lateral herniations

**Is a lumbar fusion typically required for treatment of a LDH?**

- No
- May be useful if spinal instability present (spondylolisthesis)
- Or iatrogenic instability- resection >50% of bilateral facets, 100% unilateral facet, excessive pars articularis resection
- Reherniation can occur

Spine 11: 16:40

**What is lumbar spinal stenosis (LSS)?**

- Decrease in space available for neural elements (spinal canal or neural foramina)
- Can be congenital, acquired (degenerative, systemic diseases, etc), or both
- Spinal canal decreases in extension

**What is a classification for LSS?**

- Central stenosis, lateral recess/ subarticular/ entry zone stenosis, foraminal stenosis

**What are some symptoms seen in lumbar spinal stenosis?**

- Back pain + leg pain/ paresthesias/ heaviness worse w/ walking, walking down hills
- Pain relieved w/ sitting (vs stopping walking w/ vascular claudication)
- Leg sxs start proximal > distal (opposite w/ vascular claudication)
- Pseudoclaudication - w/ central stenosis

- Possible radicular sxs- w/ lateral recess + foraminal stenosis

**What are some positive physical exam findings seen w/ LSS?**
- Positive lumbar extension test
- Weakness / LE abnormalities may be present (but not always)

**What are some non-op treatment options for patients w/ LSS?**
- Acetaminophen, NSAIDs, PT, ESI
- Transforaminal nerve blocks

**Where does the facet joint get its innervation from?**
- Medial branch of dorsal primary rami and sinuvertebral nerve

**What are the surgical indications and options for patients w/ LSS?**
- No improvement w/ non-op
- Decompress the stenosed area
- Laminectomy + partial medial facetectomy commonly performed
- Laminotomy + hemi-laminectomy also options
  - Fusion may not be needed if no signs of instability or significant deformity
- Foraminal stenosis- possible medial facetectomy + resection of SAP
- SPORT trial- surgery resulted in better pain relief, function + patient satisfaction at 4-8yr follow up

**(Lurie, 2014)**

**What are the main types of spondylolisthesis?**
- Isthmic, degenerative, dysplastic, traumatic, pathologic, iatrogenic

**What is degenerative spondylolisthesis?**
- Anterior translation of cephalad vertebral body- disc degeneration > facet joint degeneration > instability
- MC in women
- Sxs: mechanical back pain better w/ rest, leg pain as well

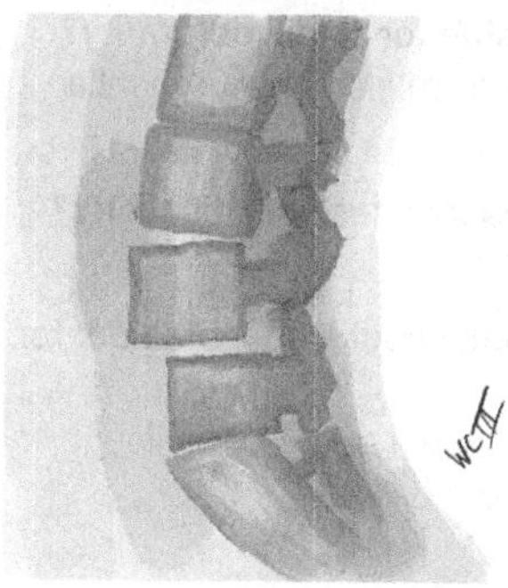

**Figure 4.17: Lateral xray of the lumbar spine showing a L4/5 spondylolisthesis.**

**What is the treatment for degenerative spondylolisthesis?**
- Non-op 1st
- Surgical options:
  - Decompression w/o fusion- assoc w/ slip progression, unclear for clinical outcome difference compared w/ fusion
  - Decompression w/ fusion- higher fusion rates w/ instrumented pedicle screw fixation

**What is isthmic spondylolisthesis?**
- Spondylolisthesis that results from a pars interarticularis defect

- Exiting nerve root affected (L5-S1 affects L5)
- Seen in adolescents
- Sxs: mechanical back pain, altered gait, +/- leg sxs
- Tx: most improve w/ non-op tx

Spine 12: 12:45

**What are some things you should note radiographically when evaluating spondylolisthesis?**

- Meyerding grade 1-5 (1-4 divided into equal percentages, 5 is spondyloptosis)
- Slip angle
- Pelvic tilt
- Pelvic incidence - most correlated with severity

**When is surgical treatment indicated for isthmic spondylolisthesis?**

- High grade slips in children + adolescents
- In situ posterolateral fusion in children w/ low grade L5-S1 slips
- Pars repair in pts w/ spondylosis, no DDD, no slip, & no discogenic pain
- Adults
  - Low grade (1-2) slips- controversy between posterolateral v circumferential fusion
  - High grade (3-4) slips- higher fusion rates w/ anterior column support. Partial reduction + transosseous fusion

## Adult Spinal Deformity

**Are most patients who have adult spinal deformity symptomatic or asymptomatic?**

- Asymptomatic
- When symptomatic, sxs can include: back pain, progressive deformity, myelopathy, radiculopathy
  - Pts may also have a history of a neuromuscular disease

**What xrays do you want to obtain when assessing for spinal deformity?**

- AP + lateral on 36 inch cassettes : to view from clavicles>pelvis/iliac crests

**Is coronal or sagittal plane deformity mostly associated with disability?**

- Sagittal

Spine 13: 5:20

**What are the sagittal measurements that should be obtained for patients with spinal deformity?**

- C7 sagittal vertical axis (C7 SVA)- distance from C7 plum line to S1 (posterior aspect of S1), normal <5cm
  - Neutral, positive, negative
- Lumbar lordosis- Cobb angle T12-S1 or L1-S1, normal ~60°
- T1 pelvic angle- Center of T1 to femoral head then to midpoint of S1 endplate angle, normal, surgical goal <14°

- Pelvic incidence- the angle of these two lines:1. midpoint of S1 end-plate to femoral head and 2. line perpendicular to S1 endplate
  - Constant + related to lumbar lordosis
- Pelvic tilt- angle between line made from midpoint of S1 to femoral head and a vertical line
  - Varies w/ position, increases w/ pelvic retroversion
- Sacral slope- line between superior end plate + horizontal

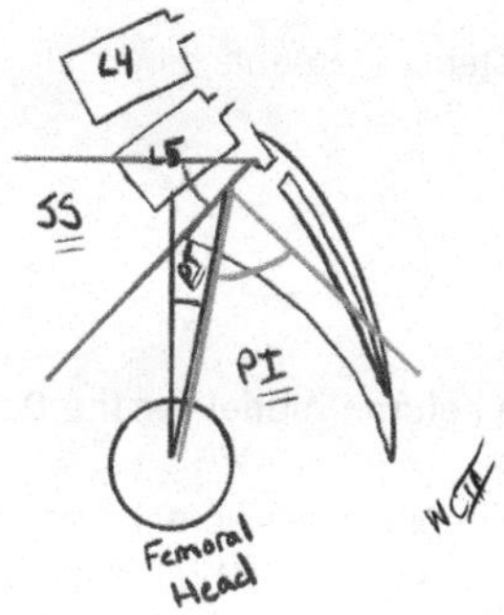


**Figure 4.18: Sagittal measurements that are commonly performed in patients with spinal deformity. Pelvic incidence remains constant while pelvic tilt and sacral slope can change with patient position. PI - Pelvic Incidence, SS- Sacral Slope, PT- Pelvic Tilt.**

### What does the pelvic incidence equal?

- Pelvic tilt + sacral slope
- Larger PI> more horizontal sacrum > greater compensatory lumbar lordosis

### What are some cervical deformity measurements?

- Chin to brow vertical angle
- Cervical lordosis, CSVA, T1 angle

### What are the surgical indications to treat patients w/ adult spinal deformity?

- Progressive coronal/sagittal deformity
- Claudication / radiculopathy w/ no non-op tx improvement
- Inability to perform ADL's

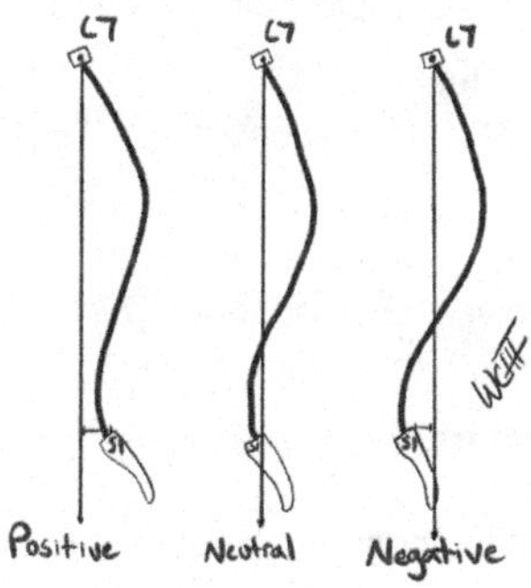


**Figure 4.19: A sagittal of the spine showing the C7 Sagittal Vertical Axis from C7 to the posterior aspect of S1. Patients can be positive, neutral, or negative.**

### What are some surgical options to treat patients w/ adult spinal deformity?

- Decompression alone (ex: radiculopathy w/ stable deformity)- could worsen post-op deformity
- Decompression w/ fusion- if some progression
- Decompression w/ deformity correction + long fusion
  - Pts w/ large scoliosis curve, degenerative deformity, apical vertebra subluxation
  - Restore sagittal balance, may require osteotomy or anterior column support

### What are some types of osteotomies that can be used in patients w/ rigid sagittal/coronal/biplanar deformities?

- Partial facet joint resection
  - 5-10° correction per level
  - Resection of inferior facet

- Complete facet joint resection
  - 10° correction per level
    - Posterior column osteotomy- facet joints + ligamentum flavor resection + others
    - Ponte osteotomy- done at unfused segment
    - Smith peterson osteotomy- done at fused segment
- Pedicle & partial body resection
  - 25-35° per level
    - Pedicle subtraction osteotomy- posterior elements, pedicles + wedge of vertebrae removed
- Complete vertebrae + disc resection

## Trauma

Spine 14: 12:15

**What are the three columns in the three column model for the Denis classification for thoracolumbar injuries?**

- Anterior column- ALL, anterior ½ of annulus + vertebral body
- Middle column- PLL, posterior ½ of annulus + vertebral body
- Posterior column- posterior ligamentous complex and bony arch

**What are the main types of thoracolumbar injuries?**

- Burst, compression, flexion- distraction, fracture dislocation

**What is the mechanism of a burst fracture?**

- Axial compression, the anterior and middle columns are involved
- Posterior column may or may not be involved- eval for bony fx (i.e. lamina)

**What is the mechanism of a compression fracture?**

- Anterior flexion + loading
- Anterior column injury, middle column intact- posterior height maintained, loss of anterior height

**What is the mechanism of a flexion-distraction (chance) fracture?**

- Flexion + distraction posteriorly- ex: body pushed forward in car accident
- Usual three column involvement, no translation

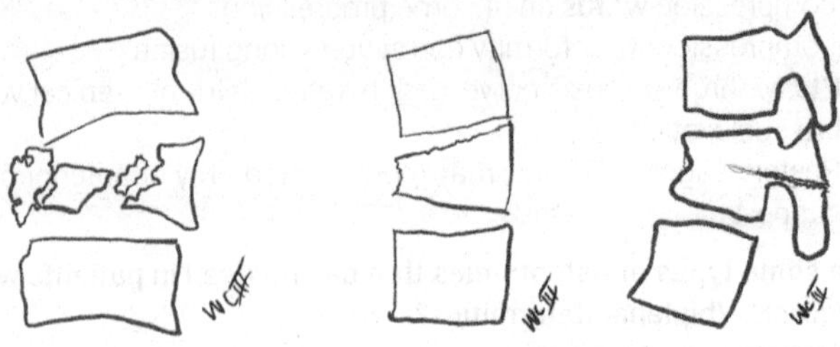

**Figure(s) 4.20, 4.21, and 4.22: Showing the difference in fracture pattern between a burst (left), compression (middle), and chance (right) fracture.**

**What is the mechanism of a fracture dislocation?**

- Mechanism varies, all columns involved + vertebral translation

**What is the treatment of most lumbar spine fractures?**

- Short period of bedrest followed by immobilization in TLSO for 12 weeks
  - TLSO helps control flexion/extension and rotation
- Single leg spica attachment sometimes used to control lumbosacral motion (L4/L5 fx)

**What are some surgical indications for lumbar fractures?**

- Cauda equina syndrome or significant neurological deficit w/ severe canal compromise
- Other things to note, w/ burst fx: loss of alignment (>30° jxn kyphosis, posterior ligamentous injury, neuro deficits)

**Spine 15: 1:05**

**What is the TLICS score and the treatment implications?**

**The Thoracolumbar Injury Classification and Severity (TLICS) Score**

| Injury Category | Point Value |
|---|---|
| Injury morphology | |
| Compression | 1 |
| Burst | 2 |
| Translation or rotation | 3 |
| Distraction | 4 |
| PLC Status | |
| Intact | 0 |
| Injury suspected or indeterminate | 2 |
| Injured | 3 |
| Neurologic status | |
| Intact | 0 |
| Nerve root involvement | 2 |
| Spinal cord or conus medullaris injury | |
| Incomplete | 3 |
| Complete | 2 |
| Cauda equina syndrome | 3 |

**Table 4.1: The Thoracolumbar Injury Classification and Severity (TLICS) Score in shown.**

- TLICS treatment implications
  - Score < 4 points
    - Nonsurgical management
  - Score = 4 points
    - Nonsurgical or surgical management
  - Score > 4 points
    - Surgical management indicated

**What is a kyphoplasty?**

- Use of a balloon impactor to restore vertebral height before a cement augmentation procedure

**What is a vertebroplasty?**

- Transpedicular injection of cement into the vertebral body
- Conflicting results for cement augmentation, may be useful in patients who fail non-op tx, metastatic disease, continued vertebral collapse, osteoporotic vertebral fx w/ cont pain

**What procedure is typically performed for lumbar fractures that meet operative indications?**

- Posterior decompression via laminectomy, w/ fixation a level above + below injury
- Possible anterior approach for decompression if neuro deficits w/ retropulsion

**What is the difference between neurogenic shock and spinal shock?**

- Spinal shock- metabolic derangement after SCI, unable to assess if SCI is complete or incomplete
  - Return of bulbocavernosus reflex shows end of spinal shock
- Neurogenic shock- injury to upper thoracic/lower cervical, loss of sympathetics- bradycardic + hypotensive

**What are the surgical indications to operate for a gunshot to the spine?**

- Abdominal organ injury

## Infections

Spine 15: 16:14

**What is the typical course of treatment after a positive pre-op nasal swab for MRSA?**

- Muporocin ointment + hibiclens body wash x5 days w/ pre-op IV vanc

**What is the most common presentation of a post-op spine infection + labs to obtain?**

- Pain
- ESR, CRP CBC
  - ESR and CRP may be elevated from initial surgery, can trend
- Blood cx if systemic infection suspected

**In what situations can a post-op infection be treated non-op?**
- Superficial infections w/o frank pus
- Follow closely

**What is the preferred treatment for post-op spine infection?**
- Surgical I&D, cultures from surgery, IV antibiotics
- Retain hardware if you can, remove bone graft (nidus for infection)

**In hematogenous spine infections, what is the typical route of the pathological organism?**
- Blood > vascular end plates > avascular disk space (nucleus pulposus) > vertebral bodies

**What is the optimal imaging choice for diagnosing infection discitis?**
- **MRI**
- Technetium -99 bone scans can also diagnose discitis, very sensitive
- Disc space narrowing may be seen on plain xrays (xray lag behind sxs for weeks)

**What is the typical treatment for most pyogenic spinal infections?**
- IV antibiotics (4-6 weeks followed by oral abx), immobilization + supportive care

**What are the surgical indications for pyogenic spinal infections?**
- Progressive neuro deficits or deformity, failure of non-op tx

**What are the surgical procedures typically performed for spinal infections?**
- Debridement, decompression, and stabilization
- Discitis + vertebral osteomyelitis typically affect anterior column > anterior approach
  - If posterior involvement > posterior approach
  - If anterior column defect s/p I&D > may need strut graft or interbody implant
  - If instability > may need arthrodesis

**What location are epidural abscesses most common and what is the most common organism?**
- Thoracic > lumbar, staph a
- Presents w/ neck/back pain
  - Progressive neuro deficits can occur from direct compression or ischemic injury from infection
  - Few patients have back pain + fever + neuro deficits

**Spine 16: 5:50**

**What is the most sensitive and specific imaging to detect an epidural abscess?**
- MRI with gadolinium

**What patients w/ an epidural abscess may undergo non-op treatment?**
- Pts w/ no neurological deficits/ poor surgical candidates, rarely indicated though
- Abx is the treatment

**What are indications for operative treatment in patients w/ an epidural abscess?**

- Neurological deficits or lack of improvement w/ non-op
- Emergent decompression w/ or w/o fusion, approach determined by location of infection

**What is the most common cause of a granulomatous (atypical/ non pyogenic) infection of the spine?**

- Mycobacterium tuberculosis
- Fungal infections may also be culprit (i.e.- aspergillus, histoplasma, etc)

**Is there any difference in the location of the nidus w/ pyogenic and granulomatous infections of the spine?**

- Yes, granulomatous infections nidus is located in peridiskal metaphysis of vertebral body, discs usually spared
- May present w/ focal kyphosis & vertebral column destruction due to indolence
- Large paraspinal abscesses are more common

**What are some additional items (in addition to those mentioned above) to note regarding the workup of these granulomatous infections?**

- Chest xray in patients where tuberculosis is being considered
- Sputum specimens may be positive in pts w/ respiratory disease (acid fast bacilli)
- May need biopsy of spinal lesion

**What is the non-op treatment for a granulomatous infection?**

- If TB- TB drugs- RIPE- rifampin, isoniazid, pyrazinamide, ethambutol, etc
- 6-12 months of tx, follow cultures for sensitivities

**What are the indications for surgical treatment for a granulomatous infection of the spine?**

- No improvement w/ non-op tx, abscesses, substantial deformity

**Don't forget to study anatomy!**

## Podcast Episodes for a Deeper Dive

- Episode 5 w/ Dr. Cyriac: Cervical Myelopathy
  https://naileditortho.com/cervicalmyelopathy/
- Episode 90 w/ Dr. Hullinger- Lumbar disc herniations
  https://naileditortho.com/ldh/
  Video: https://youtu.be/6bDaK8DUToQ

## Specific Articles Mentioned in the Podcast

Johansen, T. O., Sundseth, J., Fredriksli, O. A., Andresen, H., Zwart, J. A., Kolstad, F., ... & Nygaard, Ø. P. (2021). Effect of arthroplasty vs fusion for patients with cervical radiculopathy: a randomized clinical trial. JAMA Network Open, 4(8), e2119606-e2119606.

Nunley, P. D., Cavanaugh, D. A., Kerr, E. J., Utter, P. A., Campbell, P. G., Frank, K. A., ... & Stone, M. B. (2018). Heterotopic ossification after cervical total disc replacement at 7 years—prevalence, progression, clinical implications, and risk factors. International journal of spine surgery, 12(3), 352-361.

Schroeder GD, Kepler CK, Kurd MF, Paul JT, Rubenstein RN, Harrop JS, Brodke DS, Chapman JR, Vaccaro AR. A Systematic Review of the Treatment of Geriatric Type II Odontoid Fractures. Neurosurgery. 2015 Oct;77 Suppl 4:S6-14. doi: 10.1227/NEU.0000000000000942. Review. PubMed PMID: 26378359.

Koivikko, M. P., Kiuru, M. J., Koskinen, S. K., Myllynen, P., Santavirta, S., & Kivisaari, L. (2004). Factors associated with nonunion in conservatively-treated type-II fractures of the odontoid process. The Journal of Bone and Joint Surgery. British volume, 86(8), 1146-1151.

Lurie, J. D., Tosteson, T. D., Tosteson, A. N., Zhao, W., Morgan, T. S., Abdu, W. A., ... & Weinstein, J. N. (2014). Surgical versus non-operative treatment for lumbar disc herniation: eight-year results for the Spine Patient Outcomes Research Trial (SPORT). Spine, 39(1), 3.

# NOTES

# NOTES

# NOTES

# FOOT & ANKLE CHAPTER 5

## Anatomy

**What ligaments make up the lateral ligamentous complex and when are the strained?**

- ATFL, CFL, PTFL
- ATFL- plantarflexion, inversion, IR
- CFL- dorsiflexion + inversion

**Where does the deltoid ligament attach?**

- Superficial deltoid- anterior to navicular, inferior to sustentaculum, posterior to talar body
- Deep deltoid- from medial mal to talar body

**What is the ankle syndesmosis?**

- Tibia-fibula articulation, the incisura fibularis + fibular facet
- Composed of ligaments: AITFL, PITFL, interosseous ligament

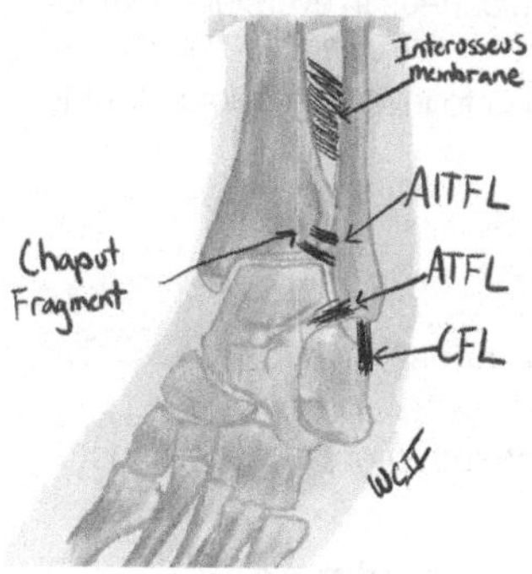


**Figure 5.1: Mortise view of the ankle with the ligaments shown. AITFL- Anteriorinferior tibio-fibular ligament, ATFL- Anterior talofibular ligament, CFL- calcaneofibular ligament**

**How many facets of the subtalar joint are there?**

- 3, the posterior facet being the largest

**What is the chopart joint?**

- The transverse tarsal joint
- Talonavicular joint + calcaneocuboid joint (works w/ subtalar joint during movement)

FA 1: 8:15

**What structure supports the talonavicular joint?**

- Spring ligament complex (superior medial + inferior calcaneonavicular ligament)

**Where does the lisfranc ligament originate and attach to?**

- Plantar aspect of medial cuneiform to base of second metatarsal
  - Composed of three layers- interosseous layer strongest, followed by plantar layer (dorsal weakest)

**What makes up the anterior compartment of the leg?**

- TA, EDL, EHL, peroneus tertius, anterior tibial artery + deep peroneal nerve

**What makes up the superficial posterior compartment of the leg?**

- Gastrocnemius- soleus complex + plantaris

- Achilles tendon fibers- rotate 90deg medially- so superficial achilles tendon fibers insert laterally on calcaneus

**What makes up the deep posterior compartment of the leg?**
- PT, FDL, posterior tibial artery, tibial nerve, FHL

**What is the knot of Henry?**
- The area where the FDL tendon crosses over FHL in midfoot

**What makes up the lateral compartment of the leg?**
- Peroneus longus, peroneus brevis, peroneal artery and the superficial peroneal nerve

**What is the main motion of the ankle (tibiotalar) joint?**
- Plantar/dorsiflexion

FA 1: 17:20

**What are the main motions of the subtalar and Chopart (transverse tarsal) joint?**
- Subtalar- inversion/ eversion of foot
- Chopart- to lock and unlock midfoot

**What are the biomechanics of the foot during heel strike and push off during gait?**
- During heel strike- joints are parallel- calcaneus in eversion- midfoot is flexible for shock absorption
- During push off- subtalar joint transitions to inversion- foot inflexible- rigid lever arm for push off

## ANKLE ARTHRITIS

**What is the most common cause of ankle arthritis?**
- Post-traumatic
- Other causes: peripheral neuropathy, inflammatory disease, talus osteonecrosis

FA 2: 2:30

**What are some of the H&P findings with ankle arthritis?**
- Pain w/ weight bearing, decreased ankle ROM

**What are some non surgical treatment options for ankle arthritis?**
- NSAIDS, PT, steroids, activity modification, shoe modifications (rocker soles), bracing (AFO)

**What are some surgical treatment options for patients w/ ankle arthritis?**
- Ankle debridement w/ anterior tibial/dorsal talar exostectomy (if impingement)
  - Pain with forced dorsiflexion
- Distraction arthroplasty (ex fix used to off load joint, controversial)
- Supramalleolar osteotomy- (mild disease w/ tibiotalar malalignment)
  - Varus deformity- medial opening wedge tibial osteotomy
  - Valgus deformity- medial closing wedge osteotomy + oblique lengthening fibula osteotomy

- Arthrodesis- end stage arthritis (arthroscopic v mini-arthrotomy v open techniques w/wo internal or external fixation)
- Total ankle arthroplasty
  - Similar outcomes to arthrodesis w/ higher revision surgery rate
  - Increased gait speed and stride length

**What is the preferred ankle position for arthrodesis?**

- Neutral or minimal dorsiflexion, hindfoot valgus 5 deg, equal rotation to other limb

FA 2: 9:20

**What can occur in patients who undergo an ankle arthrodesis with the ankle in plantarflexion?**

- Knee recurvatum to allow heel to touch ground during strike

**What is a common H&P finding seen in patients with subtalar arthritis?**

- Pain on uneven surfaces, limited hindfoot inversion/eversion

**What are some types of shoes that can be used in the treatment of subtalar arthritis (non-op)?**

- Shoes w/ rocker soles (stiff shoes)
- University of california biomechanics laboratory arthrosis
- Ankle- foot orthoses - AFO

**What are some surgical options to treat patients w/ hindfoot arthritis?**

- Arthroscopy w/ debridement
- Lateral calcaneal exostectomy (in pts w/ subfibular impingement)
- Arthrodesis
  - Selective (i.e. subtalar or talonavicular) for isolated disease
  - Triple arthrodesis- stage III PTT
  - Distraction subtalar bone block arthrodesis- (pts w/ anterior ankle impingement and loss of heel height)

**Fusion of which hindfoot joint leads to the most limited motion?**

- Talonavicular fusion can limit hindfoot motion up to 90% (subtalar 50%, CC25%)

**What structural changes are seen in the foot in patients with TMT arthritis or an untreated lisfranc fracture dislocation?**

- Loss of longitudinal arch and forefoot abduction

## First Ray + Toes

**What is hallux valgus (bunion)?**

- Lateral deviation of proximal phalanx
  - Assoc w/ medial deviation of 1st metatarsal
- MC in women, related w/ narrow toe box shoes

Ep 77 w/ Dr. Tsai

**What is the pathoanatomy behind hallux valgus?**

- Valgus deviation > metatarsal varus > Sesamoid complex lateral to 1st metatarsal head > medial MTP capsule attenuation > adductor accentuates deformity > EHL pulls toe lateral > pronation occurs > transfer metatarsalgia

**What are some types of adult hallux valgus?**

- Congruent, incongruent, degenerative
- Goal is congruent 1st MTP joint at end of procedure

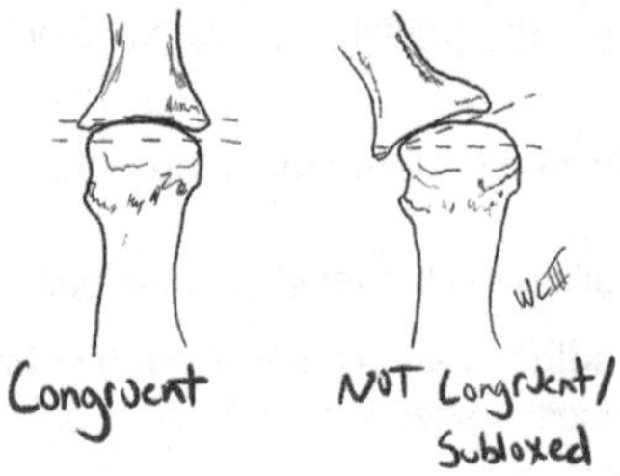


**Figure 5.2: Imaging shows the appearance of a congruent (left) and an incongruent 1st MTP joint (right).**

FA 3: 4:50

**What are some things you should note on (weight bearing) xray when evaluating for hallux valgus?**

- Intermetatarsal angle (IMA)- normal <=9
- Hallux valgus angle- normal <=15
- DMAA- normal <=15
- Proximal phalangeal articular angle - normal <=10

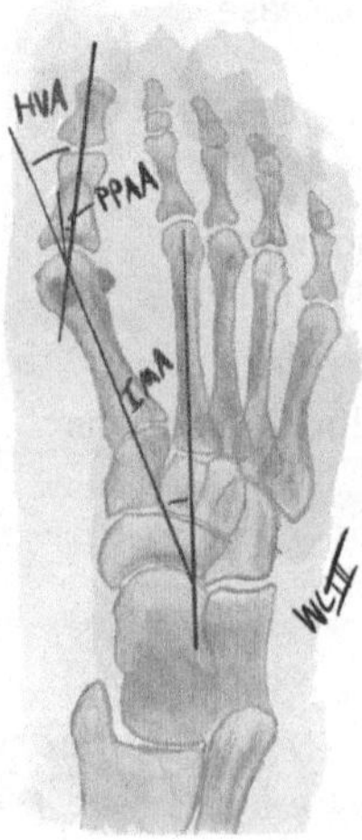


**Figure 5.3: AP of the foot showing common angles used to evaluate patients with hallux valgus. PPAA- proximal phalangeal articular angle, HVA- hallux valgus angle, IMA- intermetatarsal angle**

**What are some non-op treatment options for hallux valgus?**

- Wide toe box shoes, metatarsal pads, orthoses

**What (in general) are some operative tx options for patients with differing degrees of hallux valgus?**

- Distal soft tissue release- release lateral structures + medial eminence resection
  - Rarely done in isolation, IMA <11, HVA <35
  - Don't excise the fibular sesamoid- excision increases risk for hallux varus
- Akin osteotomy- closing wedge osteotomy of prox phalanx
  - Rarely done in isolation, high PPAA
- Distal metatarsal osteotomy- osteotomy + lateral metatarsal head translation
  - IMA<13, HVA<30
  - If DMMA >15- consider biplanar closing wedge osteotomy also

- Proximal metatarsal osteotomy- osteotomy metatarsal shaft moved laterally
    - IMA>13, HVA>25
- Lapidus fusion- fusion of metatarsal + cuneiform
    - Use w/ 1st ray hypermobility
- MTP fusion
    - Useful if arthritis or inflammatory conditions present

**What is the most common cause of hallux varus?**

- Hallux valgus repair

FA 3: 16:10

**What is hallux rigidus?**

- Arthritis of the 1st MTP joint
- Can be due to trauma / metabolic / inflammatory arthritis

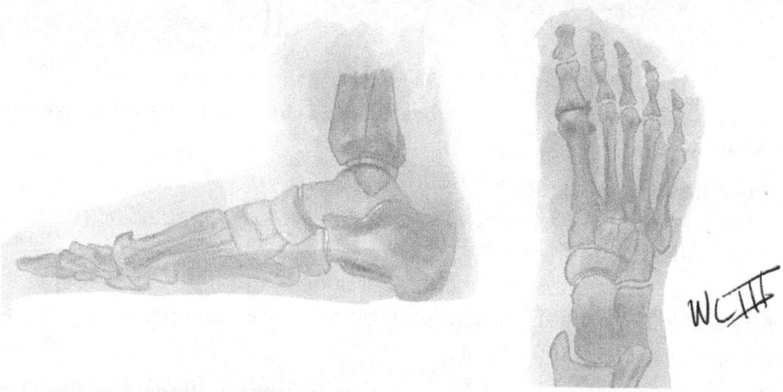

**Figure 5.4: Lateral and AP of the foot showing the appearance of hallux rigidus of the 1st MTP. The dorsal osteophyte and loss of joint space can be seen on the lateral and AP images.**

**What is something important to note on PE when examining a patient w/ hallux rigidus?**

- 1st MTP ROM
    - Pain at extremes only- limited arthritis, dorsal osteophytes may be present
    - Pain at midrange of motion- more advanced arthritis

**What are some non-op treatment options for hallux rigidus?**

- NSAIDs, steroids, activity modifications, orthoses
    - Carbon fiber footplate w/ Morton extension- limits hallux dorsiflexion
    - Extra depth shoes- (more room)

**What are some treatment options with hallux rigidus?**

- Mild - joint debridement w/ dorsal cheilectomy (shaving metatarsal head)
    - +/- microfracture of metatarsal head cartilage

FA 3: 12:20

- +/- dorsiflexion osteotomy (Moberg) of proximal phalanx (may improve ROM)
- Moderate/ severe
  - Interposition arthroplasty (w/ EHB, or some other substitute)
  - Synthetic implant - polyvinyl alcohol implant (can be used w/ dorsal cheilectomy)
  - 1st MTP arthrodesis (w/ screw + dorsal plate)
    - Fuse at ~15 dorsiflexion, 15 valgus

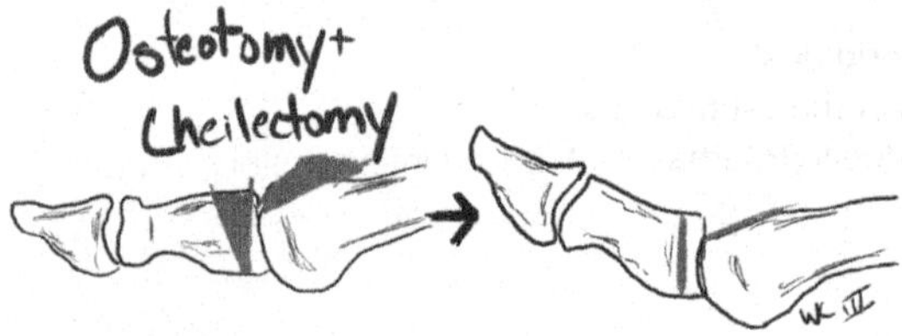


**Figure 5.5: Image showing hallux rigidus treated with a cheilectomy and a Moberg dorsiflexion osteotomy.**

**What is a freiberg infraction?**
- Infraction of the metatarsal head that commonly affects 2nd metatarsal head > eventual collapse
  - Central resorption of subchondral bone > arthritis
- Pts have pain w/ WB, can be seen on xrays, MRI can make diagnosis & osteonecrosis can be seen

**What are some non-op and operative treatment options for freiberg infarction?**
- Early stages- offloading, casting, carbon fiber insert w/ morton's extension
- Recalcitrant cases- surgery
  - Dorsal closing wedge osteotomy w/ resection of diseased bone (also shortens metatarsal)
    - Rotates plantar cartilage dorsally
  - Partial head resection, isolated debridement, osteochondral autograft

FA 4: 4:40

**What do most lesser toe deformities have in common?**
- Hyperextension of the MTP joint
- Deformities start w/ plantar plate dysfunction
- Extrinsic muscles overpower intrinsics (EDL> MTP extension, FDL> PIP/DIP flexion)

**What is the pathophysiology behind crossover toe?**
- MTP joint instability, plantar plate disruption, LCL attenuation > migration of 2nd digit towards hallux > tertiary claw toe

**What is a mallet toe deformity and treatment options?**
- Hyperflexion of DIP
- Non-op - shoes w/ high toe boxes
- Operative
  - If flexible deformity- FDL tendon release
  - Fixed deformity- middle phalanx condyle resection + extensor tendon repair + pinning

**What is a hammer toe deformity and its treatment options?**
- Flexion of PIP and extension of DIP + MTP
- Non-op- shoes w/ high toe box / silicone toe sleeve
- Operative
  - Flexible-resection of proximal phalanx condyles +/- FDL tenotomy + pinning
    - Or Girdlestone taylor FDL to extensor tendon transfer
  - Fixed: PIP arthrodesis/arthroplasty +/- EDL lengthening

**What is a claw toe deformity and its treatment options?**

FA 4: 11:20

- MTP extension w/ hyperflexion of PIP and DIP (due to plantar plate deficiency)
- Causes callus and pain due to IP joints rubbing against shoe
- Non-op: shoe wear modification, padding
- Operative
  - Flexible: EDL lengthening, EDB tenotomy, +/- FDL to EDL tendon transfer (girdlestone-taylor)
  - Fixed: Extensor tendon lengthening, distal oblique metatarsal shortening osteotomy (Weil osteotomy), +/- FDL to EDL tendon transfer (girdlestone-taylor)
    - Plantar plate repair
    - Proximal phalanx condyle resection, FDL tenotomy + pinning

**What is a bunionette and the different types?**
- Prominence of the 5th metatarsal head
- Type 1- enlarged 5th metatarsal head
- Type 2- 5th metatarsal diaphyseal bowing
- Type 3- increase 4th/5th IMA (>8 is pathologic)

**What are some treatment options for bunionettes?**
- Non-op: shoe wear modification, wide toe box shoe + padding
- Operative
  - Type 1- Lateral condylectomy
  - Type 1/2 - Lateral condylectomy
  - Distal chevron osteotomy- IMA<12 / bowing is present
- Type 2/3- Oblique diaphyseal rotational osteotomy- IMA>12 or large bow

**In what tendon do the sesamoids sit?**
- FHB, they help transmit WB pressure
- Also increases pulley function of FHB and helps protect FHL

**What are some PE and radiograph findings that may be seen in patients w/ sesamoid pathology**

- TTP, pain w/ 1st ray ROM
- Axial view- eval articulation w/ metatarsal head
- MRI- shows osteonecrosis, stress fractures/fracture

FA 4: 18:24

**What are some operative treatment options for sesamoid nonunions?**

- Partial/ complete excision
- Bone grafting also, may not work as well

**What are some potential complications w/ sesamoid excision?**

- Hallux varus/valgus (w/ lateral / medial excision) + cock up deformity

**What is turf toe and the common mechanism of injury?**

- Injury to periarticular structures around MTP of hallux
  - Plantar plate avulsion from proximal phalanx + sesamoid migration proximally
- MTP hyperextension (forced dorsiflexion) + axial load on a plantar-flexed foot

**What are some things you can see on xray in a patient w/ a turf toe injury?**

- Proximal migration of sesamoids on AP foot

**What are some non-op treatment options for turf toe?**

- Rest, NSADs, toe taping, stiff insoles
- Walker boot- if severe injury
- Partial tears- no sports for 2 weeks

**What are some indications for operative tx for turf toe?**

- Rarely indicated
- Complete plantar plate tear w/ proximal retraction
- Dorsal dislocations that are irreducible due to volar plate interposition
- Sesamoid fx w/ diastasis, sesamoid retraction, loose fragments in joint
- Tx: plantar plate repair +/- partial/complete sesamoid excision

**What is the most commonly injured ligament seen with ankle sprains?**

- ATFL

**What is the typical treatment for an acute ankle sprain?**

- RICE
- Functional rehab + proprioceptive training

**What should you be worried about in patients with continued feelings of their ankle giving away after sustaining an ankle sprain 3 months ago and going through rehab?**

- Ankle instability, can also help diagnose w/ stress radiographs

FA 5: 3:40

**What are some operative treatment options for patients with ankle instability?**

- Anatomic repair- modified brostrom lateral ligament recon - reinforced w/ inferior retinaculum

    - 90-95% successful
- Non anatomic repair- peroneal tendon sacrificing procedure - i.e.: Chrisman Snook
- If cavovarus foot- may need dwyer closing wedge calcaneal osteotomy

**What is the most common complication seen with ankle arthroscopy?**

- Neurological damage
- Intermediate branch of superficial peroneal nerve injury during anterolateral portal placement
- A synovial cutaneous fistula is also common w/ ankle arthroscopy

**What structures are at risk w/ posterolateral portal placement for ankle arthroscopy?**

- Sural nerve + lesser saphenous vein
- Portal is between achilles tendon + lateral malleolus

**What are some symptoms, radiographic findings, and some treatment options for patients with anterior ankle impingement?**

- Pain w/ ankle ROM, limited dorsiflexion
- Xrays- distal tibia osteophytes +/- dorsal talus spurring
- Tx options: arthroscopic removal of bone spurs + synovectomy (if significant arthritis is present, not really effective)

**What are some symptoms, radiographic findings, and treatment options for patients with posterior ankle impingement?**

- Hindfoot pain w/ plantarflexion
- Xrays/CT shows- os trigonum, posterior talar process fx, hypertrophy of posterior talar process
- Arthroscopic resection (stay lateral to FHL)

**What is the typical location of a talus osteochondritis dissecans lesion due to trauma?**

- Anterolateral
- Posteromedial lesions typically avascular lesions, can also be congenital

**What are some operative treatment options for talus osteochondritis dissecans lesions diagnosed on MRI?**

- Debridement w/ microfracture
- Retrograde drilling
- Larger lesions- OATS, de-novo, mosaicplasty
- Better results w/o malleolar osteotomy

**What are some intraoperative tests that can be used to assess syndesmosis stability?**

- Cotton test, external rotation stress test
- Arthroscopic evaluation helpful also

**FA 5: 17:40**

# Ankle + Foot Trauma

**What population has the highest incidence of ankle fractures?**
- Elderly women

**What happens to the fibula as the ankle is dorsiflexed?**
- Externally rotates through the syndesmosis (AITFL, PITFL, IOM)
- Accommodates the talus (wider anteriorly than posterior)

FA 6: 3:10

**What ligaments prevent talus inversion and anterior translation in regards to the fibula?**
- Anterior + posterior talofibular ligaments
- Calcaneofibular ligaments

**What ligament is the primary restraint to talar anterolateral displacement?**
- Deep deltoid ligament

**What are the components of the medial malleolus and what attaches to each?**
- Anterior malleolus +intercollicular groove + posterior malleolus
  - Anterior mal is larger + more distal
  - Anterior mal- superficial deltoid ligament
  - Posterior mal + intercollicular groove- deep deltoid

Ep 1 w/ Dr. Stewart

**What are the classifications for ankle fractures?**
- AO / Weber / Lauge Hansen

**What is the weber classification?**
- Based on fibula fracture location in relation to the syndesmosis
- Weber A- infrasyndesmotic (more likely stable)
- Weber B- transyndesmotic (most common)
- Weber C- supra syndesmotic (usually unstable)

**What is the Lauge- Hansen classification?**
- Fractures according to injury mechanism
- Based on: foot position + deforming forces applied
  - Foot in supination- lateral injury first
  - Foot in pronation- medial injury first
- Supination adduction (vertical medial mal fx)
- Supination external rotation (most common, short oblique weber B fx)
- Pronation abduction (transverse / comminuted Weber C +/- lateral articular impaction)
- Pronation external rotation (oblique Weber C)

**What are the Ottawa ankle rules?**
- Rules to see if ankle xrays are needed
- Get xrays if the patient has pain over the malleoli plus 1 of these;
  - Inability to bear weight

- 55+ y/o
- TTP over the posterior edge/ tip of a malleoli

**What xrays should be obtained and what are you looking for when evaluating for ankle injuries?**

- AP/Mortise/Lateral
- Stress views (gravity / ER stress)- isolated fibula fx
- Joint congruity
- Medial clear space <5mm
- Tib fib clear space <6mm
- Talocrural angle (assess fibula length)

**FA 6: 13:40**

**What intra-op xrays can be taken to evaluate for syndesmotic disruption?**

- Contralateral ankle xrays
- External rotation stress test- external rotation of talus + measure tibfib clear space (normally <6mm) + overlap (normally >6mm)
- Modified cotton test- lateral translation of fibula

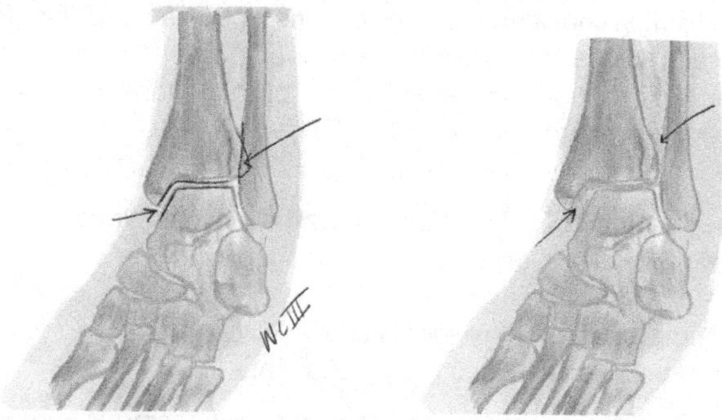


**Figure(s) 5.6 & 5.7: Mortise view of the ankle shows the even medial clear space (left) as well as normal tib-fib overlap. The image on the right is concerning for a syndesmosis injury given the medial clear space widening and decrease in tib-fib overlap.**

**What is avulsion of the AITFL called?**

- Avulsion from tibia- Chaput (fx) tubercle
- Avulsion from fibula – Wagstaffe (fx) tubercle

**What is a common laceration pattern with an open bimal ankle fracture?**

- Transverse laceration

**What ankle fractures can be treated non-op?**

- Stable fractures: i.e isolated lateral mal, medial mal avulsion fx, low transverse medal mal fx
  - Cast 4-6 weeks
- Select unstable fractures in poor surgical candidates (has disadvantages)

**FA 7: 2:20**

**What ankle fractures are considered unstable?**

- Any fractures w/ lateral talus displacement
- Bimalleolar + bimalleolar equivalent

- Trimalleolar + trimal equivalent
- Tibio talar incongruity present

**What are some fixation considerations and options for lateral mal fx?**

- Fix fibula first- can help restore length + ankle stability
- 1/3 semitubular plates, or distal fibula locking plates, 90/90 mini frag plates
- Bridge comminuted ankle fx
- Posterior antiglide plate for some oblique/spiral fx
  - Can lag through plate
  - Can also place distal screws from PA
  - Associated w/ peroneus brevis tendon injury

**What are some fixation considerations for medial mal fracture?**

- Partially threaded screws for transverse/oblique fractures
- Buttress plating for vertical shear fractures
- Hook plates, many fixation options

**What are some fixation considerations and options for posterior malleolus fx?**

- Involvement >25% articular surface is associated w/ instability
- Percutaneous fixation vs open approach (posterolateral approach)
  - Sometimes postero medial approach needed
  - Anterior > posterior screws (perc)

**What are some fixation considerations for syndesmosis injuries?**

- One or two 3.5 or 4.5 Cortical screw fixation (can be 3 or 4 cortices of fixation)
  - Screws may break with weight bearing
- Suture buttons- inc price, dec re-operation rate

**Is there a common agreement on when to remove syndesmotic screws?**

- No, controversial
- Screws should be left for at least 3 months

**Is syndesmosis malreduction very rare when treating syndesmosis injuries?**

- No, iatrogenic malreduction rates can be as high as 50%
- Fibula unstable w/ A-P translation

(Sernandez, 2021)

**Does early weight bearing and mobilization s/p ORIF ankle fracture worsen functional outcomes?**

- No, associated w/ improved functional outcomes

**What are some potential complications when fixing ankle fractures?**

(Ramsey, 1976)

- Nonunion – tx w/ ORIF + bone grafting
- Malunion – Can be iatrogenic, large posterior mal + wide medial clear space predictive of poor outcome
- Wound healing issues
- Infection
- Post-traumatic arthritis

**What are some factors that lead to increased risk of complications in patients with ankle fractures?**

- Diabetics + smokers (some may need supplemental fixation)

**What is a tibia plafond fracture?**

Ep 6 w/ Dr. Dixon

- Intra- articular distal tibia fracture
- Seen w/ axial loads such as MVC, fall from height
- Axial or torsional loads, or both seen

**Is there a commonly used classification system for tibia plafond fractures?**

- No, more attention paid to fracture characteristics
- OTA/AO classification exists, + historic Rüedi-Allgöwer classification

**What is the Rüedi-Allgöwer classification for tibia plafond fractures?**

(Rüedi, 1969)

- Depends on comminution + displacement of articular surface
- Type I- nondisplaced
- Type II- displaced w/ minimal comminution
- Type III- high comminution + displacement

**What should be paid attention to when examining patients w/ pilon fractures?**

- Soft tissue damage (i.e.- presence of open wounds, fracture blisters, abrasions, areas of skin blanching)

**What is a classification system that can be used to grade the soft tissue injuries that can be seen in plafond fractures?**

- Tscherne
- Grade 0- closed fracture w/o soft tissue injury
- Grade 1- abrasions/ contusions of skin + subcutaneous tissue
- Grade 2: deep abrasion w/ muscle involvement
- Grade 3- extensive soft tissue damage + severe muscle injury

**Should you get a CT of the ankle when assessing tibial plafond fractures?**

- Yes, if planning for external fixation, typically it is ordered post ex-fix

**Is non-op treatment the typical standard of care when treating pilon fractures?**

- No, non- op treatment is rare. May be indicated in non-displaced fractures/ non-ambulatory patients
- Surgery is indicated for displaced fx (>2mm)

**What are some treatment options for plafond fractures?**

- Soft tissue management is key
- Staged management w/ temporary ex fix followed by ORIF (w/ damaged soft tissues)
  - Plating of fibula at ex fix time often performed to restore length + alignment
  - Return to OR 10-20 days later
- Ex fix + articular fragment stabilization w/ lag screws
- ORIF w/ plate & screws (If soft tissues allow)

### What are some approaches used for ORIF pilon fractures?

(Zelle, 2019)

- Anterolateral
  - Incision lateral to anterior compartment tendons- SPN at risk
  - Helpful in valgus
- Anteromedial
  - Next to anterior tib tendon, avoid soft tissue stripping
- Posterolateral
  - Between achilles and peroneal tendons- sural n at risk

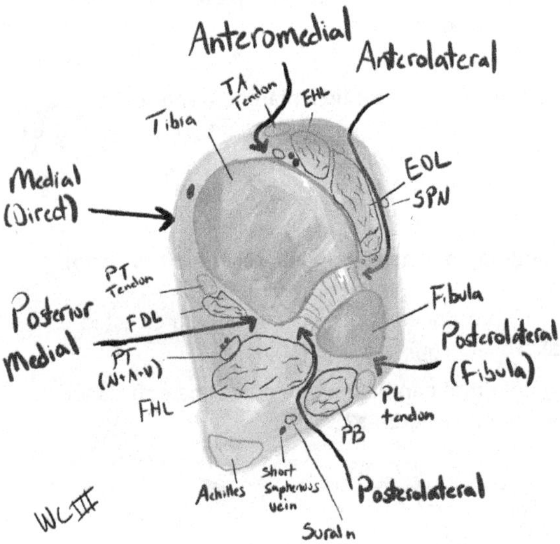


**Figure 5.8: Axial cut of the ankle showing different approaches used for the ankle. EHL- extensor hallucis longus, TA- tibialis anterior, EDL- extensor digitorum longus, PL- peroneus longus, PB- peroneus brevis, FHL- flexor hallucis longus, FDL- flexor digitorum longus**

### What are some techniques used to decrease wound problems w/ ORIF of pilon fractures?

- Temporary ex-fix placement
- Minimal incisions + soft tissue stripping
- >5cm (some say 7cm) distance between ankle incisionss
- Precontoured anteromedial + anterolateral plates helpful for percutaneous insertion

### What are some complications seen in treating plafond fractures?

- Plafond injuries can significantly affect patient quality of life
  - Worse than AIDS, MI, diabetes, or being a polytrauma patient
- Post-traumatic arthritis- may be seen in 75% of patients
- Malunion
- Nonunion – open fx, comminuted fx, devascularized fx increase nonunion rate
- Infection + wound problems- may require multiple procedures, devastating, staged treatment

### Can patient socioeconomic factors be predictive of outcomes in pilon fractures?

- Yes

### What is the injury known as the “snowboarder’s ankle” and the treatment?

- Lateral process fracture of the talus

- Nondisplaced- cast + NWB
- Displaced – ORIF (large fragments) v excision

**What artery provides most of the blood supply to the talar body?**
- Artery of tarsal canal (branch off post tib artery)
- Deltoid artery- supplies medial portion of body of talus

**What arteries provide most of the blood supply to the talar head + neck?**
- Artery of tarsal sinus (branch from AT + peroneal a)

**What is the classification for talar neck fractures?**
- Hawkins classification
  - I- Nondisplaced
  - II- Subtalar dislocation
  - III- Subtalar + tibiotalar dislocation
  - IV- Subtalar + tibiotalar + talonavicular dislocation

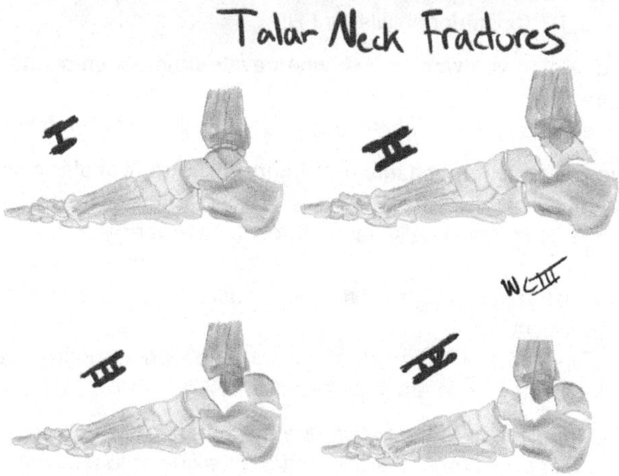


**Figure 5.9: Lateral images of the foot showing the Hawkins classification of talar neck fractures.**

**What is a risk that is increased with increasing Hawkins severity?**
- Talar osteonecrosis, due to disruption of blood supply

**Which fractures of the talar neck can be treated nonoperatively?**
- Hawkins I – cast + NWB
  - Hawkins I fractures can also be treated with percutaneous P-A screws

**What talar neck fractures should typically be treated operatively ?**
- Hawkins II- IV
  - Tx w/ ORIF, crossed A-P screws +/- plate

**What is Hawkins sign and what does it indicate?**
- Subchondral lucency on xray seen around 6-8 weeks
  - Indicates vascularity > a good sign

**What is the most common complication for patients with talar neck fx?**

- Subtalar arthritis

**What are some other complications seen with talar neck fx?**

- Tibiotalar arthritis
- Varus malunion (tx: medial opening wedge neck osteotomy)
- Osteonecrosis (tx: TTC fusion)

**What direction of subtalar dislocation is most common?**

- Medial
- Lateral- likely to be open
- Tx: closed reduction + casting

**What structures may be interposed in patients with irreducible medial and lateral subtalar dislocations?**

- Medial- EDB interposed, head of talus
- Lateral- PT (posterior tibialis) or FHL

**What is a question you want to ask when evaluating patients with calcaneal fractures?**

- Are they a smoker or diabetic (increased complications in this cohort)

Ep 29 w/ Dr. Dowd

**What is the typical mechanism of injury for intra-articular calcaneus fractures?**

- Axial load > oblique shearing force to calc > primary fx line and 2 primary fragments
  - Superomedial fragment- includes sustentaculum "constant fragment"
  - Superolateral fragment- articular component through posterior facet - posterolateral tuberosity

**What is the importance of the secondary fracture line?**

- Lets you know whether there is joint depression or tongue type fx
- Joint depression- superolateral fragment + posterior facet separated from posterolateral tuberosity or not
- Tongue type- superolateral fragment + posterior facet are attached to tuberosity posteriorly

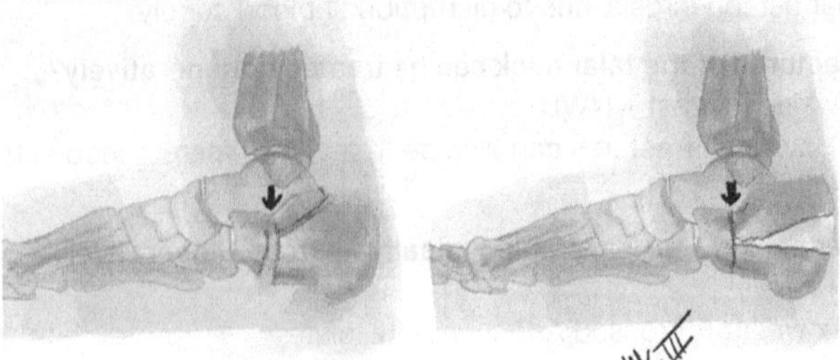

**Figure(s)5.10 & 5.11: Lateral view of the foot showing a joint depression type (left) and tongue type (right) calcaneus fractures.**

**What structure lies underneath the "constant" (sustentacular) fragment?**
- FHL tendon- can be damaged w/ screw placement too medial

**What are some xray markers that can be used when evaluating patients w/ calcaneus fractures?**
- Bohler's angle- 20-40- (flattened angle = posterior facet collapse)
- Angle of Gissane- 130-145- (inc angle = posterior facet collapse)

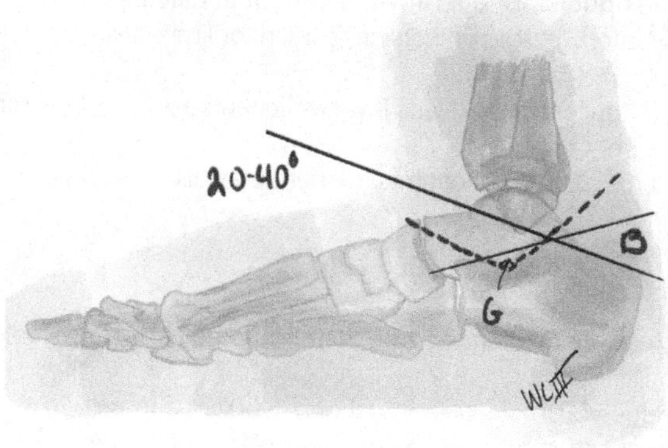


**Figure 5.12: A lateral of the ankle showing Bohler's angle (B) and the angle of Gissane (G).**

**What is the Sanders classification system for calcaneus fractures based on?**
- Coronal oblique cut of the CT scan of the widest portion of the subtalar joint + the # of fracture fragments of the posterior facet

**What is the Sanders classification system?**
- Type I- non displaced
- Type II- posterior facet in two fragments
- Type III- posterior facet in three fragments
- Type IV- comminuted w/ 3+ fragments
- All are subdivided in regard to fracture line orientation (a>c)
- Degrees of shortening, widening, lateral wall impingement (peroneal tendons) also important

**What type of calcaneus fractures should undergo immediate operative reduction and fixation?**
- Displaced tongue- type fx (extra articular)
- High risk of posterior skin necrosis

**What calcaneus fractures are indicated for non-op treatment?**
- Sanders I
- NWB 6-8 weeks
- Type II and III- controversial- can be treated non op

**What calcaneus fractures are indicated for operative treatment?**

- Sanders II, III- ORIF
  - Typically delayed ~2 weeks for skin to wrinkle
- Sanders IV- ORIF + primary subtalar arthrodesis

**What are the goals w/ ORIF calcaneus fx?**

- Articular reduction + correct heel varus + shortening

**What are some options for operative treatment of calcaneus fx?**

- ORIF w/ lateral extensile incision (sural n) or limited sinus tarsi approach
  - Less complications w/ less invasive techniques (ex: sinus tarsi)
  - Equivalent outcomes
  - Injectable calcium phosphate cement may allow early weight bearing
- Percutaneous fixation
- +/- arthroscopy

(Tufescu, 2001)

**What factors are associated with poor outcomes after ORIF calcaneus fx?**

- Inc age >50, male, obesity, laborer, workers comp
- Complication rates are as high as 40%

**In calcaneus malunions, what can be noted in regards to the position of the calcaneus?**

- Loss of height, varus malalignment, subfibular impingement / peroneal tendon irritation, talar declination

**What is a treatment option for a calcaneus malunion that is shortened and in varus alignment?**

- Distraction bone block subtalar arthrodesis

**What areas do avulsion fractures of the navicular occur?**

- Dorsal lip- deltoid ligament during eversion
- Medial avulsion- tibialis posterior
- Plantar- spring ligament
- Tx: immobilization +/- delayed excision of painful fragments
- Tx: ORIF large fragments involving 25% articular surface

**What is the treatment of a symptomatic nonunion of the navicular tuberosity?**

- Excision + tibialis posterior tendon reattachment
- Nonunion of navicular bone- ORIF w/ w/o bone grafting (ex: stress fx > non-union)

**What is the treatment for a non-displaced navicular stress fx?**

- NWB
- ORIF w/ displacement, CT may be needed before returning to play

**Where does the lisfranc ligament insert and attach to?**

- 2nd metatarsal to the medial cuneiform

**Which tarsal bone is known as the "keystone" of the foot?**

- 2nd metatarsal (base)
- The lateral TMT joints – 10 degrees motion
- Medial TMT joints- limited motion

**What is the typical mechanism for TMT fracture dislocations?**

- Direct – a dorsal force/ crush injury
- Indirect- axial load + twisting on plantarflexed foot

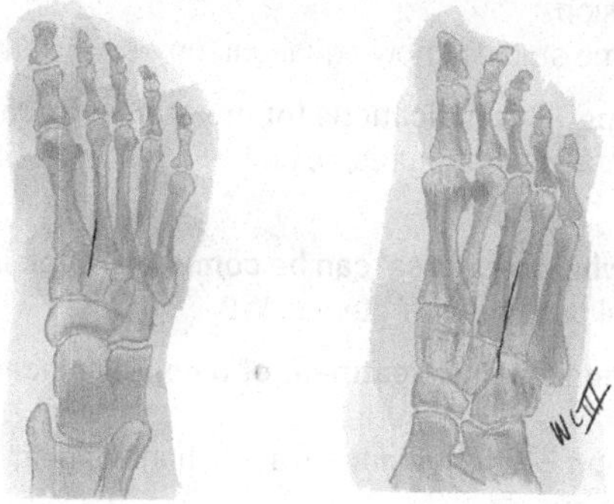

**Where should the medial aspect of the 2nd and 4th metatarsal line up on xrays?**

- Medial aspect of middle cuneiform and medial aspect of cuboid bone respectively

**Figure 5.13: AP and oblique imaging of the foot showing a line of the normal bony alignment**

**What is the fleck sign?**

- Avulsion of Lisfranc ligament from base of 2nd metatarsal- seen on xray

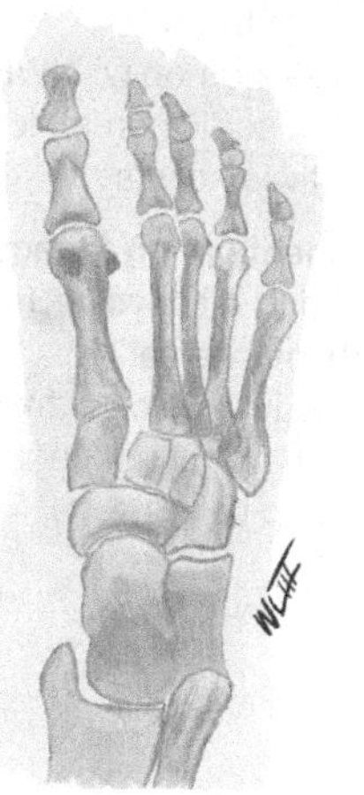

**What xrays should you get if you have a suspicion for a Lisfranc injury but the normal xrays seem inconclusive?**

Ep 16 w/ Dr. Hogan

- Weight bearing films
- Abduction stress films may also help

**Figure 5.14: AP of the foot showing a lisfranc injury and widening between the medial and middle cuneiform.**

**What is the treatment for a displaced Lisfranc / midfoot fracture dislocation?**

- ORIF
- 1 or 2 dorsal incisions
- Fix w/ threaded screws or bridging plates
- 4th/5th metatarsals (lateral column)- K-wires typically used

**What are the indications to treat a Lisfranc injury with non-op treatment?**
- No displacement- w/ WB + stress films
- NWB x 6 weeks

**What is a treatment option if intercuneiform instability is noted?**
- Reduce + fix w/ screw

(Ly, 2006)

**What is a treatment option for patients with a purely ligamentous Lisfranc injury?**
- Primary fusion
- Though some studies show equal outcomes to fixation

**What are some operative indications for metatarsal fractures?**
- Multiple metatarsal fractures, open fractures, 1st + 5th metatarsal fractures

**Stress fractures to what metatarsal can be commonly seen in dancers?**
- 2nd metatarsal base, tx w/ protected WB

Ep 72 w/ Dr. Behrens

**What is the mechanism and treatment of a non-displaced, Zone 1 5th metatarsal fx?**
- Foot inversion – avulsion due to lateral band of plantar fascia +/- peroneus brevis
- Typically WBAT in boot if not displaced

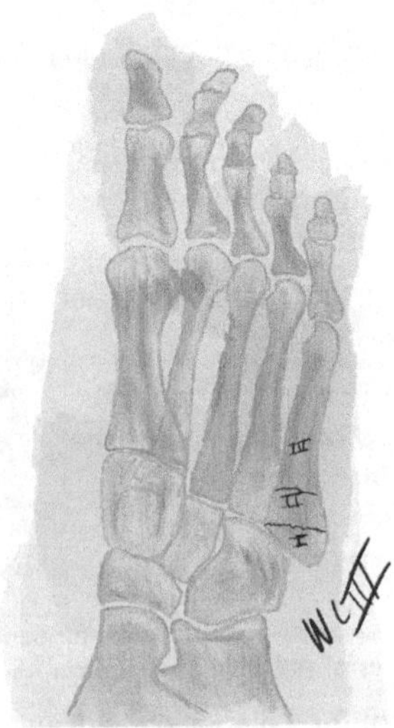

**Figure 5.15: Oblique of the foot showing the different zones of 5th metatarsal fractures. Zone II fractures are known as Jones fractures.**

**What is the treatment for Zone II (Jones) fractures in an athletic patient?**
- Percutaneous screw fixation
- Assoc w/ faster healing and return to sport
- Can treat non-op w/ NWB in cast in some non-athlete/ non-active patients

**What is a treatment option for acute Zone 3 (proximal diaphysis) fractures of the 5th metatarsal?**
- Intramedullary screw fixation, high risk of nonunion w/ non-op tx
- Can be due to repetitive microtrauma w/ athletes

## Other foot conditions

**What is Morton's neuroma?**

- A compressive neuropathy of interdigital nerve
- Pain with squeezing medial/lateral metatarsals while pushing tissue dorsal
- Sometimes along with a click (created by bursal tissue)

**What is the treatment for Morton's neuroma?**

- Shoe wear modification + metatarsal pads
- Cortisone injections may help, but may not
- Operative- removal
  - Dorsal approach w/ incision of transverse metatarsal ligament
  - Plantar approach- common for recurrent neuroma

**What is a tarsal coalition?**

- Seen when there is a failure of differentiation + no joint formation
- An abnormal connection between two bones

**What are some things you may note on radiographs with tarsal coalitions?**

- C sign- talocalcaneal coalition
- Drunken waiter sign - subtalar coalition
- Internal oblique xray- calcaneonavicular coalition

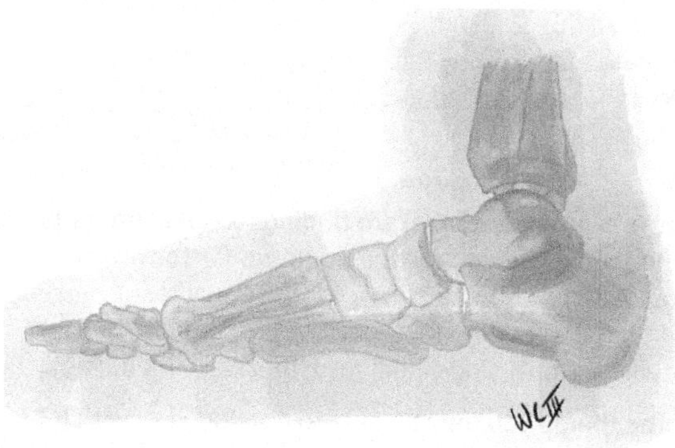

**Figure 5.16: Lateral of the foot showing a "C sign", which is commonly seen in patients with talocalcaneal coalition.**

**What is a treatment option of a symptomatic tarsal coalition?**

- In teenager- resection + bone wax or fat interposition
- If degenerative subtalar joint w/ 50%+ joint involvement > arthrodesis

**What are the contents of the tarsal tunnel?**

- PT, FDL, posterior tibial artery+ vein + nerve, tibial nerve, FHL
- Contents posterior + inferior to medial mal

**What are some causes of tarsal tunnel syndrome?**

- Soft tissue trauma, space occupying lesions- ganglion cysts, lipomas, varicose veins, ankle + foot malalignment

**What are some symptoms and PE maneuvers for patients with tarsal tunnel syndrome?**

- Burning at bottom of foot w/ paresthesias + tinel sign, discomfort w/ eversion and dorsiflexion
- NCV tests may be useful in diagnosis (sensory NCV may be abnormal)

**What are some non-op and operative treatment options for tarsal tunnel syndrome?**

- Immobilization, NSAIDs, COX-2 inhibitors, steroid injections,SSRI's, orthotics w/ medial posting
- Operative- tarsal tunnel decompression 5cm proximal to flexor retinaculum, distally- to deep fascia of abductor hallucis (1st branch of lateral plantar nerve released)
- Space occupying mass excision- best results

Ep 65 w/ Dr, Geaney

**Where does the posterior tibial tendon insert, and what does activation of this tendon allow?**

- Three limbs
  - Anterior limb attachment- navicular tuberosity + 1st cuneiform
  - Middle limb- 2nd and 3rd cuneiform, cuboid + 2nd-5th metatarsals
  - Posterior limb- sustentaculum tali
- Locking of transverse tarsal joints- creating level arm for toe-off phase of gait

**What are some of the physical exam findings seen in patients with posterior tibial tendon insufficiency (adult acquired flatfoot)?**

- Hindfoot valgus, abducted forefoot (too many toes), medial longitudinal arch collapse, +/- achilles/gastroc contracture
- Inability to perform single heel raise (flexibilt v rigid deformity)

**What are some things you may be able to note on xray with PTT?**

- Increase in Meary's angle, uncovering of the talus (due to forefoot abduction), valgus heel alignment

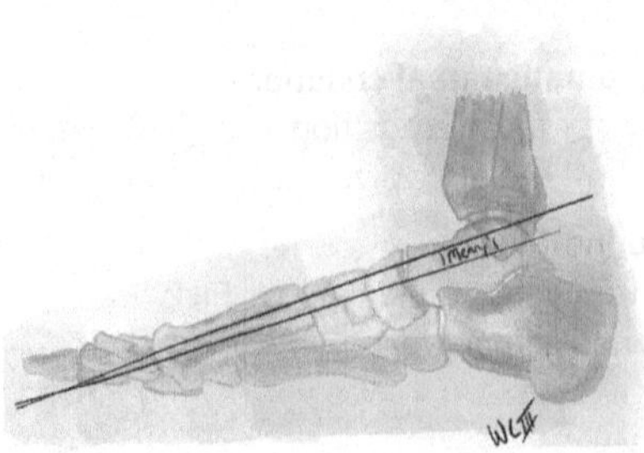

**Figure 5.17: Lateral of the foot showing Meary's angle. A line down the axis of the talus and a line down the axis of the 1st metatarsal are drawn. This can be increased in patients w/ PTT.**

**What are some non-op treatment options for PTT?**

- Medial heel wedge, UCBL, lace up ankle brace, AFO, physical therapy (good for stage 1 & 2)

**What are some operative treatment options w/ PTT?**

- Stage 1- tenosynovectomy
- Stage 2- flexible- FDL to navicular transfer
    - + medial slide calcaneal osteotomy if hindfoot valgus and <40% TN uncovering
    - + lateral column lengthening if >40% TN uncovering (evans opening wedge calcaneal osteotomy)
    - Once corrections are done > evaluate for forefoot varus/supination (can be done w/ a flat plate)
    - Stable medial column > cotton osteotomy (opening dorsal wedge of cuneiform)
    - Unstable medial column on xray > medial column fusion
- Stage III- hindfoot arthrodesis (triple)
- Stage IV- flexible- + deltoid recon w/ stage 2 + 3 surgeries
    - Rigid- ankle arthrodesis or TTC / Ankle arthroplasty + previous stage procedures

**What is the silfverskӧld test?**

- Assess for gastroc/ contracture
- w/ knee flexion- improved ankle dorsiflexion = gastroc tightness - could benefit from gastroc recession
    - If not improved w/ knee flexion- achilles is tight- negative test- could benefit from achilles lengthening
- Evaluate in patients w/ PTT

**What are some possible causes of pain in the achilles tendon area?**

Ep 45
w/ Dr.
Bitterman

- Insertional achilles tendinopathy (may have bony prominence/ haglund deformity)
- Noninsertional achilles tendinopathy
    - Paratendonitis (no tendon involvement) vs tendinosis
- Achilles tendon tear
- Retrocalcaneal bursitis

**What are some treatment options for patients with achilles tendon disorders?**

- Insertional achilles tendinopathy-
    - Debridement, haglund deformity removal +/- FHL transfer if 50% tendon involved
- Noninsertional achilles tendinopathy-
    - Eccentric strengthening, brisement (injection)
    - Debridement + tubularization. If >50 involvement- FHL transfer
- Retrocalcaneal bursitis-
    - Haglund resection + bursectomy

**What should you be concerned about in a 40M w/ ankle pain who heard a pop and had ankle pain while playing basketball? He thought someone kicked his heel.**

- Achilles tendon rupture

**What are some treatment options for acute achilles tendon ruptures?**

- Non-op treatment
  - Accelerated functional rehab w/ early ROM- faster return to mobility than casting
- Op treatment
- Open v percutaneous procedures- similar outcomes
  - Perc- may have higher sural n injury rates w/ less wound complications

**Is there any difference between non-op v op treatment for midsubstance achilles tendon ruptures?**

- Controversial, studies show similar outcomes with both
- Traditional studies show inc re-rupture rates and dec strength w/ non-op treatment
- Inc complications noted w/ surgical group

**What are some treatment options for insertional achilles tendon ruptures (avulsion from calc)?**

- Surgical repair typically recommended

**In what patients are peroneal tendon tears more common?**

- Cavovarus foot deformities
- Anatomic variants that may contribute- low lying peroneus brevis muscle, peroneus quartus muscle

**What is some imaging that may be useful to diagnose peroneal tendon tears and some operative treatment options?**

- MRI- longitudinal tears in tendon- sometime false positive results
- Ultrasound useful- can do dynamic exam of tendons
- Tenosynovectomy + repair- <50% tendon involvement
- Tenodesis/ tendon transfer- >50% tendon involved
- +/- lateral slide calcaneal osteotomy if hindfoot varus present

**What may be seen in patients with peroneal tendon instability and some treatment options?**

- Superior peroneal retinaculum rupture
- Operative: tendon debridement + SPR repair +/- fibular groove deepening (shallow peroneal groove may be present)

**What is a cavovarus foot and causes?**

- High medial arch
- Forefoot equinus + pronation (1st MT plantarflexion)
- Unilateral- poliomyelitis, spinal cord tethering
- Bilateral (progressive)- Charcot Marie Tooth, Hereditary Sensory Motor Neuropathies

- Inherited disorders of peripheral + CNS

**What is Charcot-Marie Tooth disease?**

- An inherited motor + sensory neuropathy (primarily in PNS)
- MC form of inheritance- AD, peripheral myelin protein duplication (PMP on chromosome 17)
- Intrinsic muscle weakness + high arch

**What is the pathophysiology behind the foot deformity (cavovarus) in Charcot-Marie Tooth disease?**

- Weak intrinsic muscles + contracture > high arch
- Tib ant affected > peroneus longus pull > first ray plantarflexion
- Hindfoot varus to balance forefoot varus

**What is the Coleman block test, and what is it used for?**

- Used to see if hindfoot is flexible and if a plantarflexed 1st ray is the reason for deformity
- Block placed under lateral side of foot + hind foot
  - If hindfoot corrects to neutral > cavovarus due to plantarflexed ray
  - If no correction > may be due to both plantarflexed ray + varus hindfoot

**What are some non-op treatment options for cavovarus foot?**

- PT- strengthen weak muscles
- Orthotics- ankle foot orthosis (AFO), lateral heel wedge orthotic

**What are some operative treatment options for cavovarus foot?**

- Soft tissue procedures-
  - PL to PB transfer- inc eversion strength + removes deforming force
  - Plantar fascia release- allows metatarsal dorsiflexion
  - PT transfer to foot dorsum - decreases varus
  - Girdlestone-taylor procedure (flexor>extensor transfer)
- If forefoot driven- 1st metatarsal dorsiflexion osteotomy
- Hindfoot driven- lateral displacement osteotomy or lateral closing wedge osteotomy of calc
- +/- lateral ankle ligament recon if ankle instability present
- Severe deformity- triple arthrodesis

**What should you be concerned about in a female patient w/ heel pain w/ worse when walking in the AM with tenderness to the plantar medial tuberosity of the calcaneus? Treatment?**

- Plantar fasciitis
- Tx:
  - Non-op stretching PF + achilles, heel inserts, injections (multiple can lead to rupture)
  - Op: open v endoscopic limited plantar fascia release +/- distal tarsal tunnel decompression (if compression neuropathy present)

**Entrapment of what nerve can be seen with plantar fasciitis that should be released at the same time as plantar fascia release?**

- 1st branch of the lateral plantar nerve (Baxter's nerve)
- Compressed between deep fascia of abductor hallucis + quadratus plantae

**What should you be worried about in a female patient who has recently started training for a marathon with heel pain and tenderness with medial/ lateral heel compression?**

- Calcaneal stress fracture
- MRI can be useful in diagnosing, a fx line/ area of increased density may be seen on xray

## Podcast Episodes for a Deeper Dive

- Episode 1 w/ Dr. Stewart: Intro to Ankle Fractures https://naileditortho.com/introtoankle/
- Episode 6 w/ Dr. Dixon: Intro to Pilon Fractures https://naileditortho.com/pilonintro/
- Episode 16 w/ Dr. Hogan: Lisfranc Injuries https://naileditortho.com/lisfrancintro/
- Episode 29 w/ Dr. Dowd: Calcaneus Fractures https://naileditortho.com/calcaneusfx/
- Episode 45 w/ Dr. Bitterman: Achilles Tendon Injuries https://naileditortho.com/achilles/
  Video: https://www.youtube.com/watch?v=I06pYvPfUMI&t=69s
- Episode 65 w/ Dr, Geaney: Flatfoot/ Posterior Tibial Tendon Deficiency https://naileditortho.com/flatfoot/
  Video: https://www.youtube.com/watch?v=f7pW1_8v1mo&t=21s
- Episode 72 w/ Dr. Behrens: 5th Metatarsal Fractures https://naileditortho.com/fifthmetatarsal/
  Video: https://www.youtube.com/watch?v=qGCrtEx5ng0&t=2s
- Episode 77 w/ Dr. Tsai: Hallux Valgus https://naileditortho.com/halluxvalgus/
  Video: https://www.youtube.com/watch?v=MoGvZ01PYl0
- Episode 93 w/ Dr. Mangone- Lateral ankle instability https://naileditortho.com/ankleinstability/
  Video: https://youtu.be/W1YVOAmo62c

## Specific Articles Mentioned in the Podcast

Sernandez, H., Riehl, J., & Fogel, J. (2021). Do early weight-bearing and range of motion affect outcomes in operatively treated ankle fractures: a systematic review and meta-analysis. Journal of Orthopaedic Trauma, 35(8), 408-413.

Ramsey, P. L., & HAMIITON, W. I. L. L. I. A. M. (1976). Changes in tibiotalar area of contact caused by lateral talar shift. JBJS, 58(3), 356-357.

Rüedi, T. P., & Allgöwer, M. (1969). Fractures of the lower end of the tibia into the ankle-joint. Injury, 1(2), 92-99.

Zelle, B. A., Dang, K. H., & Ornell, S. S. (2019). High-energy tibial pilon fractures: an instructional review. International orthopaedics, 43(8), 1939-1950.

Tufescu, T. V., & Buckley, R. (2001). Age, gender, work capability, and worker's compensation in patients with displaced intraarticular calcaneal fractures. Journal of orthopaedic trauma, 15(4), 275-279.

Ly, T. V., & Coetzee, J. C. (2006). Treatment of primarily ligamentous Lisfranc joint injuries: primary arthrodesis compared with open reduction and internal fixation: a prospective, randomized study. JBJS, 88(3), 514-520.

# NOTES

# NOTES

# NOTES

# ADULT RECONSTRUCTION KNEE

# CHAPTER 6

## Knee Arthritis

**What are some risk factors for knee osteoarthritis?**
- Inc age, female, obesity

**What are some history and physical exam findings seen in patients with knee OA?**
- Pain w/ activity, decreased ROM, joint line tenderness, varus/valgus deformity

**What is an increased adductor moment?**
- Increased knee adduction with ambulation > leads to inc medial compartment loads > medial compartment OA

**In addition to normal standing AP and lateral films, what are some other films that may be useful in evaluating knee arthritis?**
- Flexion PA view, sunrise

**If you are considering unicompartmental arthroplasty, in addition to xrays, what other imaging can be obtained to evaluate for compartmental disease?**
- Triple phase bone scan
- MRI used also

(Baker, 2020)

**What are some treatment options for knee arthritis?**
- Knee strengthening + aerobic conditioning and neuromuscular training
- NSAIDs (oral & topical)
- Weight loss if BMI >25
- Other options: acetaminophen/opioids, steroid injections, bracing, HA, growth factors, acupuncture, lateral wedge insoles

**What are some strong recommendations for the non-operative treatment of knee osteoarthritis from the AAOS (3rd edition)?**
- Strong for: Topical NSAIDs, supervised exercise/ aerobic program, self management programs, patient education programs, oral NSAIDs, oral Acetaminophen, tramadol
- Strong against: Lateral wedge insole use

(AAOS, 2021)

**What are some operative treatment options for knee arthritis?**
- Arthroscopy (early OA)
- Osteotomy (early OA)

AR 1: 16:50

- Unicompartmental knee arthroplasty
- Total knee arthroplasty

**What are some arthroscopic treatment options for patients with arthritis?**
- Subchondral drilling or microfracture - fibrocartilage produced
- Debridement of loose cartilage, synovium, meniscus
- Chondroplasty - damaged cartilage removed

**In what patients with arthritis would an osteotomy be an option for?**
- Young active patient with isolated compartment disease

**What are some osteotomy options for young patients with medial compartment OA and a varus alignment?**
- Valgus producing high tibial osteotomy- lateral closing wedge, medial opening wedge, and dome osteotomy
- Problem is typically proximal tibia varus

**What are some potential risks associated with a high tibial lateral closing wedge osteotomy?**
- Peroneal nerve injury, proximal tib/fib joint injury, loss of posterior slope, patella baja

**What are some potential risks associated with medial opening wedge osteotomy?**
- Collapse, nonunion, loss of correction, patella baja

**AR 2: 7:31**

**What are some contraindications to perform a valgus producing tibial osteotomy?**
- Flexion contracture >15°
- Ligamentous instability (ex varus thrust)
- Inflammatory arthritis
- ROM <90°
- Multicompartmental disease + medial compartment bone loss

**What are some osteotomy options in patients with lateral compartment OA?**
- Varus producing femoral osteotomy
- Lateral femoral condyle typically hypoplastic > distal femur valgus

**What are some contraindications to performing a varus producing femoral osteotomy?**
- Medial OA
- Flexion contracture >15°
- ROM <90°

**(Chalmers, 2019)**

**Is the survivorship of TKA affected by prior osteotomy?**
- No, excellent long term results

**Which of the varus producing femoral osteotomies has the least displacement?**
- Dome osteotomy

**What are some advantages to unicompartmental knee arthroplasty?**

- Fewer early complications
- Quicker recovery compared w/ TKA + osteotomy
- Smaller incision
- Higher INITIAL success rate (long term not comparable to TKA)

**What are some contraindications for unicompartmental arthroplasty?**

- Tricompartmental arthritis
- ACL deficiency
- Inflammatory arthritis
- Flexion contracture >15°

**What are some technique principles that should be maintained when performing unicompartmental arthroplasty?**

- Avoid overcorrection > can lead to failure and arthritis progression
    - Undercorrect mechanical axis by 2-3°
- Avoid extensive releases
- Caution w/ prox tibia guide pin placement > could lead to tibia stress fx

**What is the treatment of a tibia stress fracture after unicompartmental arthroplasty?**

- Stable implant- rest + WB restriction
- Unstable implant- revision + ORIF, possible conversion to stemmed TKA if compromised bone

**What are some reasons for failure after unicompartmental arthroplasty?**

- Opposite compartment degeneration - can be seen w/ overcorrection
- Component loosening, poly wear/failure, osteolysis- can be seen w/ undercorrection
- Patella impingement
- Implant subsidence - can be seen in cases w/ poor metaphyseal bone

# TKA Implants 101

**What are the different types of unconstrained implants and important things to note about them?**

AR 3: 3:15

- PCL- retaining TKA (Cruciate retaining CR)
    - Retained PCL allows for some femoral rollback (poly should be flat or slightly dished to allow rollback)
    - Tight PCL may cause poly wear >> osteolysis
    - Excess PCL recession > can lead to late failure due to flexion instability
- PCL- substituting TKA (Posterior stabilizing PS)
    - Use in patients w/ inflammatory arthritis / PCL insufficiency/ patellectomy
    - Polyethylene post + cam- allows rollback during flexion
        - Can have impingement between post + femoral box
- Ultracongruent or anterior stabilized

- Congruent liner w/ anterior lip buildup- allows no box
- Medial pivot TKA
  - High congruency on medial aspect, less laterally
  - Use of CR style femur
- High flexion TKA
  - Implant designed to allow greater arc of motion... though studies don't necessarily show clinical post-op ROM increase

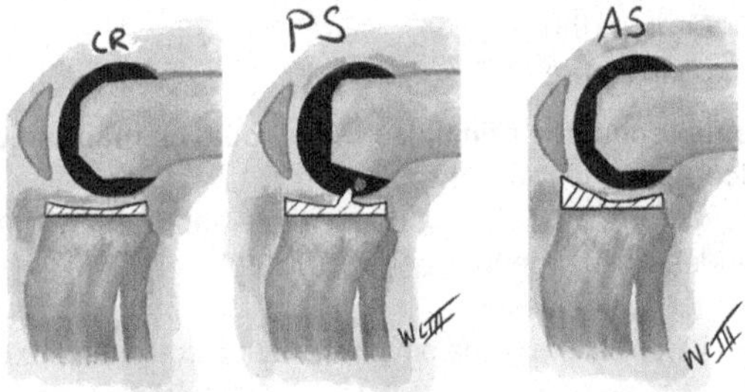


**Figure(s) 6.1 & 6.2: Lateral of the knee showing cruciate retaining (CR), posterior stabilizing (PS), and anterior stabilized (AS) knee implants. Note the cam and post in the PS knee engaging during flexion and the raised polyethylene anteriorly in the AS implant.**

### Are there any differences in outcomes between PS and CR TKA designs?

- No

### What is a constrained, non hinged implant?

- Implant w/ large poly post (+/- metal reinforcing pin) and deeper femoral box- increase varus/valgus constraint and rotation
- May be useful for revision TKA and primary TKA w/ severe pre-op deformity
- Inc stress across component + bone- may lead to aseptic loosening + poly wear

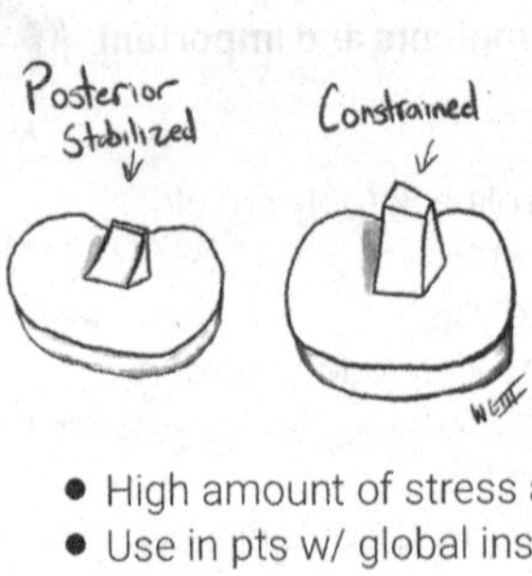


**Figure 6.3: Image showing the polyethylene post on a standard and constrained polyethylene. The constrained implant is larger and increases varus/valgus constraint.**

### What is a rotating hinge implant?

- Implants are hinged together, complete varus/valgus and Anterior/posterior constraint
- High amount of stress at bone cement interface
- Use in pts w/ global instability / extension instability

### What is a mobile vs fixed bearing TKA?

- Mobile bearing- motion between tibial polyethylene and the top of the tibia base plate

- Articular portion of implant is congruent through ROM
- Fixed bearing- no motion
  - Reduces stress on poly

**What are some long term problems seen with standard poly (in comparison w/ cross linked)?**

- Oxidation, osteolysis, putting, delamination
- Increasing use of cross-linked poly to help minimize these

**When can polyethylene spinout be seen?**

- Mobile bearing rotating platform
- Also seen w/ loose flexion gaps

## TKA Principles

**What are some indications for total knee arthroplasty (TKA)?**

- Knee arthritis causing pain
- No active infection

**What are some strong recommendations/evidence for surgical management of OA of the knee?**

(AAOS, 2021)

AR 4: 1:50

- Pre-op: Obese patients have less improvement w/ TKA
- Periop: use of peri-articular local anesthetic decreases opioid use, peripheral nerve block dec post-op pain, tourniquet use increases post-op pain, TXA decreases blood loss and need for post-op transfusions
- No diff in outcomes between: PS + CR knees, all polyethylene or modular tibial components, pain w/ patella resurfacing or not, cemented v cementless tibial component, surgical navigation or not, patient specific instrumentation or not, not using a drain, CPM use does not improve outcomes
- Post-op: rehab day of surgery reduces hospital stay length

**What are some nerve blocks commonly used in knee arthroplasty?**

- Femoral nerve block (motor + sensory)- posterior knee not covered, KI used post-op due to patient unable to extend knee + knee buckling
- Adductor canal nerve block (sensory only)- posterior knee not covered, earlier post-op ambulation compared w/ femoral n block
- IPACK- infiltration between popliteal artery and capsule of the knee- blocks sensory fibers of sciatic n

**What are some different approaches used for knee exposure for arthroplasty?**

- Medial parapatellar, lateral parapatellar, mid-vastus, subvastus
- No differences in outcomes
- Malalignment noted more often w/ quad-sparing approaches (ex: mid vastus)

**What are some different extensile approaches to the knee for arthroplasty?**

- Quadriceps snip, quadriceps turndown, banana peel, tibial tubercle osteotomy

**What is the anatomic axis of the femur?**

- A line split down the medullary canal of the femur

**What is the mechanical axis of the femur?**

- Line from center of femoral head to center of distal femur

Ep 42 w/ Dr. Harb

**What do these lines (anatomic and mechanical femur axis) have to do with TKA?**

- Anatomic axis- starting point of intramedullary guide
- Mechanical axis- distal femur cut is perpendicular to this axis

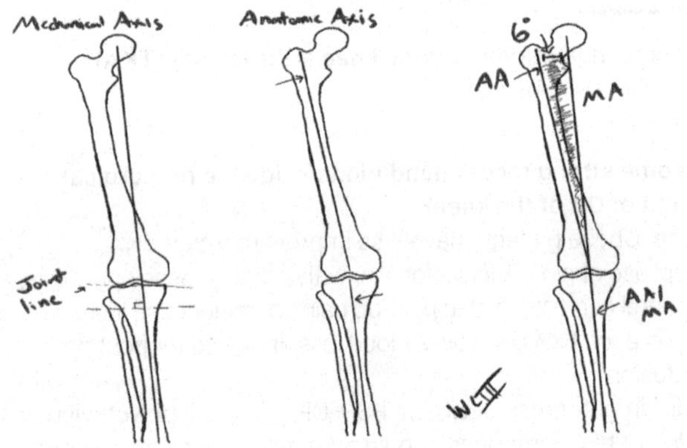


**Figure 6.4: On the left is the mechanical axis (MA) of the limb, from the femoral head to the middle of the ankle. The joint line is in slight varus. The middle image is the anatomic axis (AA) of the femur and tibia. The mechanical and anatomic axis of the tibia are the same. There is a 6° (5-7°) difference between the anatomic and mechanical axis of the femur.**

**What are the limb alignment principles seen in total knee arthroplasty?**

- Mechanical alignment- restoring neutral mechanical alignment of the limb through cuts
- Contrarian/Kinematic- recreates the coronal and sagittal alignment of the joint line (same limb alignment pre op as post op)
    - Ex: varus knee pre-op > varus knee post-op
- Anatomic alignment- tibia is cut in more varus and femur cut in more valgus
- Mechanical alignment currently is widely accepted

**What alignment is the test mostly going to ask about?**

- MECHANICAL ALIGNMENT, so we will talk about that from now on

**What is the alignment aiming to be restored with mechanical alignment and why?**

- Line from the center of the hip to the center of the ankle, also goes through the center of the knee

- Leads to even load distribution along prosthesis

**What is the angle between the anatomic and mechanical axis of the femur typically?**

- 5-7°
- This is also the valgus cut angle for distal femur cut
    - An intramedullary guide is placed in femur (anatomical axis), and the jig is set to the valgus cut angle (5-7°), thus the cut will be perpendicular to mechanical axis

**Do taller or shorter people typically have more valgus in the femur?**

- Shorter people, taller people have less valgus
- So, the valgus cut is less in taller people and more in shorter

**What is the anatomic axis of the tibia?**

- A line split down the medullary canal of the tibia

**What is the mechanical axis of the tibia?**

- Line from center of proximal tibia to center of ankle

**What is the angle between the mechanical and anatomic axis of the tibia?**

- Usually zero... lines are the same
- If not, the angle created between the two, is the tibial cut angle

**Why is the mechanical axis of the tibia important in regards to the cut?**

- The proximal tibia cut is perpendicular to mechanical axis > even load distribution across prosthesis

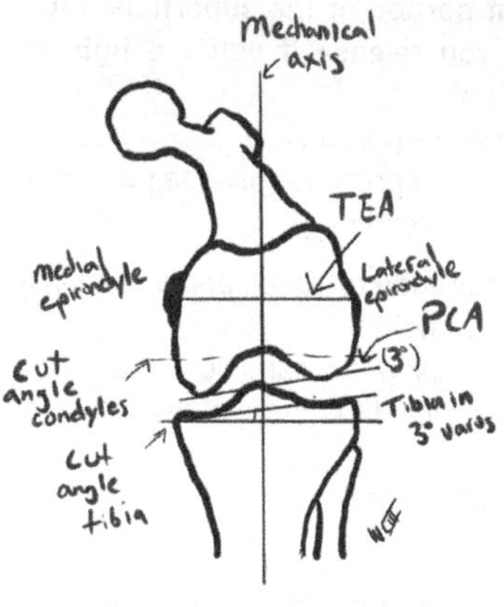


**Figure 6.5: The knee viewed in flexion. On the femur, the posterior condylar axis (PCA) is 3° from the transepicondylar axis (TEA). In order to make a box cut, the cutting guide is adjusted to account for this. On the tibia, the joint line is around 3° of varus. The cut is made perpendicular to the mechanical axis of the tibia.**

**What are some situations where the mechanical and anatomic axis of the tibia may not be the same and you have to make an angled proximal tibia cut?**

- Old tibia shaft fracture treated non-op with an angular deformity

**How much bone should be resected when making femur and tibia cuts?**

- Enough for femoral + tibial components to be placed along w/ thinnest poly
- Typically around 8-10mm off the highest part of femur/tibia
- Ideally bone + cartilage cut = implant thickness
    - Helps w/ maintaining joint line + ligament tension

**What is the maximum alteration of the joint line that is typically allowed?**

- 8mm

**Is it important for the medial/lateral ligaments to be balanced for proper knee function?**

- Yes, hence ligamentous balancing
- Also important that the sagittal plane be balanced as well (extension/flexion)
- Goal: equal tension in flexion/extension in medial + lateral compartments

**How is this typically done in the coronal (varus/valgus) plane?**

- Release the tight side and fill the loose side
- Ex: varus- release MCL

AR 5: 18:20

**What are the releases performed sequentially in a varus knee?**

- Osteophyte > Subperiosteal release of deep MCL > posterior medial corner(capsule + semimembranosus)> superficial MCL / epicondylar osteotomy
  - Component can also be downsided and moved laterally

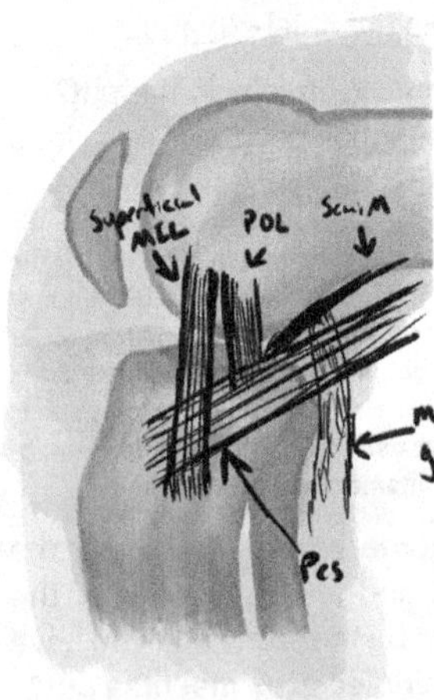


**Figure 6.6: A lateral view of the knee showing the medial sided structures that can be released during ligamentous balancing. The pes tendons, superficial MCL, posterior oblique ligament (POL), and semimembranosus tendon are shown. (capsule not shown)**

**What portion of the superficial MCL can you release if you are tight in flexion?**

- Anterior portion
- Release posterior oblique portion if tight in extension

**What are the releases performed in a valgus knee?**

- Osteophytes > capsule > popliteus/ IT band > LCL (last)
- Key is to release the tight structures
- Important not to perform aggressive medial release
- Peroneal nerve palsy can occur

**If you are tight laterally in extension, what structure can you release?**

- IT band (because its tight in extension)
- Popliteus is tight in flexion

**Where does the popliteus sit in relation to the LCL?**

- 18 mm distal and anterior to the LCL

**What are some surgical options for patients with a large coronal deformity in the distal ¼ femur or proximal ¼ tibia?**
- Osteotomy w/ TKA w/ diaphyseal press fit spline stem
- McPherson's ¼ rule

**What are some releases that can be performed in patients w/ a flexion contracture (unable to fully extend)?**

**AR 7: 2:25**

- After posterior condyle cut > removal of posterior osteophytes > strip capsule/ posterior capsule release > gastrocnemius release
- Can also make a larger distal femur cut if you do not think soft tissue releases are going to solve the problem

**What is a general rule of thumb when balancing flexion/extension gap?**
- Find out where you are loose/ tight
- Assess whether it is a symmetric problem or asymmetric

**What are bone cuts that you can make that will affect both the flexion and extension gap (tight)?**
- Cutting proximal tibia (do this if tight in both)

**What are some things you can do if you are loose in both extension and flexion?**
- Add something to the tibia
  - Increase polyethylene insert thickness
  - Add metallic augments

**What are some things you can do if you are loose only in flexion?**
- Increase femoral component size
- Translate femoral component posterior + add augment (metal or cement)
- Add posterior femur
- Or add tibia (inc poly / metallic augments) then re-address the tightness in extension

**What are some things you can do if you are only loose in extension?**
- Add distal femur
- Distalize femoral component + add augment
- OR, add tibia (inc poly/ metallic augment) then re-address the tight flexion gap

**What are some things you can do to increase your extension gap only and leave the flexion gap alone (i.e.- tight in extension only)?**
- Remove more distal femur (~2mm bone ~ 10° correction)
- Release posterior capsule

**What are some things you can do to increase your flexion gap only while leaving the extension gap alone?**
- Increase posterior slope on tibia
- Remove posterior femur
- Partial PCL release off intercondylar notch if doing PCL retaining TKA
- Downsize femoral component

**When cementing components, what are some technical aspects that are important?**

- Use of vacuum suction/centrifuge (minimize voids)
- Cancellous bone cleaned w/ lavage
- Cement penetration of 3mm
- No superiority between cement on implant vs cement on bone prior to implantation

**Why is it important to not notch the femur when making femoral cuts?**

- This lessens the load to failure > can lead to fracture

AR 8: 3:15

**What are some technical errors while performing TKA that can lead to patellar maltracking?**

- Internal rotation of the femoral and tibial components (this is bad)
  - Femoral implants should be 3° ER to transepicondylar axis
  - If anything put femoral component more lateral > keeps patella centered
  - Tibia component should line up w/ middle ⅓ of tibia
- Placement of patellar component lateral (this is bad)

**What surgical technique can be performed if some patella maltracking is observed after component placement?**

- Lateral retinaculum release
  - May injure the superior lateral genicular artery > possible osteonecrosis of patella
  - Can also make lateral arthrotomy which can lead to pooling of blood in subcutaneous tissues and wound issues post op, so look for lateral arthrotomy and close superficially so that synovial space is a closed environment

## TKA Complications

**What are some complications seen after TKA?**

- Instability, stiffness, HO formation, infection, fracture, wound issues, vascular injury

**What patients are at highest risk for peroneal nerve palsy s/p TKA?**

- Patients w/ valgus and contracted knees

**What is the first step if you suspect peroneal nerve palsy in the post-op area after TKA?**

- Take off compressive wrap + flex knee
- +/- AFO use

**What is a treatment option for a patient s/p TKA 6-8 weeks ago w/ ROM 0-75°?**

- Manipulation under anesthesia
- Can be performed up to 12 weeks post op- later manipulation can lead to fracture

**What is the most common type of metal hypersensitivity?**

- Nickel (Type IV T cell hypersensitivity)

**What is important to check in a patient that has a TKA with a new patella fracture?**

Ep 66 w/ Dr. Chen

- If the implant is stable, and if the patient has an extensor lag
- If significant lag >10° + unstable- revise component if enough bone (>13mm)
- If lag >10° + stable- extensor mechanism repair

**What is the treatment of choice for periprosthetic TKA femur fracture?**

- Implant loose > revision TKA + ORIF fx
- Implant stable > ORIF fx (locked lateral plating, IMN)
  - Can't use IMN w/ closed box implant
- Highly comminuted + osteoporotic bone/ limited activity > endoprosthesis

**What are some post-op symptoms associated with a loose flexion gap?**

- Trouble getting up from a chair, problems w/ stairs, instability, pain

**What is femoral cam jump?**

AR 9: 7:30

- This can be seen in PS knees when the flexion gap is loose and the cap jumps over the polyethylene post>> may require revision TKA
- Can also be seen w/ over-release of popliteus + anterior portion of MCL

**What is patellar clunk syndrome?**

- A clunk: hear as knee extends
- Scar tissue superior to patella gets caught into the box (PS knee)
- Tx: scar removal via open v arthroscopic
- Prevent by doing synovectomy at time of quad tendon

**What are some implant related risk factors for patellar clunk syndrome?**

- Wide (patella settles) and tall (overstuffed) femoral boxes
- Small patella implant

**What type of impingement can be seen with hyperextension in a PS knee?**

- Wear between the anterior post and the superior edge of the femoral box
- Also seen w/ flexion of femoral component or excess posterior tibial slope

# Revision TKA

**What are some causes of knee pain s/p TKA to have on your differential diagnosis?**

Ep 43 w/ Dr. Cody

- Infection (global pain, get inflammatory markers, aspiration, >3000 is +)

- Other joint pain (hip*, lumbar back pain)
- Loosening (radiolucent lines around implant/cement)
- Malalignment (get CT scan to assess rotation)
- Instability
- Osteolysis
- Hypersensitivity (Nickel is MC, order lymphocyte T cell proliferation test)
- Chronic regional pain syndrome

**Is early implant loosening associated more with non-cemented or cemented TKA?**

- Non-cemented TKA

**What are some causes of early failure vs late failure of TKA?**

- Early- infection, malalignment, instability, arthrofibrosis
- Late- Polyethylene wear

**How do patients with aseptic loosening after TKA present?**

- Mild knee discomfort, normal inflammatory labs, negative aspiration w/ lucency seen around implant or cement on xray

**How do patients with osteolysis after TKA present?**

- 7+ years after TKA, knee pain, normal inflammatory labs, negative aspiration, round lytic lesions around implant on xray (posterior femur common)

**What is the pathophysiology behind osteolysis?**

AR 9: 7:30

- TNFa, IL6, IL1 released > up regulate RANKL > osteoclast mediated bone resorption > cystic lesions in periarticular bone
- Macrophage cells absorb smaller particles <10mm

**What are some polyethylene factors that are associated with the rate of wear?**

- Sterilization +manufacturing method, motion between insert/tray, malalignment, cement debris

**Is sterilization of polyethylene in free air the preferred method?**

- No, this leads to free radical formation > oxidative degradation > poly wear
- Oxidation -increases poly stiffness and decreases strength

**In what technique(s) can be used to minimize free radical formation?**

- Sterilize in an inert atmosphere- ethylene oxide or gas plasma
- Remelting - poly changed from crystalline to amorphous state (reduces fatigue toughness)
- Annealing- poly heated to temp below melting point (keeps crystallinity but leaves more free radicals than remelting)

**What technique(s) are used to increase cross linking of polyethylene?**

- Gamma or electron beam irradiation > thus improving wear properties
- Cross linking increases resistance to adhesive wear but decreases fatigue strength

**Is there any difference between ram extrusion or compression molding when processing the poly?**

- Similar wear rates, compression molding has lower susceptibility to fatigue cracking/ crack propagation

**Doing what to the Q angle will result in patellar maltracking?**

- Increasing the Q angle

**What are the component positions that can lead to increased Q angle and patellar maltracking?**

- Tibial component IR (bad)- implant should be in line w/ medial ⅓ of tubercle
- Femoral component IR (bad)
- Lateralization of patella component (bad)
- (overstuffing the patellofemoral joint can also lead to patella maltracking- check patellar height)

**What is something you should note about setting rotation in a valgus (hypoplastic LFC) knee?**

- Using posterior condylar axis to set rotation > implant too internally rotated

**What are some approaches used in revision TKA?**

- Medial parapatellar arthrotomy (many go through prior incision)
- Scar tissue removal, lateral retinacular release,proximal medial tibia subperiosteal dissection
- Extensile: rectus snip, quadriceps turndown, banana peel, tibial tubercle osteotomy
    - TTO is used best in cases w/ adequate bone stock

**What are some techniques to deal with constrained and unconstrained bone defects with revision TKA?**

- Contained
    - Small defects- fill w/ cancellous bone graft or cement
    - Large defects- highly porous ingrowth cone (meta-diaphyseal fiber metal trabecular cone- implant cemented inside cone)
- Non-contained
    - Metal augments / cones
    - Massive bone loss > endoprosthesis

## TKA Infection

**What is one of the most common causes for early failure after TKA?**

- Infection

**What are some risk factors for periprosthetic TKA infections?**

- Smoking, diabetes, malnutrition, increasing age >70, autoimmune diseases, immunocompromised state,

Ep 37 w/ Dr. Vickers

Immunosuppressive drugs (mab's, glucocorticoids), post-op wound complications, history of infection, excessive anticoagulation

**What is the difference between an early vs a late infection when it comes to PJI?**

- Early- weeks to months after TKA
- Late- months to years
- (within 1 year of TKA it is considered a surgical site infection)

AR 11: 4:35

**What are the first steps in working up a TKA with increasing pain?**

- Physical exam + serum biomarkers (ESR, CRP), joint aspiration
- IL-6 cytokine is sometimes used as well- returns to normal w/i 2/3 days

**What is alpha defensin?**

- An antimicrobial peptide release by neutrophils
- Can send joint fluid for this test as well
- Assoc w/ PJI

**What are some radiographic signs of PJI?**

- Endosteal bone erosion around implant (in comparison to scalloping w/ osteolysis)
- Generalize bone resorption

**What are some other imaging studies that may be useful when diagnosing PJI?**

- Technetium Tc- 99m - detects inflammation
- WBC labeled Indium In-111- detects leukocytes in periprosthetic tissue
- Triple phase bone scan
- Fluorinated deoxyglucose PET scan (FDG-PET) - travels to area of high metabolic activity

(Parvizi, 2011)

**What is the musculoskeletal infection society definition of a PJI?**

- Major criteria:
  - Presence of a draining sinus that communicates to the JOINT
  - Two positive cultures with the same organism
- Minor criteria
  - Elevated ESR (chronic >30) + CRP (Acute >100, Chronic >10)
  - Inc synovial WBC (Acute >10,000, Chronic >3000) or +++ leukocyte esterase test strip
  - Elevated synovial PMN% (Acute >90%, Chronic >80%)
  - Positive histological analysis of periprosthetic tissue

**How long does it take for bacterial biofilm to be formed and established?**

- Around 4 weeks or so
- Bacterial ECM adhere to implant surfaces + defends against antibiotics and host immune system
  - Highest in titanium alloy > stainless steel > titanium > tantalum
- Early/ acute hematogenous infections less likely to be assoc w/ biofilm formation

**Is the biofilm gone when the implants are retained in a presumed PJI?**

- No
- Implant + all foreign material must be removed (screws, cement fragments, etc) when biofilm present

**What is the treatment for PJI?**

- Acute <3 / 4 weeks- I&D, modular bearing exchange, IV antibiotics, implant retention
  - Assuming no biofilm
- Chronic >3 / 4 weeks
  - 1 vs 2 stage exchange arthroplasty (2 stage is test answer)
  - 2 stage
    - 1st stage- Implant removal, antibiotic spacer placement (ideally articulating), IV antibiotics
    - 2nd stage- implant placement (amputation, arthrodesis, implant retention also options)
- Antibiotic impregnated cement also used (ex: vancomycin, gentamicin, tobramycin, voriconazole)

**What type of soft tissue flap could be useful in a TKA patient with an anterior or medial wound issue?**

- Medial gastrocnemius flap (medial sural artery is blood supply)
- For lateral wounds- lateral gastroc flap (risk peroneal n palsy)

**What is SP-ONK?**

- Spontaneous osteonecrosis of the knee- MFC common
  - Sxs: sudden onset knee pain w/o trauma, crescent sign on xray
  - Tx: No collapse- Non-op, arthroscopy, osteotomy
    - Collapse- arthroplasty (UKA/TKA)
    - TKA assoc w/ inferior outcomes than TKA for arthritis

**What is SECONK?**

- Secondary osteonecrosis of the knee
  - LFC common
- Sxs: gradual onset knee pain, crescent sign on xray
- Tx: no collapse- non-op, core decompression, arthroscopy
  - Collapse- TKA
  - TKA assoc w/ inferior outcomes than TKA for arthritis

**What is PA-ONK?**

- Post-arthroscopy osteonecrosis of knee (idiopathic/ atraumatic/ maybe assoc w/ steroid use)
  - Seen s/p arthroscopy, sudden onset knee pain
  - Similar tx options as SECONK and SPONK

# HIP

## Hip Arthritis

AR 12: 11:45

**What are some common hip pain symptoms and their associated hip pathology?**

- Groin pain > hip arthritis
- "C" sign > labral tear
- Lateral hip pain > trochanteric bursitis / abductor muscle tendinitis/dysfunction
- Buttock pain w/ radiating symptoms down leg in dermatomal fashion > spine pathology
- Thigh/ buttock pain w/ activity relieved by rest > claudication / iliac artery atherosclerosis

**What is an antalgic gait?**

- Shortened stance phase on the affected leg

**What is a trendelenburg gait?**

- Patient leans towards affected hip - sign of abductor weakness/ pathology

**What are some conditions that may lead to hip arthritis?**

- Femoroacetabular impingement (CAM/Pincer lesions)
- Acetabular dysplasia
  - Most have a mix of the two
- Post-traumatic

**What are some acetabular changes seen in DDH?**

- Poor coverage of femoral head
- Hip center of rotation lateralization
- Decrease acetabular depth/ shallow hip socket (cartilage stress at superolateral rim > labral tears > femoral head subluxation)
- +/- increased anteversion

**What are some femoral changes seen in DDH?**

- Femoral head/neck changes
- Valgus neck/shaft angle
- Decreased offset
- +/- increased anteversion

AR 13: 1:35

**What are some things to note on x-ray in patients with DDH?**

- Lateral center edge angle (Wiberg)- normal >25°
- Tonnis/Sourcil angle - normal <10°
- Acetabular/head index

**What is a treatment option for a young patient with DDH and minimal hip arthritis with hip pain?**

- Bernese periacetabular osteotomy
- Reorients socket into a more horizontal position - reducing contact stress on cartilage

**What is the Crowe classification?**

- Used to classify severity of adult DDH
- I: <50% subluxation
- II: 50-75% subluxation
- III: 75-100% subluxation
- IV: high dislocation

**What is a surgical technique option for patients undergoing THA with Crowe IV hips?**

- Subtrochanteric shortening osteotomy (possible sciatic n palsy when lengthened >2-4 cm)

**What conditions can be associated with hip osteonecrosis?**

- Hematologic disorders, cytotoxins, alcohol use, chronic steroid use, trauma, sickle cell, etc

**What is important when predicting future collapse of hip osteonecrosis (AVN)?**

- Lesion size + location

**What are some signs of AVN on Xray?**

- Mixed sclerosis + subchondral cysts in femoral head (earlier stages)
- Crescent sign (subchondral lucency- represents cartilage delamination- poor prognostic sign)
- Femoral head collapse + DJD (late stages)

**What is the Kerboul method?**

- Add widest area of osteonecrosis on AP +lateral- angle helps predict eventual collapse
- MRI now used- high risk of collapse if combined angles >240°, low risk of collapse if angles <190° (modified Kerboul)

(Ha, 2006)

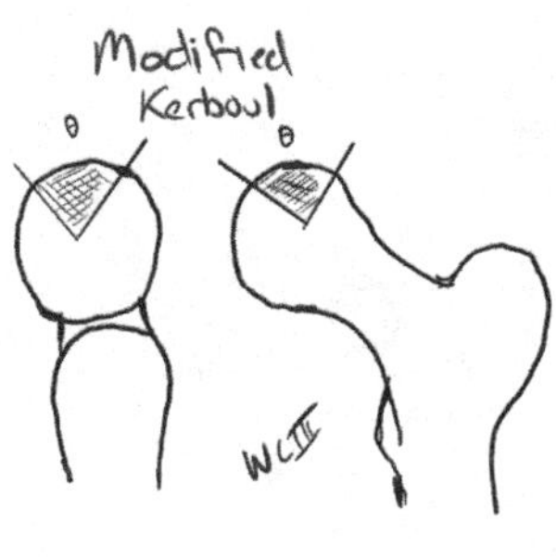


**Figure 6.7: Images showing the Kerboul angle, which is measured on coronal and sagittal images of the femoral head, showing the areas of necrosis. A combined angle >240 indicates a high risk of collapse.**

**What are some treatment options for osteonecrosis of the femoral head w/o collapse?**

- Bisphosphonates (mixed results)
- Core decompression (multiple techniques, 1 v multiple holes)

- Decompression + vascularized fibula grafting
- Decompression + nonvascularized grafting

**What are some treatment options for osteonecrosis of the femoral head with collapse?**

- Total hip arthroplasty - main treatment
- Other options: resurfacing hemiarthroplasty, total hip resurfacing arthroplasty

**What should be on your differential in a 40 F w/ hip pain, with no traumatic event, and osteopenia on xrays?**

- Transient osteoporosis of the hip
- MRI changes can be seen in femoral head down to intertrochanteric region
- Surgery typically not necessary

## Hip Biomechanics/ Templating

AR 14: 1:50

**What is the hip offset?**

- Distance from femoral head to anatomical axis of femur

**What is the relationship between the hip, abductors, and a person's body weight?**

- Hip acts as fulcrum - allows equilibrium between body weight and opposing abductors
- Distance between femoral head + abductors - less than distance between head + body weight
    - Abductors thus generate larger force & JRF is > body weight

**Let's ask that another way to drive the point home:**

**When assessing joint reactive forces, what are the two lever arms to pay attention to?**

- Distance from hip center to center of body weight
- Distance from hip center to greater trochanter-abductor mechanism
- Body lever arm is typically 2.5x longer than abductors, so abductors need to be 2.5x stronger than body weight

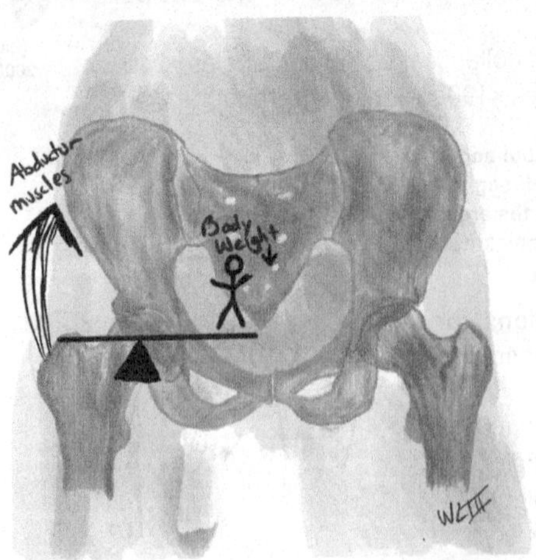


**Figure 6.8: Imaging showing the joint reactive forces for the hip.**

**What is a difference between varus and valgus hips in regards to hip biomechanics?**

- Valgus - improved mechanical advantage of abductors (due to inc tension on abductor mechanism)
- Varus hips- generate greater forces across hip center

**What are some of the biomechanical changes seen in hip OA?**

- Femoral head collapses > neck shortens > abductors lose tension > increased joint reactive forces (hip pain + arthritis)

**What happens when you increase the hip offset (femoral head - femur axis distance)?**

- Abductors work less to keep equilibrium
- Joint reactive forces decrease

**What happens when you medialize the hip center of rotation?**

- Longer lever arm for abductors > decrease work of abductors needed

**What are some things done in surgery to help assist with optimal joint reactive forces?**

- Again, medialization of acetabular cup + restoring femoral offset to maximize abductor tension + leg length for normal gait

**In regards to sagittal balance, what is the goal orientation of the hip center in relation to the spine?**

- The hip center is ideally under the center of the spine to keep the body upright

**What pelvis parameters change with the position of the body?**

- Pelvic tilt and sacral slope
  - Their sum = pelvic incidence, which is a fixed number

**What sagittal balance changes occur with standing?**

- Lumbar lordosis increases (sacral slope increases) > pelvis flexes (pelvic tilt decreases)

**What sagittal balance changes occur with sitting?**

- Pelvic tilt is increased (pelvis extended- which brings hip center more anterior)
- Increasing tilt > inc acetabular anteversion > prevents anterior impingement
  - Think - pelvic tilt is the degree of pelvic extension

**Why is pelvic tilt/ sacral slope important in THA?**

- Lumbo-pelvic motion is important to minimize THA dislocation risk
- Sitting after THA can risk posterior dislocation due to anterior impingement
- Hx of lumbar fusion > decreases lumbopelvic motion > higher dislocation risk

**When templating, where is the ideal location for the acetabular cup?**

- In the center of the hip
- Medial border- ilioischial line
- Inferior border- teardrop

**When templating, what is the ideal location for the femoral stem?**

- Stem center should line up with GT tip (length)
- Canal should be filled w/ stem and bottom of stem should be in middle of canal (basic)

**Ideally after THA, where do you want the center of the stem and acetabulum to be in relation to each other?**

- At the same point, the dots should overlap

**What is a good way to think about the changes that will happen when templating?**

- Once you reduce the femur to the cup- those are the changes that will occur (explained better on podcast)

## THA/ Implants 101

Ep 33 w/ Dr. Schuett

**What are some common approaches used in THA?**

- Anterior approach
- Direct lateral approach (Hardinge)
- Anterolateral approach (Watson-Jones)
- Posterior approach (Southern)

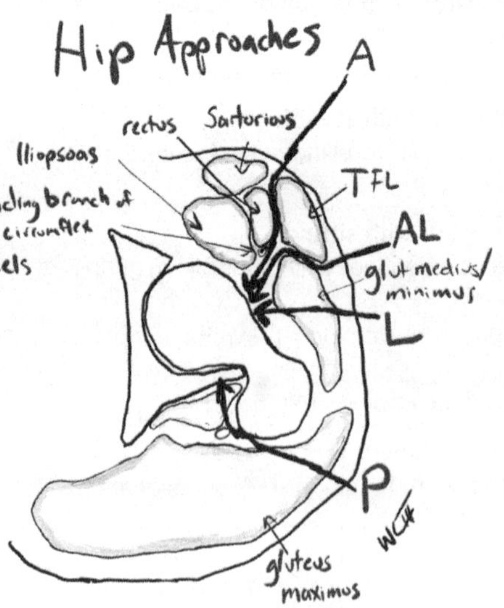


**Figure 6.9: Image showing various approaches to the hip. A-anterior, AL- Anterolateral, L-Lateral, P- Posterior.**

**What are the intervals for the anterior approach + structures at risk?**

- Superficial: sartorius (femoral n) / TFL (superior gluteal n)
- Deep: rectus / glut medius
- Ascending branch of lateral circumflex artery at risk + LFCN injury
- Pros: early recovers (internervous plane)
- Cons: limited acetabular exposure, some say limited femoral exposure as well

**What is the interval for the anterolateral Watson Jones approach?**
- TFL/ gluteus medius
- Cons: may denervate the TFL

**What is the lateral, modified Hardinge approach to the hip?**
- Split the gluteus medius + vastus lateralis
- Cons: prolonged muscle recovery

**What is the posterior, Southern, approach to the hip?**
- Gluteus maximus is split + external rotators are tenotomized
- Cons: some instability

**What typically makes up the acetabular component?**
- Metal shell (smooth on inside, porous coated on outside) + liner (polyethylene, sometimes a metal/ceramic)
- This is for a press fit design (cementless)

**What are some different fixation options for acetabular cups?**
- Cemented or cementless
- Cementless cup use is most common (w/ or w/o screws)
- Titanium cups common
- Polyethylene cups can be used as well (used to be cemented)

**What are some complications that can occur with use of acetabular cups?**
- Acetabular fracture during impaction
  - If incomplete > add screws
  - If complete > ORIF acetabulum
- Periacetabular osteolysis
  - If holes present > retro acetabular osteolysis common
  - If no holes present > proximal femoral osteolysis

**What are some material options for the acetabular liner?**
- Polyethylene (most common), ceramic, metal (cobalt chrome, etc)

**What is the minimum the polyethylene liner thickness should be to prevent fracture?**
- 6mm thick (measured by inner diameter)
- A shell can accommodate multiple poly sizes, and different head sizes (cup size = femoral head size + poly thickness)

**What are some different types of liners?**

AR 16: 3:55

- Standard liner- neutral, hemispherical design
  - Inner diameter = femoral head size, outer diameter = shell size
- Lateralized liner- extra poly on medial side added that increases offset (may use w/ protrusio / revision THA)
- Elevated liner- raised lip of poly (10-20° or so)- increases jump distance before dislocation
- 10° face changing liner- cup is angled to change version in case surgeon doesn't like version of the shell
- Dual mobility- bipolar head in cup

- Constrained liner- femoral head locked into the poly

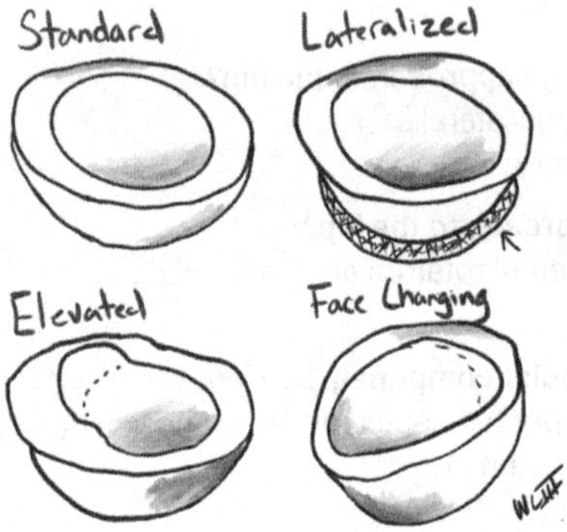


Figure 6.10: Image showing various types of polyethylene used in total hip arthroplasty.

**What is the trunnion?**
- The junction of the femoral head and stem
- Also called a morse taper (typically larger diameter towards the stem and decreases towards the femoral head- i.e. 12/14)

**What are some different options for materials used for the femoral head?**
- Cobalt chromium (can articulate w/ poly or metal)
- Ceramic also commonly used- smoothest material w/ lowest wear properties (assoc w/ squeaking)
- Titanium- scratches easily, leads to abrasive wear w/ poly (better used for acetabulum)

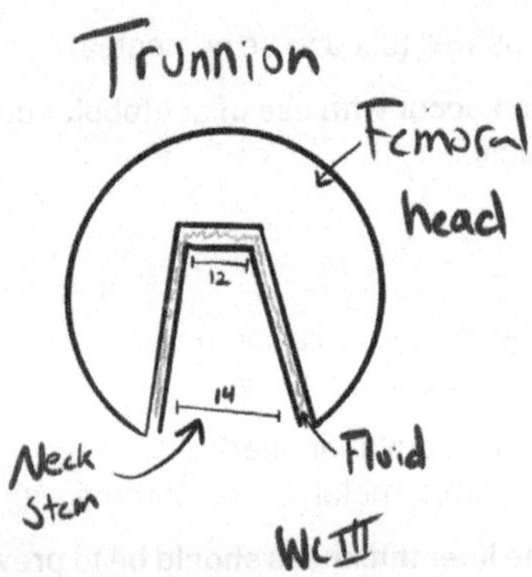


Figure 6.11: Image showing the trunnion. The taper on the neck can be appreciated.

**What is the jump distance?**
- The distance the femoral head displaces before dislocation

**What are some things that limit hip ROM?**
- Lipped liners
- Constrained liners
- Skirts/collar use

**What are some advantages to increasing the femoral head size?**
- Increased head/neck ratio > larger arc of motion before impingement > decreases chance to dislocate
- Increases jump distance before dislocation occurs
  - 32mm head size is good

**What are some disadvantages to increasing the size of the femoral head?**
- Increased volumetric wear of liner
- Increases forces across trunnion due to increase in head/neck ratio

**What is the Door classification and why is it important?**

- Type A- thick cortex + narrow canal "champagne flute"
- Type B- normal
- Type C- thin cortex w/ wide canal, loose fit "stove pipe"
- Describes relation between proximal femur anatomy + femoral diaphysis
  - Helps w/ stem selection for press fit

**What are some different fixation options for femoral stems?**

- Cemented or cementless (press fit)
- Cementless is more common as well (cemented cups fail before cemented stems)

**What are some situations where you may cement a femoral stem?**

- Elderly patients, hip fractures
- Excellent results

Ep 84 w/ Dr. Cohen-Rosenblum

**What type of stem design leads to worse outcomes when cementing the femoral stem?**

- Precoated/ rough components- produces osteolysis + abundant wear debris
  - Causes cement bone interface to fail early
- Flexible stems- stresses the cement mantle more (cobalt chrome or stainless steel used to prevent this)
- In contrast... smooth, highly polished stems don't bond to cement- some micromotion- little wear debris

**What are some techniques used when cementing a femoral stem?**

- Vacuum mixing- decreases porosity + increases fatigue strength
- Use of pulsatile lavage
- Pressurization - highest pressures seen during stem insertion

**What are some different types of press fit (non cemented) stems?**

- Metaphyseal fitting (broach to prepare metaphysis)
- Meta-diaphyseal fitting- (broach + ream to prepare metaphysis and diaphysis)
- Diaphyseal fitting (broach + ream)

**What are some different techniques used for canal preparation for the stem?**

- Broaching + placing a slightly oversized stem- hoop stress prevents motion
- Line- to- line- canal + stem are perfect size in match, rough stem coating creates friction to prevent motion (Scratch fit)

**What is the difference between ingrowth and ongrowth?**

- Ingrowth- bone grows into the implant (beads, mesh, porous metals, etc)
  - Porous coating, pore size between 50-150μm
- Ongrowth- bone grows on to roughened implant surface
  - Surface plasma sprayed or grit blasted, hydroxyapatite can be used as well
  - No pores

**What is the chemical formula for hydroxyapatite?**

- $Ca_{10}(PO_4)_6(OH)_2$
- An osteoconductive plasma sprayed surface coat
- Coats roughened and porous surfaces

Ep 84 w/ Dr. Cohen-Rosenblum

**What are some design features of non-cemented femoral stems?**

- Tapered- proximal to distal taper to allow implant fit w/ cylindrically porous coated in metaphyseal region
    - This can be a dual taper or a single taper
- Cylindrical- typically fully coated (proximal + distal)
    - Assoc w/ thigh pain + stress shielding
- Anatomic- fills metaphyseal region in coronal + sagittal plane
- Modular (Wagner)- more than one piece
    - Ex: different stem + neck
- Also: ingrowth v ongrowth, proximal v distal fixation, fully v partially coated

AR 17: 20:08

**What are some situations where a modular femoral stem (Wagner or diaphyseal fit) may be used?**

- Hip dysplasia, revision hip arthroplasty, difficult anatomy- allows more freedom to restore hip biomechanics
- At modular junction pain, corrosion, + pseudotumor formation can occur

**What are some bearing surface options seen in THA?**

- Metal on poly- most frequent
- Ceramic on poly- lower in vitro wear rates than metal on poly + increased costs
- Ceramic on ceramic- lowest wear rates, squeaking can occur + liner fracture
- Metal on metal- low wear rates, larger head use w/ lower dislocation rate

**What metal has the highest Young's modulus?**

- Ceramic > cobalt chrome > stainless steel > titanium alloy > cortical bone

**Do metals with a closer modulus of elasticity to bone have more or less stem related thigh pain?**

- Less thigh pain and stress shielding
- Titanium implants common

**What are some femoral stem properties that could lead to higher incidence of stress shielding?**

- Stiffer metal (i.e. cobalt chrome)
- Distally fixed fully coated stems
    - Proximal osteopenia/bone loss and distal sclerosis and spot welds may be present

**What is the ideal component positioning for THA?**

- Acetabulum
    - 30-50° of abduction ~40°

- 10-40° of anteversion~ 20°
- Femur
  - 5-25° of anteversion ~15°
- Combined anteversion
  - 35-45° degrees

## THA Wear

**What is wear?**

- Loss of material due to relative motion between surfaces

**What are the modes of wear?**

- Wear between:
- Mode 1- articulating between bearing surfaces (head+ poly liner
- Mode 2- articulation between primary bearing and surface not intended to be the bearing surface (head + metal acetabular shell)
- Mode 3- articulation between the indented bearing surfaces w/ 3rd body wear (head + poly liner w/ cement in between)
- Mode 4- two non-bearing surfaces rubbing together

**What are some different types of wear?**

- Abrasive wear- hardness difference between two metal > third body wear
- Adhesive wear- bonds between surfaces need to break to allow movement > weaker material breaks 1st
- Seen in osteolysis - seen w/ metal on poly
- Volumetric / Linear

**What was the relationship between femoral head size and wear?**

- In past, larger head size produced an increased rate of volumetric wear
- BUT... with emerging techniques and use of highly cross-linked ultra molecular weight polyethylene acetab liners- wear decreased- femoral head size doesn't matter as much

**What occurs during osteolysis?**

- Macrophages phagocytose submicron polyethylene particle > release osteolytic factor > bone resorption by osteoclasts
- Around 0.1mm/year

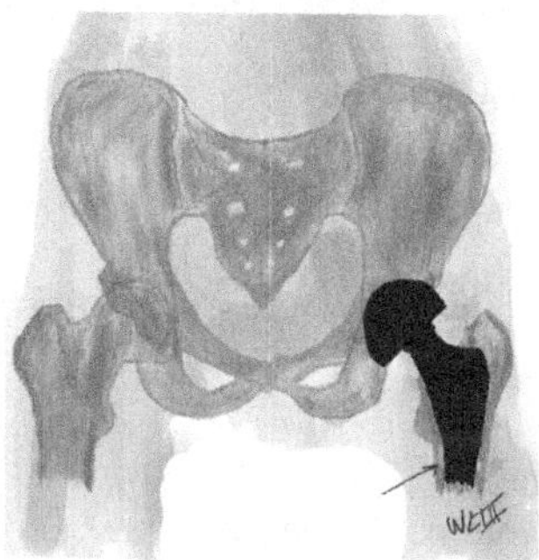

**What does osteolysis look like on xrays?**

- Endosteal scalloping + osteopenia

**Figure 6.12: The arrow is pointing to endosteal scalloping of the femur, which can be seen in osteolysis.**

**What were some advantages to metal on metal bearings?**

- Larger diameter head use- dec dislocation

- Low wear rates IF you have:
  - Good implant position
  - Fluid radiograph lubrication
  - Polar contact > equatorial contact

**What were some disadvantages to metal on metal bearings?**

- Inc cobalt + chromium > cleared by kidney (kidney disease)
- Crosses placenta barrier
- Not linked with cancer though

**What are some indications for hip resurfacing?**

- Young patient,highly active, male, + hip arthritis w/ preserved proximal femur bone stock
- Advantages- preserves prox femur
- Disadvantages- post-op femoral neck fx ~0-4%, lack of modularity, metal debris

**What is the difference between boundary and fluid film lubrication?**

- Boundary- load bearing surfaces are non deformable- fluid partially separates the articulating surfaces
- Fluid film- articulating surfaces separated by lubricant
- Increasing femoral head size- more fluid trapped in between the two surfaces- less wear (entrainment)
  - Clearances of 100-200μm maximize fluid film thickness

**What are some causes of edge wear?**

- Inc contact pressure at the edge of the metal cut > lubrication breakdown
- Impingement, microseparation, edge loading
- Cup positioning is important w/ metal on metal prosthesis

**What are some adverse local tissue reactions (ALTR) seen with metal on metal bearings?**

- Perivascular infiltrate of lymphocytes - Type IV delayed hypersensitivity
- Aseptic, **lymphocyte** dominated vasculitis associated lesion (ALVAL)
- **Lymphocyte**- dominated immunologic answer (LYDIA)
- Pseudotumor formation (histopathology similar to ALVAL)
- All lead to osteolytic responses (from metal debris) + pain +/- tissue necrosis

**What is the workup for a painful metal on metal THA?**

- PE, Xrays (note implant position, any osteolysis), labs (ESR,CRP, serum cobalt + chromium)
  - Ion levels >7-10 ppb
- Metal artifact reduction sequence MRI (MARS)- to evaluate for ALTR
- Aspiration

**What is trunnionosis?**

- Corrosion at the femoral head/neck taper
- Can lead to metal ion release + pseudotumor formation

- Cobalt > chromium elevated 5:1

**What are the types of corrosion that occurs at the trunnion?**
- Crevice corrosion- small gaps allow fluid to enter- corrosion at morse taper junction, dominant type in trunnionosis
- Fretting corrosion- micromotion at femoral head-neck interface, disrupts protective oxide layer
- Galvanic corrosion- presence of fluid + metal alloy mismatch (ex titanium trunnion w/ cobalt chrome head)

**What are some risk factors for trunnionosis?**
- Larger femoral head size
- Small diameter + shorter tapers

**What is passivation and which material is self-passivating?**
- Formation of a protective oxide coat
- Titanium

# THA Complications/ Revision

**What are some benefits (and disadvantages) seen with hip hemiarthroplasty?**
- Increased stability
- Disadvantages: protrusio, chondrolysis, poorer function (compared w/ THA)

**What are some "classic" history findings when working up patients with a painful THA?**

**AR 18: 7:00**

- Anterior thigh pain- femur issue
- Groin/buttock pain- acetabular issue
- Lateral hip pain- trochanteric bursitis, abductor weakness/tendinitis, trochanteric impingement
- Delayed onset pain/ early antibiotic treatment/ prolonged drainage- infection
- History of hip dislocation- instability
- Pain w/ active hip flexion- psoas tendon irritation or anterior impingement

**What are some signs of loosening seen on xray?**
- Increasing radiolucency
- Absence of spot welding
- Component subsidence
- Pedestal formation (femur)

**What are some other things to notice on xray when evaluating for painful THA?**
- Implant position (cup position- vertical vs horizontal)
- Uneven poly wear

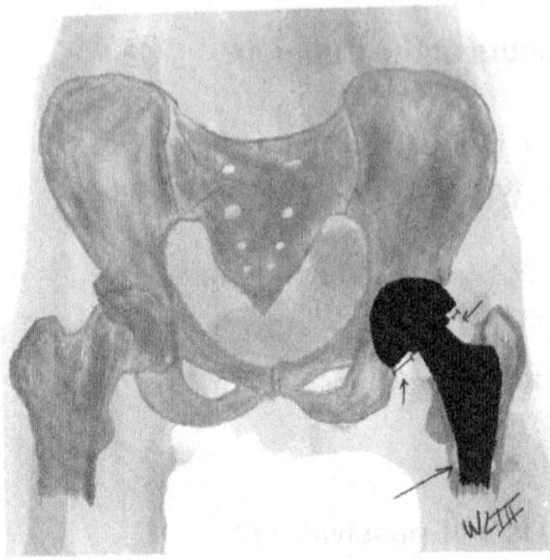

**Figure 6.13: Arrows are pointing to the uneven spacing between the femoral head and the acetabular shell, indicating that there is uneven polyethylene wear.**

**What THA complication may be seen in patients who undergo irradiation?**

- Cementless cup loosening

**What are some potential complications seen with total hip arthroplasty?**

- Poly wear
- Dislocation
- Heterotopic ossification
- Leg length discrepancy
- Impingement
- Aseptic loosening
- Infection
- Trunnionosis

**What are some signs on xray of THA poly wear?**

- Eccentric position of the femoral head + osteolysis

AR 19: 1:05

**What is the treatment for a THA w/ poly wear?**

- If metal shell is fixed + has good positioning > head/liner exchange
- If large lytic lesion w/ instability > THA revision +/- bone grafting
- Post- op instability can occur after revision*

**What are some risk factors/ potential causes of THA instability?**

- Female
- Prior hip surgery
- Implant positioning (version, vertical cups, soft tissue tension mismatch)
  - Ideal cup version- 5-25°, ideal cup abduction- 30-50°
  - Ideal combined version 30-40°
- Decreased offset/ leg length
  - Abductors - reduced moment arm decreases efficiency
  - Femoral neck impingement against acetabulum
- Limited spine mobility (hx of lumbar fusion or OA)
- History of femoral neck fx or AVN
- Neuromuscular disorder

**What is the treatment of a THA dislocation?**

- Closed reduction
- If dislocation 3+ times- THA revision

**What are some surgical treatment options/techniques for revision THA due to instability?**

- Revisie w/ components in correct position (if malposition)
- Increase offset, leg length, or perform trochanteric advancement (if poor soft tissue tension)
- Revise to a constrained liner (useful if abductor insufficiency)
  - Reduces ROM to impingement- assoc w/ higher failure rates
- Increase size of femoral head / head neck ratio (increases ROM till impingement)

**Is heterotopic ossification (HO) after THA more common in males or females?**

- Males
- Tx: prophylactic w/ low dose radiation 24 hrs pre op or 48 hrs post op, or indomethacin
- If HO develops + patient has severely limited ROM > remove HO

**Is operative limb lengthening or shortening more common w/ THA?**

- Lengthening
- If lengthened >4cm - may cause nerve issues - sciatic nerve

**What are some techniques during THA that could lead to increased leg length?**

- Higher cut on femoral neck
- Leaving femoral stem proud

**What are some symptoms of impingement after THA?**

- Pain /weakness w/ resisted hip flexion
- Decrease in pain after ultrasound injection
- On cross table lateral- prominence of anterior edge of cup may be seen as well

**What is the surgical treatment for impingement after THA?**

- Iliopsoas tenotomy
- THA cup revision if cup is prominent

**What is the #1 cause of late THA revision ?**

- Aseptic loosening

**What is the #1 cause of early THA revision?**

- Infection

**What are some classic symptoms of aseptic loosening?**

- Start up pain
- Groin pain - cup, thigh pain- stem

**What are some signs of aseptic loosening on xray?**

- Progressive radiolucency
- Implant subsidence
- Pedestal formation

**What are some types of revision THA stems?**

- Extensively coated cylindrical stem (cobalt chromium- 4cm of isthmus required + difficult to control version)
- Tapered fluted modular stem (titanium- 2cm of isthmus required)

AR 20: 9:20

**What is the Paprosky classification and treatment for femoral bone loss?**

- Type I- metaphysis diaphysis intact (tx: noncemented v cemented implant)
- Type II- metaphyseal bone loss + intact diaphysis (Tx: porous coated or ongrowth tapered stem)
- Type III- metaphyseal + diaphyseal bone loss (Tx: diaphyseal engaging tapered stem)
  - IIIa- >4cm intact diaphysis
  - IIIb- <4cm intact diaphysis
- Type IV- deficient metaphyseal bone + nonsupportive diaphysis (Tx: proximal femur replacement)

**What are some types of revision THA acetabular cups**

- Augments on a hemispherical cup (used for rim defects)
- Jumbo cups- size bigger than 66 men 62 women (used w/ large cavitary defects)
  - Assoc w dislocation
- Antiprotrusio cage- treat large contained lesions
- Cup-cage - jumbo cup w/ cage added for extra fixation- used
- Triflange cup (used when rim not intact, and some cases of pelvic discontinuity)

**What is the Paprosky classification for acetabular defects and the treatment?**

- Type I- Acetabular rim intact, small contained areas of bone loss (Tx: cementless THA revision w screws)
- Type II- acetabular rim distortion w/ deficiencies that support acetab cup fixation
  - IIa- superior migration < 3cm above obturator line
  - IIb- superior migration > 3cm but medial to kohler's line
  - IIc- superior migration > 3cm and lateral to kohler's line
  - Tx: standard or jumbo cup, possible graft, augment, or cage for 2B and C
- Type III- superolateral acetabular bone loss + greater than one third of rim deficiency
  - IIIa- deficient superior or superolateral coverage
  - IIIb- superior plus medial component migration, possible pelvic discontinuity
  - Tx: structural allograft or cage or triflange

**How much of the acetabular rim should be intact for a rim fit?**

- 2/3
- 50% bone stock required for cementless hemispherical cup

**What are the zone for acetabular screw placement (safest to dangerous)**

- Posterior superior (sciatic n plus gluteal NV bundle at risk)
- Posterior inferior (sciatic n, gluteal NV bundle, pudendal NV bundle at risk, screws less than 20mm)
- Anterior = danger zone
  - Anterior inferior (obturator NV bundle)
  - Anterior superior (external iliac vessels)

**What is the Vancouver classification of periprosthetic femur fractures?**

Ep 47 w/ Dr. Decker

- A- trochanteric fracture (G,L) ’ non-op, operate on displaced GT fx (Cable plate vs hook plate)
- B- diaphyseal fracture at level of implant
  - B1- implant stable - ORIF
  - B2- loose implant w- good bone stock- ORIF plus revision to diaphyseal engaging tapered stem plus or minus allograft strut
  - B3- loose implant w- poor bone stock - proximal femur replacement- allograft prosthesis
- C- fracture distal to implant- ORIF

**What is the treatment of an intra op calcar fracture?**

- Check extent of fx, cerclage cables

## THA Infection

**See section above (knee) for more on infections**

**What is the most common organism seen in PJI?**

AR 21: 1:54

- Staph a- most common organism
- Staph epi- biofilm production, seen in late THA infections (biofilm at 4 weeks)

**What is the treatment of THA PJI?**

- Early- within 4 weeks, I&D w/ head + liner exchange
- Late/- chronic- 2 stage revision is gold standard
  - 2 stage =implant removal, thorough I&D cultures, cement spacer placement, IV antibiotic treatment for 6 weeks, then implant removal and place final implants
  - (Single stage revision done in Europe, but likely not test answer on OITE/Boards)
- Hematogenous - acute- I&D + poly/liner exchange

**What number is considered positive for THA PJI after hip aspiration?**

- Looks these up it changes every couple years
- Per orthobullets:
  - WBC >3k and 80%PMN
  - WBC >4350 for MOM hips

**What is the workup for suspected THA PJI?**

- ESR plus CRP

- If elevated aspirate
- If they have been on abx, stop abx then reaspirate

**Does a transfusion increase your risk for PJI?**

- Yes

**What medications/procedures decrease the risk for post op infection after THA?**

- TXA decreases risk for post op transfusion (PO, IV, and topical)
- Hypotensive epidural/spinal anesthesia

**What is the mechanism of action of TXA?**

- Inhibits plasminogen by binding to the lysine binding site

## Podcast Episodes for a Deeper Dive

- Episode 33 w/ Dr. Schuett: Intro to total hip arthroplasty https://naileditortho.com/introtohip/
  Video:
  https://www.youtube.com/watch?v=7C2s8vnQYJo&t=2245s
- Episode 42 w/ Dr. Harb: Introduction to total knee arthroplasty https://naileditortho.com/introtka/
  Video: https://www.youtube.com/watch?v=_bL_pbTwGuU&t=729s
- Episode 43 w/ Dr. Cody: Evaluation of a painful TKA
- www.naileditortho.com/painfultka
  Video: https://www.youtube.com/watch?v=P0bCxISGlhA&t=270s
- Episode 37 w/ Dr. Vickers: Periprosthetic infection
- Episode 47 w/ Dr. Decker: Periprosthetic hip fractures https://naileditortho.com/prosthetichip/
  Video: https://www.youtube.com/watch?v=7ISL7RbKDy8
- Episode 66 w/ Dr. Chen: TKA extensor mechanism failure https://naileditortho.com/extensormechanismfailure/
  Video:
  https://www.youtube.com/watch?v=cu8VBTJZAuQ&t=2421s
- Episode 84 w/ Dr. Cohen-Rosenblum: THA Cementless Design Explained https://naileditortho.com/thadesign/
  Video: https://youtu.be/glh0oG7aWjo

## Specific articles/sources mentioned in this podcast

Baker, J. F., Caborn, D. N., Schlierf, T. J., Fain, T. B., Smith, L. S., & Malkani, A. L. (2020). Isolated patellofemoral joint arthroplasty: can preoperative bone scans predict survivorship?. The Journal of Arthroplasty, 35(1), 57-60

https://www.aaos.org/globalassets/quality-and-practice-resources/osteoarthritis-of-the-knee/oak3cpg.pdf

Chalmers, B. P., Limberg, A. K., Tibbo, M. E., Perry, K. I., Pagnano, M. W., & Abdel, M. P. (2019). Total knee arthroplasty after high tibial osteotomy results in excellent long-term survivorship and clinical outcomes. JBJS, 101(11), 970-978.

Parvizi, J., Zmistowski, B., Berbari, E. F., Bauer, T. W., Springer, B. D., Della Valle, C. J., ... & Zalavras, C. G. (2011). New definition for periprosthetic joint infection: from the Workgroup of the Musculoskeletal Infection Society. Clinical Orthopaedics and Related Research®, 469, 2992-2994.

Ha, Y. C., Jung, W. H., Kim, J. R., Seong, N. H., Kim, S. Y., & Koo, K. H. (2006). Prediction of collapse in femoral head osteonecrosis: a modified Kerboul method with use of magnetic resonance images. JBJS, 88(suppl_3), 35-40.

Bolognesi MP, Ledford CK. Metal-on-Metal Total Hip Arthroplasty: Patient Evaluation and Treatment. J Am Acad Orthop Surg. 2015 Dec;23(12):724-31. doi: 10.5435/JAAOS-D-14-00183. Epub 2015 Oct 22. PMID: 26493972.

# NOTES

# NOTES

# NOTES

# HAND CHAPTER 7

## Wrist + Hand Anatomy

**What are the compartments of the forearm?**

- Dorsal (superficial + deep)
- Volar (superficial + deep)
- Mobile wad

**What is the anatomy of the extensor tendons as it enters the hand/fingers?**

- Extensor tendon trifurcates at P1
  - Central portion inserts dorsal base of P2 (central slip)
  - Lateral slips- joined w/ oblique fibers of extensor hood from interossei and lumbrical muscles> forms lateral bands
    - > Forms terminal tendon + inserts on P3 dorsal base

**What is the function of the sagittal bands?**

- Stabilize the extensor tendon at the dorsal MCP joint
  - (They originate from MCP volar plate and base of P1)

**What ligaments help stabilize the lateral bands to prevent volar subluxation?**

- Triangular ligament

**What ligaments help stabilize the lateral bands to prevent dorsal subluxation?**

- Transverse retinacular ligaments

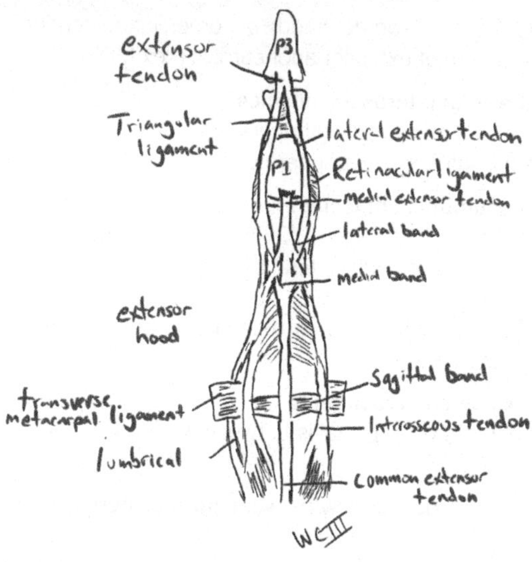


**Figure 7.1: Image showing the anatomy of the extensor tendon. Note the triangular ligament and transverse retinacular ligaments helping to stabilize the tendon.**

**What is the function of the pulleys and where are they?**

- To maximize efficiency of joint rotation and force transmission
- 5 annular pulleys + 3 cruciform pulleys

  - A1,A3,A5- over palmar surfaces of MCP, PIP, and DIP joints
  - A2,A4- over P1 and P2 (both are most important biomechanically)

**What comprises the pulley system of the thumb?**

- A1, oblique, A2 pulley
  - A1- at MCP joint
  - Oblique- proximal phalanx
  - A2- at IP joint
- A1 + oblique pulley most important biomechanically
- *Radial digital nerve at risk during trigger thumb release

**Does the FDS or the FDP bifurcate?**

- FDS, the FDP attaches to the base of P3

**Where does the FDS bifurcate and what is its course to its insertion?**

- FDS bifurcates laterally + dorsally at level of A1 pulley> then divide into medial + lateral slips
  - Medial slips > cross dorsal to FDP + rejoin as campers chiasm at distal P1 and PIP volar plate
  - Lateral slips> insert at base of P2

**What is the vascular supply for the flexor tendons?**

- Direct vascular supply via vinicular system
- Synovial diffusion for avascular zones- canaliculi system

**What is the function of the dorsal interossei muscles?**

- Abduct digit + flex MCP (interossei originate from metacarpals)
- Bipennate muscle
  - Superficial muscle> becomes medial tendon>attaches at proximal phalanx
  - Deep muscle> passes over sagittal hood> becomes lateral tendon> inserts transverse fibers of extensor aponeurosis (flex MCP)

**What is the function of the volar interossei muscles?**

- Flex MCP + adduct index, ring + middle fingers
  - One muscle> inserts into extensor apparatus

**What is the function of the lumbrical muscles?**

- Extend DIP + PIP joints
- Originate from FDP + insert on radial lateral band of extensor apparatus
- Lumbricals pass DEEP to transverse intermetacarpal ligament (interossei pass dorsal to ligament)

**What are the wrist portals named in relation to?**

- Extensor compartments (ex: 4,5 portal is between 4th + 5th compartments)

**What are some structures at risk and with what portals during wrist arthroscopy?**

- 1,2 portal- superficial branch radial n + radial artery at risk

- 3,4 portal (1 cm distal to lister's tubercle)- superficial branch radial n at risk
- 6R portal (radial to ECU)- dorsal sensory branch of ulnar n
- 6U portal- dorsal sensory branch of ulnar n

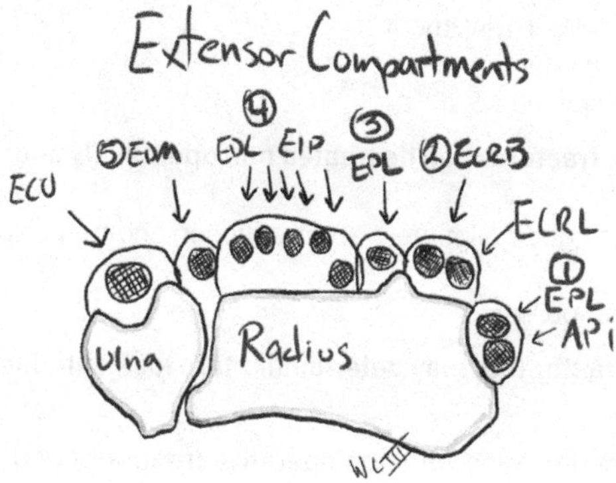


**Figure 7.2: Image showing the 6 extensor compartments of the wrist.**

## Wrist + Hand Trauma

**What are some common eponyms for distal radius fractures?**

- Colles- dorsally displaced
- Smiths- volarly displaced
- Barton- volar shear (can be used for dorsal shear pattern too)
- Chauffeur - radial styloid
- Die punch fx- lunate facet

**Ep 7 w/ Dr. Ficke**

**What are the normal radiographic parameters you should note when discussing distal radius fractures?**

- Volar tilt 11°
- Radial inclination 23°
- Radial height- 11mm

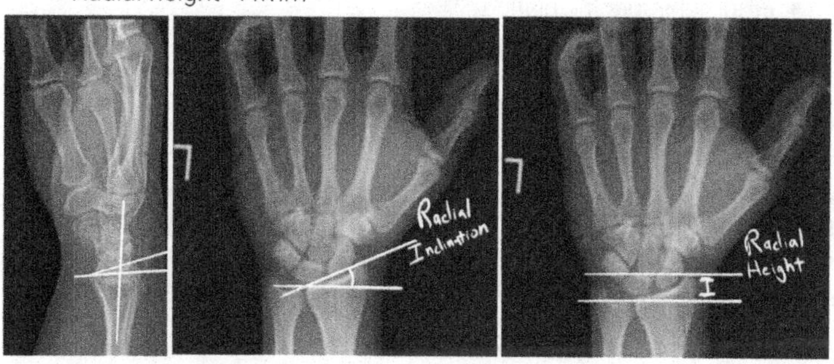


**Figure(s) 7.3, 7.4 & 7.5: Lateral xray of the wrist showing the volar tilt of the distal radius (left). Radial inclination (RI) and radial height are also shown.**

**What are some characteristics of unstable distal radius fractures?**

(Lafontaine, 1989)

- Lafontaine criteria
- Age> 60 may have greater than 50% risk of reduction loss
- Distal ulna injury
- Intra articular involvement
- Fx comminution
- Dorsal angulation > 20°

**What distal radius fractures can be treated non operatively and what is the treatment?**

- Fractures with good alignment after reduction and non displaced fractures
- Reduce + immobilize

**What is the main factor that may determine future loss of reduction?**

- Age

**What is a complication seen with non operative treatment of distal radius fractures?**

- Late EPL rupture (around 4-6 weeks after injury)
- Tx with EIP to EPL transfer

**What are the operative indications for distal radius fx?**

- Intra articular displacement greater than 2mm
- Dorsal angulation greater than 10°
- Radial shortening greater than 3mm (after reduction)
- Loss of reduction
- Unstable volar shear fractures

**Is there any difference between operative vs non op tx in the elderly patient with distal radius fx?**

(Arora, 2011)

- Op tx have improved grip strength and xrays

**What are some operative options for distal radius fractures?**

- Dorsal plating
- Locked volar plating
- Fragment specific plating
- Dorsal bridge plate
- Intramedullary nail
- K-wire fixation
- External fixation

**What should you be worried about in patients w/ distal radius fx and median nerve symptoms?**

- Acute carpal tunnel syndrome associated w/ fx
- Seen in 5-8% of distal radius fx

**What is the treatment for acute CTS in patients w/ distal radius fx?**

- Open carpal tunnel release

**What are some indications and complications seen with dorsal plating of distal radius fractures?**

- Indication: dorsal shear fractures
- Complications: tendonitis and tendon rupture

**What are some advantages and complications seen with volar plating of distal radius fractures?**

Ep 80 w/ Dr. Orbay

- Advantages: Early ROM + soft tissue coverage
- Complications:
  - Plate too distal- FPL tendon rupture + intra-articular hardware
  - Screws too long- EPL tendon rupture
- Soong Classification

(Soong, 2011)

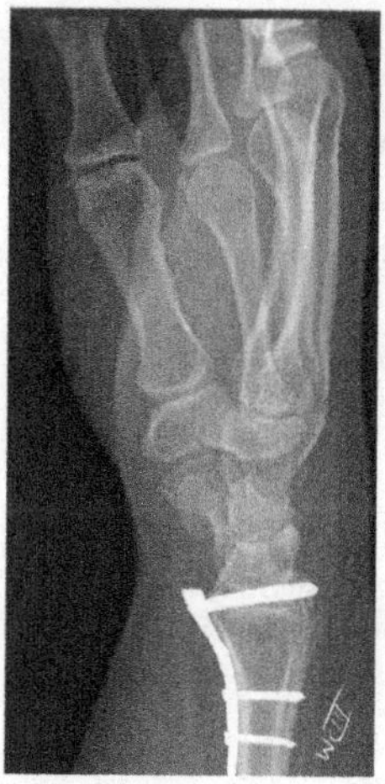

**Figure 7.6: Xray showing a distal radius fracture after fixation with the plate placed a little to distal with possible long intra-articular screws.**

**What are some complications seen with external fixation of distal radius fractures?**

- Fracture subsidence
- Stiffness of fingers
- Pin site infections
- Injury to superficial radial nerve (make full incision)

**What are some indications and advantages for dorsal bridge plating for distal radius fracture?**

- Indications: High fracture comminution, polytrauma, significant diaphyseal extension
- Advantages- increases axial load stiffness
- Dorsal bridge plate usually a 3.5mm plate attached to radius + 3rd (or 2nd) metacarpal

**What type of distal radius fracture would bridge plating be contraindicated in?**

- Palmar lunate facet fractures (volar marginal rim fx)

**What is a radial styloid fracture called?**

- Chauffeur fracture
- May be associated w/ SL ligament injury
- If intra articular displacement >2mm, can ORIF (screws v plate v pin)

**What is the TFCC and where are its attachments?**

- Triangular fibrocartilage complex
- Radioulnar ligaments
- Superficial fibers- styloid
- Deep fibers- fovea (plays greater part in DRUJ instability v superficial)

**What are the types of ulnar styloid fractures?**

- Tip, midportion, base, base oblique
- Base fx: most common- most tx non-op if DRUJ stable

- W/ base oblique fractures- inc incidence of foveal disruption and DRUJ instability

**What is the treatment of a DRUJ dislocation?**
- Closed reduction + immobilization
- Dorsal dislocation - immobilize in supination
- Volar dislocation- immobilize in pronation

**What percent of axial force is transmitted to the ulna at the wrist (neutral variance)?**
- 20%
- Inc ulnar variance by 2mm - 40% transmitted to ulna (malunion)

**What are acute TFCC tears associated with?**
- Avulsions at ulnar periphery
- May be able to be repaired (similar to peripheral meniscus tears)

**What condition are chronic TFCC tears associated with?**
- Ulnar impaction syndrome

**What is possible diagnosis for a patient w/ ulnar sided wrist pain w/ wrist extension and ulnar deviation?**
- Ulnar impaction syndrome (seen in ulnar positive wrists)
  - Also can be seen in patients w/ distal radius fx malunion
- Dx w/ true PA xray, MRI, arthroscopy
  - May see edema in lunate if damaged

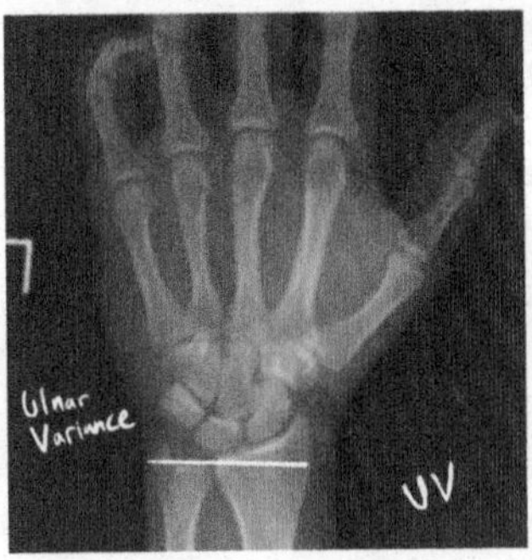


**Figure 7.7: Xray of the wrist showing neutral ulnar variance. In ulnar positive wrists the distal end of the ulna will be distal to the drawn line.**

**What are some treatment options for ulnocarpal impaction?**
- Non-op
- Surgical
  - Wrist arthroscopy w/ TFCC debridement (assoc w/ chronic TFCC tears)
  - Arthroscopic distal ulna removal
  - Ulnar shortening osteotomy (contraindicated w/ arthritis)

## Carpal fractures

**What is the most commonly injured carpal bone?**
- Scaphoid (waist)

**What is the most common mechanism for scaphoid fractures?**
- Wrist extension + radial deviation

Ep 55 w/ Dr. Roberts

**What physical exam findings may be positive in patients with scaphoid fractures?**

- Snuffbox + tubercle tenderness + pain with axial load

**What xrays may be useful in diagnosing scaphoid fractures?**

- Scaphoid view (wrist extended + ulnar deviated)

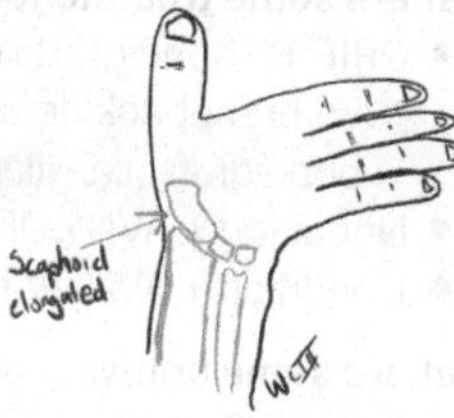


**Figure 7.8: Image showing a scaphoid view, taken with the wrist in extension and ulnar deviation.**

**What are some other imaging that could be used to diagnose a scaphoid fracture?**

- MRI- sensitive + specific
- CT scan- good to evaluate bony morphology / displacement

**How much of the scaphoid is covered by cartilage?**

- Around 80%

**How does the scaphoid receive its blood supply?**

- Via retrograde flow
- Mostly via dorsal ridge vessels (70% or so)
- Proximal pole of scaphoid has limited blood supply

**How much displacement is considered "displaced" in scaphoid fractures?**

- 1mm

**What fracture characteristic contributes to the healing capacity of scaphoid fractures?**

- Fx location
- Distal pole can heal in cast in 8 weeks
- Proximal pole fx may take up to 6 months to heal

**What are some non-op treatment options for non-displaced scaphoid fractures?**

- Cast
- No difference in outcomes w/ short vs long vs spica vs no spica cast

**(Doomberg, 2011)**

**What is the difference in healing rate for operative vs non op treatment of NONdisplaced scaphoid fx?**

- None
- Operative patients: inc complications, quicker return to work, inc grip strength

**What are the operative indications to fix a scaphoid fracture?**

- Displacement >1mm (nonunion rate around 50%)
- Fx associated w/ perilunate dislocation
- Some proximal pole fx

**What are some approaches used to treat scaphoid fx?**

- Dorsal - may be used for proximal pole fx, more central screw placement

- Volar- may be useful for distal fx
  - Screw may be trans-trapezial in order to be parallel to bone
  - May help in pts w/ humpback deformity
- No diff in union or functional outcome between the two
- Arthroscopic assisted also an option

**What are some treatment options for patients with a scaphoid nonunion?**

- ORIF +/- bone graft
  - w/ humpback deformity- volar approach useful w/ a structural bone graft (i.e.- iliac crest)
- Nonunion + AVN - ORIF + vascularized bone graft
- Nonunion + AVN w/ humpback deformity- volar ORIF + graft (MFC)

**What are some non-vascularized graft options for scaphoid fractures?**

- Iliac crest graft
- Volar distal radius graft
- Osteochondral rib autograft
- These may be useful when structural support is needed

**What are some vascularized grafting options (and their blood supply) for scaphoid fracture nonunion where AVN may be present?**

- Dorsoradial distal radius - 1,2, intercompartmental supraretinacular artery
- Volar DR graft based on volar carpal artery
- Medial femoral condyle- descending genicular artery (shorter time to union than 1,2 intercompartmental supraretinacular artery)
- \+ many more options

**What is SNAC?**

- Scaphoid nonunion advanced collapse
- A form of post-traumatic arthritis of the wrist

**What are the stages of SNAC?**

- I- radial styloid arthritis
- II- radioscaphoid involvement
- III- radioscaphoid + scaphoid-capitate + capitolunate involvement
- IV- pancarpal arthritis

**What are some operative treatment options for SNAC?**

- Distal scaphoid pole excision
- Radial styloidectomy
  - Excision >4mm can lead to radioscaphocapitate ligament injury
- Wrist denervation (complete or partial)
- Proximal row carpectomy
  - (Traditionally, capitate degeneration was a contraindication, but with newer techniques not necessarily)
- 4 corner fusion (excise scaphoid + fuse capitate, lunate, hamate + triquetrum
- Complete wrist arthrodesis (an option in pts w/ pancarpal disease)

- Total wrist arthroplasty (not best for young patients)

**What is a common mechanism for hook of hamate fractures and the treatment?**

- Direct blow (ex: baseball)
  - Dx via xray (45° supinated), carpal tunnel view xray, or CT
- Can be missed initially and present w/ continued pain months later (think nonunion)
- Tx: cast, ORIF, or excision
  - Symptomatic nonunion- excise (assoc w/ ulnar n injury + grip strength loss)

## Wrist ligament injuries

**What is the primary stabilizer of the scapholunate joint?**

- Scapholunate interosseous ligament (SLIL)**
  - Composed of 3 portions: membranous, dorsal (strongest), palmar (rotational constraint)
- Scaphotrapezial interosseous ligament (STIL)- distal scaphoid stabilizer
- Other wrist ligaments are secondary stabilizers

**What is the difference between carpal instability nondissociative (CIND) and dissociative (CID)?**

- Nondissociative - radiocarpal joint instability or instability between proximal + distal rows
  - Ex: volar extrinsic ligament injury or radial styloid fx
- Dissociative- instability within proximal or distal carpal row
  - Ex: scapholunate injury

**What are some other categories of carpal instability?**

- Carpal instability adaptive
  - Unstable secondary to extra-articular issue (distal radius malunion)
- Carpal instability complex
  - Combination of CID and CIND (ex: perilunate injury)

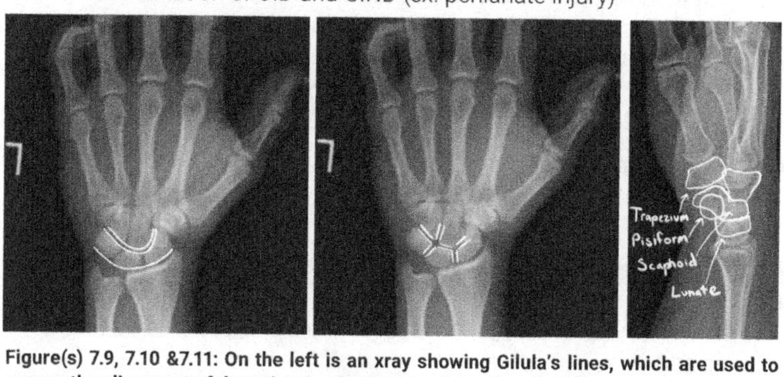


**Figure(s) 7.9, 7.10 &7.11: On the left is an xray showing Gilula's lines, which are used to assess the alignment of the wrist. On the right is a lateral xray of the wrist outlining some of the bones that can be seen.**

**What portion of the lunotriquetral ligament is the strongest?**

- Palmar

**What is the natural tendency of the proximal row bones?**

- Scaphoid - palmar flexion
- Triquetrum - extension (dorsiflexion)
- Lunate- depends on what ligaments are injured- it will go along with scaphoid (flex) or triquetrum (extend)

Ep 50 w/ Dr. Rose

**What are the wrist pathomechanics associated with a scapholunate ligament injury?**

- Unopposed extension of lunate (with triquetrum) due to injury > dorsal intercalated segment instability (DISI)
- During wrist flexion- dorsal subluxation + abnormal scaphoid motion > scapholunate advanced collapse arthritis
- SL injury can be seen w/ trauma + inflammatory arthropathy (i.e. rheumatoid)

**What is a positive scaphoid shift test?**

- Pain / clunk when the wrist is moved from ulnar to radial deviation when examiners thumb is over scaphoid tubercle
- Differing degrees of positivity with instability grade

**What xray can be obtained in patients with suspected SL injury but negative PA wrist xray?**

- Clenched fist PA
- Advanced imaging including MRI can also be obtained
- Wrist arthroscopy is also useful in diagnosing these injuries

**What is the treatment for scapholunate injury (acute + chronic)?**

- Acute:
  - Open repair w/ stabilization (suture anchors/ drill holes, K-wire stabilization, cast, etc)
- Chronic:
  - If reducible (and quality tissue)- open repair
  - Soft tissue reconstruction(differing results)
    - Dorsal capsulodesis, FCR tenodesis, ligament reconstruction, etc
  - If irreducible- proximal row carpectomy, fusion,
  - If arthritis- partial denervation (AIN/PIN), fusion, PRC

**What is the wrist deformity seen with lunotriquetral injuries?**

- Volar intercalated segment instability (decreased SL angle / increased LT angle)

**What are some physical exam tests that can be used to diagnose LT injuries?**

- LT shuck + shear test (stabilize lunate + translate triquetrum palmar/ dorsal)
- Arthroscopy also useful in diagnosing these injuries

**What are some treatment options for LT injuries?**

- Acute- ligament repair
- Chronic - soft tissue reconstruction, arthrodesis

**What is the Mayfield classification used to describe?**

- Perilunate instability
- Mechanism: wrist extension, ulnar deviation, axial load + midcarpal supination

**What are the Mayfield classification stages?**

- I- scapholunate dissociation or scaphoid fracture
  - If wrist is radially deviated during injury> likely to lead to scaphoid fx
  - LRL + SRL maintain lunate position
- II- capitolunate dissociation
- III-lunotriquetral dissociation or triquetral fracture
- IV- lunate dislocation

**What is the treatment for perilunate injuries?**

- Acute: closed reduction
- Early ORIF
  - Doral approach- fix SL injury +/- screws/wires across SL interval
  - Volar approach- fix LT injury + address carpal tunnel

## Hand fractures

**What are the deforming forces seen in metacarpal base fractures?**

- 2nd- ECRL
- 3rd- ECRB
- 5th- ECU (diaphysis is displaced proximally and ulnar

**What is a xray to evaluate metacarpal base fractures?**

- Oblique films (30° pronated)

**Are CMC fracture dislocations associated with higher or lower energy mechanisms?**

- Higher, associated w/ wrist injuries

**What is the treatment for metacarpal base fx?**

- Non-displaced - cast
- Displaced - ORIF v CRPP

**What is the acceptable angulation for metacarpal shaft fractures?**

- 5-10° for index + long finger
- 10-40° for ring and small finger
- Transverse IMC ligaments + IO muscles help resist shortening
- If operative indicated, can treat with ORIF, intramedullary screw, or K-wire

**How much shortening in metacarpal fractures is associated with a 7° extensor lag?**

- 2mm shortening

**What is the acceptable angulation for metacarpal neck fractures?**

- Index + long . <20°
- Ring <40°
- Small <60°

**What is the most common deformity noted with metacarpal neck fractures?**

- Apex dorsal (pull of intrinsics)

**What is the treatment for most metacarpal neck fx?**

- Closed reduction, splint/casting, ROM at 3 weeks

**What is the treatment of choice for a patient with a 2nd metacarpal head fx after punching someone in the face with a small wound over the hand?**

- I&D +/- fixation (fix if displaced fx)
- Fight bite

**What is the most common direction for a MCP dislocation?**

- Dorsal
- Index finger most common

**How do you reduce a simple MCP dislocation?**

- Flex wrist + fingers to relax flexors & push proximal phalanx distal + dorsal
- Don't hyperextend and use traction

**What may be the issue of a MCP dislocation does not reduce with closed efforts?**

- Interposed volar plate (or sesamoids)
  - Need to go to OR to remove plate from blocking reduction
  - Volar approach- risks digital nerve injury
  - Dorsal approach can also be used

**What makes a phalanx fx unstable (radiographically)?**

- Angulation >10°, <50% apposition, >2mm shortening, or malrotation
- Tx: CRPP, ORIF, ex fix
- Stable fx can be tx non op (ex: buddy tape)

**What is the most common location for a PIP dislocation?**

- Dorsal, often assoc w/ volar plate avulsion or fracture
- Tx: closed reduction, stiffness* is a complication (mobilize early)

**What injury may occur with a volar PIP dislocation and what position do you want the PIP in to heal?**

- Central slip injury
- PIP joint extension (extension splint)
- Complication: boutonniere deformity

**What is the tx of a stable PIP dorsal fx dislocation (middle phalanx articular surface is involved)?**

- Dorsal extension block splint
- Tx of unstable fx: ORIF, pinning, hemi hamate arthroplasty, volar plate arthroplasty

**What is a mallet finger and the non-op treatment?**

- Injury to dorsal distal phalanx "baseball finger", can be due to extensor tendon injury
  - Patients present w/ extensor lag + deformity
- Tx: splinting

**What are some operative indications for mallet finger?**

- Distal phalanx subluxation, articular fragment >40% + articular gap >2mm (debated)
- Tx options, ORIF, CRPP, suture repair, tendon grafting, fusion, amputation

**What is an epiphyseal injury to the distal phalanx in the pediatric patient called?**

- Seymour fracture (open fx), nail matrix and plate injury may be present
- Inc infection risk, tx w/ I&D + reduction

## Thumb Injuries

**What is a Bennett fracture and the deforming forces seen in this fracture?**

- Fx of the base of the 1st metacarpal
- Volar oblique ligament- stays attached to volar ulnar fragment of metacarpal base*
- Abductor pollicis longus- displaced distal metacarpal proximally
- Adductor pollicis- adducts metacarpal

**What is the treatment of a Bennett fracture?**

- CRPS, ORIF

**What is a Rolando fracture?**

- More complex articular injury to 1st metacarpal base

**What is the typical closed reduction maneuver for 1st metacarpal base fractures?**

- Traction, pronation, external rotation

**Where does the true thumb UCL insert and attach to?**

- Metacarpal head (more dorsal) > proximal phalanx (more volar)
- Accessory UCL is more superficial

**What is the difference between a skier's thumb and a gamekeeper's thumb?**

- Acute UCL disruption - skiers thumb (most common to rupture off prox phalanx)

- Chronic UCL attenuation- gamekeeper's thumb

**What is a Stener lesion?**

- Avulsed ligament is above the adductor aponeurosis (prevents healing of UCL)

**What thumb UCL injuries can be treated nonoperatively?**

- Partial tears + tears w/ firm endpoint - splint (~6 weeks) + PT
  - True thumb UCL ligament tested at 30 degrees of flexion**

**Which thumb UCL injuries are indicated for operative treatment?**

- Complete tears (no end point on PE), displaced avulsion fx, Stener lesion
- Tx options: primary repair, reconstruction, tendon transfer/advancement, arthrodesis

**What is the treatment for thumb RCL tears?**

- Mostly non-op (no aponeurosis to prevent healing)
- Operative tx in select cases (chronic instability)

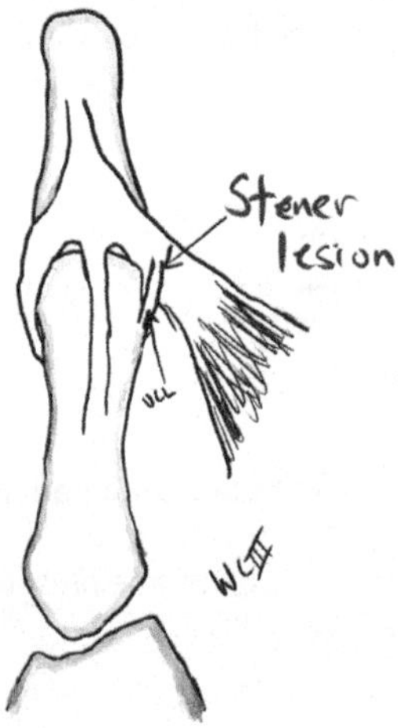


**Figure 7.12: Image showing a Stener lesion and the avulsed thumb UCL ligament.**

## Tendon Injuries

Ep 58 w/ Dr. Dacus

**What are some general considerations with treatment of flexor tendon injury?**

- Strength of tendon repair is proportional to # suture strands across repair site
- Lacerations >60% tendon- tx w/ simultaneous core + epitendinous repair
- Minimum of 4 strand repair allows active motion w/ therapy
- A2 + A4 pulleys most important for function (oblique pulley in thumb)

**What are the different zones for flexor tendon injury?**

- Zone I- distal to FDS (FDP avulsion, jersey finger)
- Zone II- proximal to FDS between palm (FDS and FDP both present- risk of adhesions)
- Zone III- palm
- Zone IV- carpal tunnel region
- Zone V- distal forearm

**What are the surgical treatment options for flexor tendon injuries (by zone)?**

- Zone I (FDP avulsion/ avulsion fx of base)

- Type I (FDP retracted to palm)- early repair preferred
- Type II (FDP retracted to PIP)- delayed repair is ok
- Type III (FDP retracted to DIP)- delayed repair ok
- Prolonged DIP flexion> dorsal lateral band subluxation> swan neck deformity

- Zone II (no man's land)- repair v reconstruction (stiffness)
  - Up to 50% of patients may require tenolysis 3mo after surgery for motion
- Zone III- direct repair
- Zone IV- direct repair + repair transverse carpal ligament
- Zone V- direct repair

**What are the different zones for extensor tendon injury?**

- Zone I & II- involve terminal insertion of extensor mechanism (may lead to mallet finger)
- Zone III- disruption of central slip (positive Elson test- inability to extend PIP w/ joint at 90°, boutonniere)
- Zone IV- proximal phalanx (thumb metacarpal)
- Zone V- directly over MCP joint (sagittal band injury, fight bite zone)
- Zone VI-VII - proximal to MCP joint

**What are the treatment options for extensor tendon injuries (by zone)?**

- Zone I- full time extension splinting of the DIP x8 weeks (pin in extension if bone fragment)
  - Tx swan neck deformity: central slip tenotomy, spiral oblique retinacular ligament reconstruction
- Zone III (acute boutonniere)- PIP joint extension splint, surgical repair
- Repair for most other zones

**What are some complications after tendon repair?**

- Tendon adhesions (Can tx w/ tenolysis after 3-6mo)
- Tendon rupture (acute- around 7 days post op, late- tx w/ tendon reconstruction)
- Joint contracture (splint, surgical release)

**What are some indications for flexor tendon reconstruction?**

- Failed primary repair, chronic untreated injuries

**What is a 2 stage tendon reconstruction?**

- Stage 1- temporary silicone rod implanted + fixed distally and allowed to glide
- Stage 2- 3mo later, rod removed + autograft placed through sheath

**What are some late complications after tendon repair?**

- Triggering
- Lumbrical finger plus (paradoxical extension of IP joints with attempted flexion)
  - Tx: release or excise lumbrical tendon
- Quadriga (uninjured fingers unable to obtain full flexion)
  - Caused by functional shortening or overtightening of FDP during repair

## Nail/Fingertip Injuries

**What are the parts to a nail?**

- Nail plate
- Sterile matrix- beneath nail plate
- Germinal matrix
- Hyponychium - between distal nail bed and skin
- Eponychium - at distal part of proximal nail fold - "cuticle"
- Paronychium- lateral margins

**What is the typical treatment for a patient with a subungual hematoma >50% of the nail?**

- Nail removal + nail matrix laceration repair
  - Potential risk: hook nail (if loss of bony support/tight repair)

**What are some of the orientation types for fingertip injuries?**

- Transverse, dorsal oblique, volar oblique

Ep 18 w/ Dr. Gottschalk

**What are some common flaps used to treat fingertip injuries with soft tissue defects?**

- V-Y advancement- useful for transverse lacs/ dorsal oblique
- Thenar flap- useful for index/ long finger in young patients (skin from palm covers digit, then flap divided after ~2 weeks)
- Cross finger flap- dorsal skin+tissue to cover volar defect of adjacent finger
- Reverse cross finger flap- dorsal tissue used to cover dorsal defect
- Moberg advancement flap- useful for volar thumb injuries (stiffness- complication)
- First dorsal metacarpal artery (FDMA) flap- useful for dorsal thumb injuries
- Groin flap (superficial circumflex iliac artery)- useful for dorsal hand injuries

**What are some absolute indications for hand/ finger replantation ?**

- Amputation of thumb
- Multiple digits
- Wrist/ forearm amputations
- Any level implant in pediatric population
- Midpalmar amputation

**What are some contraindications to replantation?**

- Severely mangled parts
- Pts w/ severe vascular disorders
- Pts w/ prolonged warm ischemia (>6 hours) w/ a major muscle
- Pts w/ prolonged ischemia in a finger (>12 hrs)
- Pts w/ severe injury/ diseases

# Nerve Injuries

**What are the main parts of a nerve?**

Ep 53 w/ Dr. Dy

- Axon (extend from dorsal root ganglion of anterior horn)> endoneurium > fascicle (multiple nerve fibers)> perineurium (surround fascicles)> internal epineurium (between fascicles)> external epineurium

**What is an important prognostic factor in nerve recovery?**

- Age, younger age = better

**What are the different types of nerve injuries?**

Ep 53 w/ Dr. Dy

- Neuropraxia
  - Stretching of nerve, temporary demyelination (endo, peri, + epineurium intact)
- Axonotmesis
  - Axons disrupted, wallerian degeneration distal to injury, + fibrillations & sharp waves on EMG
- Neurotmesis
  - Complete nerve injury (axon > epineurium disrupted)
  - Worst prognosis

**How does regeneration work in neurotmesis + axonotmesis?**

- Wallerian degeneration distal to injury> products phagocytized> Schwann cells proliferate + endoneurial tube formed that will receive axons
- Structural protein production increases> nerve growth 1 mm/ day

**What is electromyography, and the findings seen with nerve injury?**

- EMG- detects axonal function at neuromuscular junction
  - Acute denervation- reduced motor unit potential recruitment pattern + fast firing rate
  - 3 weeks- abnormal spontaneous activity- fibrillations, positive sharp waves
  - Early reinnervation - polyphasic motor unit potentials
  - Chronic denervation - decreased insertional activity, absent motor unit potential recruitment

**What does a nerve conduction velocity test examine?**

- Large myelinated nerve fibers, it determines location + how severe injury is
- Demyelination - dec amplitude, inc latency, decreased conduction velocity
- Transected nerve- no response

**What is the indication to operate for nerve injuries?**

- Open trauma w/ concern for nerve injury, sharp nerve transections, direct trauma w/ suspected nerve injury

- (Neuropraxia can be monitored for return of function)

**What are some different surgical options for nerve injuries?**

- Neurorrhaphy (repair)
- Nerve conduits
- Nerve grafting

**What are some different types of neurorrhaphy and technical considerations?**

- Epineurial repair, individual fascicular, group fascicular (none superior to the other)
- Tension free repair is important, wound should be clean
- Microscope can be useful to align fascicles

**What is a nerve conduit and when can it be used?**

- A tube (biocompatible) to allow nerve to regenerate
- Useful for sensory nerves <10mm gap, some use in gaps up to 25mm

**What are the treatment options in patients w/ nerve injuries w/ large gaps, i.e. >3cm?**

- Nerve grafts
- Autograft (i.e. sural n) + decellularized allograft options (less donor site morbidity)

**After what period of time after nerve injury does the number of regenerating axons and response to growth factors decrease?**

- 6 months
- Distal motor endplates degenerate

**How long until there is irreversible muscle fibrosis after nerve injury?**

- 18-24 months

**What are some principles of nerve transfers?**

- Use of an expendable motor nerve close to denervated target muscle (shorter distance may be better)

**What are some different types of nerve transfer techniques?**

- End to end- cut ends of nerve are slightly overlapped
- End to side- donor nerve inserted into recipient opened perineurium "Supercharges" the recovery

**What are some common nerve transfers and what are they used for?**

- AIN >> Ulnar motor fascicle (loss of hand intrinsics)
- Ulnar fascicle of FCU or median fascicle to FCR/FDS >> musculocutaneous branches of biceps (loss of elbow flexion)
- Spinal accessory nerve >> suprascapular nerve (shoulder abduction + ER loss)
- Median branch to FCR/FDS >> PIN (loss of wrist/ finger extension)
- Radial n branch to triceps or medial pectoral >> axillary nerve (loss shoulder flexion, ER, abduction)

**What are some positive physical exam findings seen in carpal tunnel syndrome?**

- Durkan's, Phalen's, Tinels
- Static 2 point discrimination >6mm, inability to detect 2.83 monofilament
- Nerve conduction studies: inc distal motor latency >4.5msec, sensory latency >3.5msec

**Ep 15 w/ Dr. Bilbrew**

**What are some treatment options for carpal tunnel syndrome?**

- Non-op: nighttime splinting, steroid injection (better for mild disease)
- Operative: open carpal tunnel release, endoscopic CTR (quicker return to work)
    - Similar long term results, pinch strength 6 weeks, grip- 12 weeks

**What are some other sites of median nerve entrapment?**

- Ligament of struthers, lacertus fibrosus, deep head pronator teres, FDS arcade

**What is a way to tell the difference between carpal tunnel syndrome and pronator teres syndrome?**

- Proximal forearm pain + sensory disturbances along palmar cutaneous n

**What are some causes of anterior interosseous nerve syndrome?**

- Compression by pronator teres, biceps bursae, accessory FPL head
- Viral (Parsonage Turner)
- Tx: mostly observe, can do tendon transfers in chronic cases

**What are some sites of entrapment of the ulnar nerve?**

- Arcade of struthers (fascial thickening), medial intermuscular septum, medial head of triceps, Osborne's ligament, FCU aponeurosis, deep flexor-pronator aponeurosis, anconeus epitrochlearis

**What are some physical exam findings seen in cubital tunnel syndrome?**

- + Tinels, elbow flexion test, compression test
- Wartenberg sign- abducted small finger (unopposed extensor digiti minimi)
- Froment sign- weak thumb adduction, FPL flexion during pinch
- Ulnar digit clawing

**Ep 67 w/ Dr. Conti Mica**

**What is ulnar tunnel syndrome?**

- Ulnar nerve entrapment at Guyon's canal (3 zones)
    - Zone 1 is proximal to nerve bifurcation (sensory + motor, ganglion)
    - Zone 2- deep motor branch (hook hamate fx)
    - Zone 3- superficial sensory branch, sensory deficit (ulnar a thrombosis)

**What are some treatment options for ulnar tunnel syndrome?**

- Non-op: NSAIDs, splinting
- Operative: decompression, if CTS, release of carpal tunnel may be enough

**Where are some sites of compression of the radial nerve?**

- Fascial band at radial head, recurrent leash of Henry, leading edge of ECRB, arcade of Frohse (proximal supinator), distal supinator

**What may be a physical exam findings seen in PIN syndrome?**

- Difficulty extending at MCP joints or extending wrist
- r/o space occupying lesion

**Where is the most common site of compression in radial tunnel syndrome (pain, no motor/sensory deficits)?**

- Arcade of Frohse

**Know the brachial plexus + relevant applied anatomy!**

## Tendon Transfers

**What are some principles for tendon transfers?**

- Similar power between donor + recipient muscle
- Similar excursion between donor + recipient muscle
- Muscle phases should be synergistic
  - I.e- wrist extension/ finger flexion, thumb adduction (and the opposite)

**What is the first and last muscle in the forearm innervated by the radial nerve?**

- Brachioradialis, EIP
- (First muscle -innervated is brachioradialis, last is EPL)

**What deficits are seen in a high radial nerve (proximal to elbow) injury?**

- Wrist extension, thumb extension, finger extension

**What are some tendon transfers for high radial nerve injury?**

- Typically donor is from median nerve
- Pronator teres > ECRB
- Palmaris longus > EPL
- FCR> EDC

**What are some tendon transfers for low radial nerve injury?**

- PL> EPL
- FCR> EDC
- Wrist extensors transfer may not be needed as ECRL preserved

**What deficits are seen in high median nerve injury?**

- Thumb IP flexion (FPL), index + long finger distal IP flexion (FDP), proximal IP flexion (entire FDS), thumb opposition (APB, opponens pollicis)

**What are some tendon transfers for high median nerve injury?**

- Brachioradialis > FPL
- Suture index FDP to long/ring/little finger FDP tendon distally
- Transfer to restore thumb opposition

- FDS opponensplasty (ring finger FDS wrapped around FCU + inserted into APB)
- EIP opponensplasty (EIP passed around ulnar arm + inserted into APB)
- Abductor digiti minimi (huber) transfer (adds muscle bulk to palm, improved cosmesis, used in peds patients)
- Palmaris longus (camitz) transfer

**What are some deficits seen in high ulnar nerve injury?**
- Loss FCU + loss of FDP to little + ring finger, loss of hand intrinsics
- Loss of intrinsics leads to little finger abduction due to pull of extensor digiti minimi (Watenburg sign)

**What may be seen with low ulnar nerve injury?**
- Clawing of little + ring fingers (intrinsic paralysis w/ preserved FDP to small/little finger)

**What are some possible tendon transfers for high ulnar nerve injury?**
- Tenodesis of FDP to long/index fingers
- FCU may cause weakness but FCR functional > no tendon transfer needed

**What are some possible tendon transfers for low ulnar nerve injury?**
- FDS split> lateral bands (intrinsics)
- ECRB > adductor policis (thumb adduction)
- EPL or EIP tendon transfer for index finger abduction (not commonly performed)

# Tendonopathy

**What condition may a patient who feels a click or a pop and pain in their fingers with finger flexion/extension have?**
- Trigger finger (stenosing tenosynovitis)

**What is stenosing tenosynovitis due to, and associated conditions?**
- Tenosynovitis of flexor tendons causing impingement at A1 pulley (inc type III collagen and chondrocytes)
- Seen in pts w/ systemic diseases (diabetes, gout, calcific tendinitis, pseudogout, amyloidosis)

**What are some treatment options for trigger finger?**
- Steroid injection, A1 pulley release

**What condition may be noted in a 45F w/ radial sided wrist pain w/ wrist pain w/ ulnar deviation while making a fist?**
- De Quervain tenosynovitis (involving APL and EPB tendons)
- Finkelstein test was described in question

**What are some treatment options for De Quervain tenosynovitis?**
- Steroid injection, 1st dorsal extensor compartment release

**What condition may be noted in a 40y/o weightlifter w/ radial sided wrist pain + TTP 6 cm proximal to radial styloid?**

- Intersection syndrome (inflammation at intersection of 1st and 2nd dorsal compartments)

**What are some treatment options for intersection syndrome?**

- Activity modification + steroid injection, 2nd dorsal compartment release

**What physical exam can help determine if ulnar wrist pain is from ECU tendinitis vs TFCC pain?**

- ECU synergy test
  - Elbow supinated, digits extended,+ patient radially deviates thumb
  - TTP about ECU = positive finding

## Hand infections

**What are some common hand infections and their treatment?**

- Paronychia (nail fold infection)- Tx: acute- abx, I&D of abscess, chronic- nail plate removal + eponychial marsupialization
- Felon (fingertip pulp abscess)- Tx: I&D
- Herpetic whitlow (vesicles, viral shedding +/- bullae)- Tx: acyclovir, abx only if bacterial superimposed infection
- Human bite wounds (think S aureus, streptococcus, Eikinella)- Tx: I&D
- Animal bite wounds (think S aureus, Pasteurella) - Tx: abx + clean wound
- Deep space / collar button abscesses- Tx: I&D + IV abx, volar+dorsal incisions for collar button
- Pyogenic flexor tenosynovitis- I&D

**What are the Kanavel signs?**

- Clinical findings seen w/ pyogenic flexor tenosynovitis
- Fusiform digit swelling, digit held in flexion, TTP along flexor sheath, sheath pain w/ passive extension

## Arthritis

**What joint in the hand is most commonly affected by OA?**

- DIP> thumb CMC>PIP>MCP

**What are some diagnoses on the list for thumb CMC pain?**

- Thumb CMC arthritis
- Radioscaphoid arthritis
- De Quervain's tenosynovitis
- Scaphotrapeziotrapezoid arthritis

**What is the difference between stage III and IV 1st CMC arthritis (Eaton)?**

- CMC + STT arthritis (stage IV)

**What are some operative treatment options for thumb CMC arthritis?**

Ep 79 w/ Dr. Gray

- Hemitrapeziectomy
- Thumb metacarpal extension osteotomy
- Trapeziectomy (lower complications)
- Trapeziectomy + interposition (i.e.- FCR/APL tendon)
    - LRTI - ligament reconstruction and tendon interposition
- Arthrodesis (young laborer)
- Implant arthroplasty (higher complications)

**What are some operative treatment options for PIP arthritis?**

- Long/ring finger w/ bone stock- arthroplasty
- Border fingers (index/small)- arthrodesis
    - Fusion angle- index- 30°, long- 35, ring-40°, small-45°

**What is a Heberden nodule?**

- Bony prominence on DIP (seen w/ DIP arthritis)
    - Mucous cysts may also be present in DIP arthritis (I&D)

**What are some treatment options for DIP arthritis?**

- Arthrodesis (10-20° flexion)- more reliable
- Arthroplasty

**What is avascular necrosis of the scaphoid called?**

- Preiser disease

**What is avascular necrosis of the lunate called?**

- Kienbock disease

**What are some treatment options for Preiser disease (+ Kienbocks)?**

- Core decompression
- Vascularized bone graft (1-2 ICSRA), (4-5 ECA for Kienbocks)
- PRC/ scaphoid excision + fusion
- Total wrist fusion

**What are some symptoms of DRUJ arthritis?**

- Chronic pain + pain w/ supination + pronation
- Tx: non op 1st- spinting/ injections
    - Operative: distal ulna resection, hemiresection w/ interposition, ulna head arthroplasty (assoc w/ instability)

## Rheumatoid

**What extensor tendons are most likely to rupture in patients with rheumatoid arthritis?**

- EDQ + EDC (Vaugh- Jackson syndrome)
- Tenosynovitis can occur also

**What flexor tendons are likely to be injured in patients w/ RA?**

- FPL or index FDP (Mannerfelt syndrome)
- Volar STT osteophyte causes attenuation

**What is caput ulnae syndrome?**

- Dorsal subluxation of the ulna (or volar subluxation of carpus)- contributes to extensor tendon injuries
- Tx: EIP to EDQ transfer or EDQ to EDC piggyback transfer (after non-op + medical tx has failed)

**What deformity is seen in the wrist in patients w/ RA?**

- Supination, palmar dislocation, radial deviation + ulnar translation
- Tx: depends on severity (partial arthrodesis, total arthrodesis, arthroplasty)

**What are some treatment options for the wrist manifestations w/ RA?**

- Early tx: medical tx, ECRL>ECU transfer (to fix radial deviation), partial fusion (radiolunate)
- Late tx: Total wrist fusion, total wrist arthroplasty

**What are some manifestations of RA seen at the MCP joint?**

- Ulnar drift (extensor subluxation), collateral ligament injury, synovitis, wrist radial deviation + volar plate disruption

**What structures extend the PIP joint?**

- Lumbricals + interossei + central slip

**What is a swan neck deformity due to?**

- Volar plate attenuation + dorsal subluxation of lateral bands
- Hyperextension of PIP w/ extensor lag of DIP

**What structure normally prevents dorsal subluxation of the lateral bands?**

- Transverse retinacular ligament (attaches volar plate to LB)
- ... thus swan neck deformity (PIP hyperextension, extensor lag at DIP)

**What is the treatment for swan neck deformity?**

- Flexible: extension splinting, central slip tenotomy +/- intrinsic release, FDS tenodesis
- Rigid: dorsal capsule release, lateral band mobilization, extensor tenolysis, collateral release
    - Or arthrodesis

**What is boutonniere deformity (PIP flexion, DIP hyperextension) due to?**

- Central slip + triangular ligament injury leading to volar subluxation of CLB when PIP flexes

**What structure normally prevents volar subluxation of the CLB during PIP flexion?**

- Triangular ligament

## Dupurtyen

**What is Dupuytren disease?**

- Abnormal thickening of palmar fascia beneath skin>> leads to eventual contractures
- High amounts of fibroblasts + contractile myofibroblasts

- Affects ulnar digits slightly more

**What type of collagen is most prevalent in the ECM in Dupuytren disease?**
- Type III

**What is the fascia structure like from the forearm > fingers?**
- Palmaris longus/ deep forearm fascia> pretendinous bands (going towards digits, superficial to tendon)> at distal palmar crease (DPC), divides into 3 layers
    - 1- Pretendinous band > sends attachment fibers from DPC to MCP
    - 2- spiral bands> both sides of pretendinous bands distally along flexor sheath
    - 3- perforating fibers from pretendinous bands to dorsal sides of MCP

**What is the difference between bands and cords?**
- Bands- normal anatomic structure
- Cords- diseased contracted structures

**Which bands(cords) displace the NV bundle superficially and proximally towards the midline?**
- Spiral cords (careful during dissection)

**What cord causes DIP contracture?**
- Retrovascular cord

**What fascia ligament is not involved with Dupuytren disease?**
- Cleland's ligament (which is dorsal to NV bundle)

**What are some indications to treat Dupuytren disease?**
- Pt unable to lay hand flat on table (Hueston test)
- MCP contracture >30°
- PIP flexion contracture

**What are some non-op treatment options for Dupuytren?**
- Collagenase injection (isolated from Clostridium histolyticum) + stretch the following day
    - May cause skin tears
- Percutaneous needle aponeurotomy - divides contracted cords
    - Provides better improvement in MCP>PIP
    - May cause neurovascular damage

**What are some operative treatment options for Dupurtyens?**
- Fasciotomy - cutting cords
- Limited fasciectomy- removal of diseased tissue of ray
- Radical fasciectomy- removal of all palmar + digital fascia (higher complications)

**What are some other operative treatment options that may be used for recurrent Dupuytrens?**

- Dermofasciectomy - removal of fascia + skin w/ coverage
- "Open palm" technique (McCash)- transverse skin incision + aponeurosis division

**Hand tumors covered in oncology section**

## Podcast episodes for a deeper dive

- Episode 7 w/ Dr. Fickle: Intro to distal radius fractures
  https://naileditortho.com/distalradiusintro/
- Episode 15 w/ Dr. Bilbrew: Carpal Tunnel Syndrome
  https://naileditortho.com/cts/
- Episode 50 w/ Dr. Rose: SLAC/SNAC wrist
  https://naileditortho.com/slac/
  Video: https://www.youtube.com/watch?v=xWpj9KR1r4w&t=2s
- Episode 53 w/ Dr. Dy: Intro to peripheral nerve injury and repair
  https://naileditortho.com/nerveinjury/
  Video: https://www.youtube.com/watch?v=Q7P9Ty-5KGE&t=4s
- Episode 55 w/ Dr. Roberts: Scaphoid fractures
  https://naileditortho.com/scaphoidfractures/
  Video: https://www.youtube.com/watch?v=BI2oVlbDsZ4&t=6s
- Episode 58 w/ Dr. Dacus: Flexor tendon injuries
  https://naileditortho.com/flexortendoninjuries/
- Episode 67 w/ Dr. Conti Mica: Cubital tunnel syndrome
  https://naileditortho.com/cubitaltunnelsyndrome/
- Episode 79 w/ Dr. Gray: 1st CMC arthritis
  https://naileditortho.com/cmcarthritis/
  Video: https://youtu.be/_5cYS_PZknI
- Episode 80 w/ Dr. Orbay: Volar plating of distal radius fractures
  https://naileditortho.com/drorbay/
  Video: https://www.youtube.com/watch?v=V2cUgFyJRYo

# Specific articles mentioned in the podcast

Lafontaine, M., Hardy, D., & Delince, P. H. (1989). Stability assessment of distal radius fractures. Injury, 20(4), 208-210.

Arora, R., Lutz, M., Deml, C., Krappinger, D., Haug, L., & Gabl, M. (2011). A prospective randomized trial comparing nonoperative treatment with volar locking plate fixation for displaced and unstable distal radial fractures in patients sixty-five years of age and older. Jbjs, 93(23), 2146-2153.

Soong, M., Earp, B. E., Bishop, G., Leung, A., & Blazar, P. (2011). Volar locking plate implant prominence and flexor tendon rupture. JBJS, 93(4), 328-335.

Doornberg, J. N., Buijze, G. A., Ham, S. J., Ring, D., Bhandari, M., & Poolman, R. W. (2011). Nonoperative treatment for acute scaphoid fractures: a systematic review and meta-analysis of randomized controlled trials. Journal of Trauma and Acute Care Surgery, 71(4), 1073-1081.

# NOTES

# NOTES

# NOTES

# PEDIATRICS CHAPTER 8

## Upper Extremity Peds

**What are some differences between adult and pediatric bones?**

- Pediatric bones- more elastic, thicker periosteum, bone remodeling due to open physis

**What is the Salter Harris classification?**

- Classification of physeal fractures
- Type I- Slip or physeal separation
- Type II- fx exits Above physis (Me-TWO-physeal)
- Type III- fx exits beLow physis
- Type IV- fx is Through metaphysis, epiphysis, and physis
- Type V- crush injury to physis

**What are some important notes in the evaluation, resuscitation, and transportation of pediatric Peds patients?**

- ABCDE's
- Intraosseous resuscitation if IV not possible
  - Kids remain hemodynamically stable then crash if not properly resuscitated
- Special transport bed w/ occiput cutout used for kids (big heads)

**What are some signs of non-accidental Peds (NAT)?**

- Skin bruises in different healing stages
- Retinal hemorrhages
- Multiple fractures in different healing stages
- Fracture in non-walking children
- Long bone/ head injuries

**What are some fracture patterns concerning for NAT?**

- Metaphyseal corner injuries (twisting/pulling leading to shear forces)
- Posterior rib fractures
- Transverse femur fractures

**What should you do if you suspect NAT?**

- Report it

**What is the likely injury when you suspect a medial clavicle fracture in a pediatric patient?**

- Physeal injury (physis doesn't close until close to 25 y/o)

**What is the treatment of a sternoclavicular dislocation?**

- Anterior - closed reduction, non- op
- Posterior - percutaneous reduction possibly w/ cardiothoracic surgeon on standby (fx impinges on vessels + mediastinum)

Ep 94 w/
Dr. Gibbons

**What is the typical treatment for a pediatric midshaft clavicle fx?**
- Non- op w/ sling
- Op- if open fx, floating shoulder, some recommend ORIF if significantly shortened (>2cm) + displaced (some studies still say non-op)

**Where is the majority of the growth of the humerus seen?**
- Proximal humerus ~80%

**What is the typical treatment for proximal humerus fractures?**
- Non op w/ sling
- Closed reduction if the fx is displaced > ⅔ of humeral diameter (biceps, deltoid, periosteum can impede reduction)
    - +/- pinning after reduction (beware pin migration + axillary n injury)
- Open reduction possibly needed

Peds 2: 1:00

**Up to what degree of angulation can be accepted for a humeral shaft fracture?**
- 30°
- Tx w/ splint/ functional brace/ sling

**What are the indications to operate on a pediatric humeral shaft fx?**
- Open fx, floating elbow

Ep 12 w/ Dr. Weiss

**What is the classification used for supracondylar humerus (SCH) fractures?**
- Gartland
- Type I- non displaced
- Type II- displaced w/ intact posterior hinge
- Type III- completely displaced w/ no hinge
- Type IV- completely displaced w/ no hinge and unstable in flexion / extension

**What are the most common nerves injured in flexion/extension type SCH injuries?**
- Extension - AIN
- Flexion - ulnar

**What are some radiographic lines used to evaluate SCH injuries?**
- Anterior humeral line (should bisect capitellum)
- Baumann angle (measures coronal plane reduction accuracy)
    - Bonus- radius should always line up with capitellum

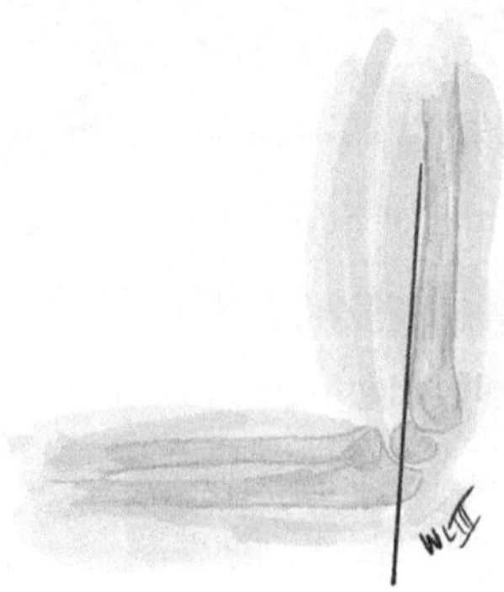

**Figure 8.1: Lateral view of the elbow showing the anterior humeral line. This should bisect the capitellum or run through the anterior ⅓.**

**What is the typical treatment for SCH fractures?**

- Type I- cast
- Type II- reduce + cast (some reduce + pin)
- Type III/IV + IV- reduce + pin

**What are the typical pin configurations and advantages to each?**

- Crossed pins (medial + lateral pins)- more biomechanically stable in a lab, + risk ulnar n injury
- Three lateral pins- comparable clinical stability

**What should you do if prior to surgery a patient had a well perfused hand w/ palpable pulse and after pinning, no palpable pulse but a pink, perfused hand?**

- Keep pins, cast + monitor

**What should you do if the extremity had pulses, and after you reduced + pinned you lost pulses and the hand is not perfused?**

- Remove pins + displace fx
- May need exploration

**What are some complications of SCH fx?**

- Cubitus varus
- Recurvatum
- Stiffness is rare (kids typically don't need physical therapy)
- Volkmann ischemic contracture (casted greater 90°)

**What should you be worried about in a kid w/ a SCH fx who is starting to need more and more pain medication?**

- Compartment syndrome

**What part of the elbow is first and last to ossify?**

- First- capitellum
- Last- lateral epicondyle

**What xray view can be used to evaluate lateral condyle fractures (in addition to AP/lateral)?**

- Internal oblique view

**What is the treatment for pediatric lateral condyle fractures?**

**Peds 3: 6:30**

- Non displaced- cast
- Minimally displaced- reduce + fixation (divergent pinning v screws) +/- arthrogram to assess joint congruity
    - Smooth pins may be preferred exam answer
- Displaced- ORIF w/ screws v plate

**Where does the blood supply to the lateral condyle come from?**

- Posterior (avoid posterior dissection)

**What are some complications seen w/ lateral condyle fx?**

- Cubitus valgus (+/- ulnar nerve palsy), capitellum osteonecrosis, lateral bone spurring

**What are the mechanisms associated with a medial epicondyle fracture?**

- Avulsions + elbow dislocations

**What is the absolute operative indication for a medial epicondyle fracture?**

- Fracture entrapped in joint
- Relative indication: throwing athlete/gymnast, displacement >5mm, elbow fx dislocation
- Tx: ORIF w/ screw fixation

**What other diagnosis should be on your mind with a suspected elbow dislocation in a patient <3y/o?**

- Distal humeral physeal fracture
- Arthrogram, MRI, or ultrasound can aid in diagnosis

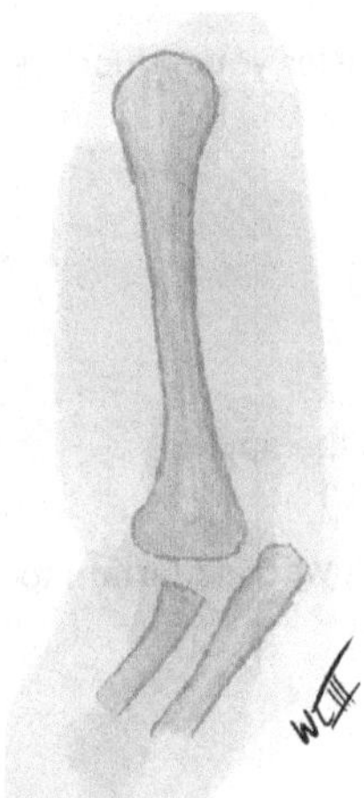

**Figure 8.2: AP view of the elbow showing a distal humeral physeal fracture. Note that the ulna does not line up with the distal humerus.**

**What is the treatment of a pediatric distal humeral physeal fracture?**

- Closed reduction + pinning
- If late diagnosis, don't close reduce - concern for physeal injury
- Associated with NAT**

**What is the typical mechanism for a pediatric proximal radius fracture?**

- Extension + valgus loading
- Elbow dislocation

**What are some closed reduction techniques for pediatric proximal radius fractures?**

- Elastic bandage- apply bandage and a spontaneous reduction may occur
- Patterson maneuver- traction + varus w/ elbow extended and supinated (+ direct pressure over radial head)
- Israeli technique- elbow flexed to 90° and taken from supination to pronation (+ direct pressure over radial head)

**What are some indications for surgical treatment of a proximal radius fracture?**

- >30° angulation, >3mm translation, <45° pronation/supination

**What are some treatment options for pediatric proximal radius fractures?**

- Wire fixation, flexible rod, ORIF if unstable fx

**What is an indication to operate on a pediatric olecranon fracture?**

- Intra articular displacement >3mm

**What is a nursemaid's elbow?**

- Subluxation of the orbicular ligament over the radial head
- Seen w/ longitudinal traction over the arm

**What is the treatment for a nursemaid's elbow?**

- Supinate forearm and flex past 90°, palpate radial head to feel reduction

**What is a greenstick fracture?**

- Incomplete diaphyseal forearm fx
- Tx: cast

**What are some indications for surgical treatment of a pediatric diaphyseal forearm fracture?**

- Angulation >15° if younger than 10
- Angulation >10° if older than 10

**What are the surgical indications for a pediatric Monteggia fracture?**

- Unstable fx (after reduction)
- Tx: IMN to maintain ulnar length, ORIF w/ plates

**What is a treatment for a chronic pediatric Monteggia fracture?**

- Ulnar osteotomy, radial head reduction + annular ligament reconstruction

**What is a buckle fracture of the distal forearm?**

- Impacted / torus fracture
- Tx: removable wrist splint vs cast

**What is the typical treatment for a distal metaphyseal forearm fracture in the pediatric patient?**

- Closed reduction + short arm casting

**What are some surgical indications for pediatric distal forearm fractures?**

- Malalignment after closed reduction
  - Metaphyseal- >20° angulation, bayonet apposition in kids >10
  - Physeal - residual displacement >50%
- Tx: percutaneous pinning

**What is a Seymour fracture?**

- Physeal fx of distal phalanx w/ nail bed laceration
- Germinal matrix becomes incarcerated
- Tx: I&D, nail removal + nail bed repair & fx reduction

## Lower Extremity Peds

**Can pediatric pelvis fractures be missed on AP pelvis?**

- Yes, 1/2 are identified on CT scan

**What are some operative indications for pediatric pelvis fractures?**

- Vertically unstable pelvis, displaced acetabular fracture >2mm, pelvic ring fx >2 cm displacement, bleeding control

**What are the pelvic avulsion fx areas and the associated muscle?**

- Iliac crest- abdominal muscles

- ASIS- sartorius
- AIIS- rectus femoris
- Ischium- hamstrings
- Lesser trochanter- iliopsoas
- Tx: non op <2 cm displacement

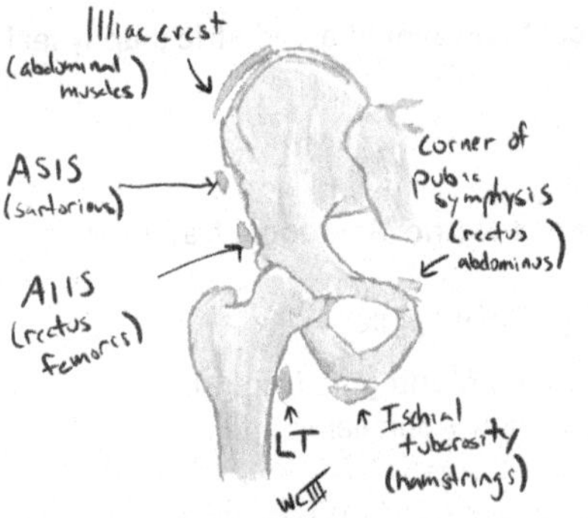


**Figure 8.3: AP of the pelvis showing common areas of avulsion fractures in adolescent patients.AIIS - Anterior inferior iliac spine. ASIS- anterior superior iliac spine.**

**What is the classification system for pediatric hip fx?**

- Delbet
- I- transepiphyseal +/- epiphyseal dislocation
- II- transcervical (MC)
- III- basicervical
- IV- intertrochanteric

**What is the typical treatment for a pediatric hip fracture?**

- Operative w/ different fixation options depending on fx severity
  - K wire fixation (type I), cannulated screws, pediatric hip screw, proximal femur locking plate (Type IV)
  - Fixation can extend across physis if needed
  - Anatomic reduction is most important*

**What are some complications s/p pediatric hip fracture?**

- Osteonecrosis, coxa vara + nonunion (when tx non op), leg length discrepancy (LLD)

**What is the majority blood supply to the pediatric femoral head?**

- Before 4 y/o- both medial/ lateral femoral vessels,
- After 4 y/o- mostly medial femoral circumflex (via retinacular branches)

Ep 34 w/ Dr. Heffernan

**What are the indications and tx for non-operative tx w/ a pediatric femur fx?**

- <6 y/o
- 0-6mo - pavlik harness
- 6mo- 5yrs- spica cast
  - Single leg spica cast assoc w/ good parent satisfaction compared w/ double spica cast
  - Shortening >3cm is relative contraindication to spica cast
  - Careful w/ applying short leg portion 1st then pulling traction- assoc w/ compartment syndrome

**What are the tx options for operative tx of a pediatric femur fx?**

- Titanium flexible IM rods- age 5-11y/o

  - Achieve 80% canal fill
  - Harder to control distal or comminuted fx
- Submuscular plating
  - Used for comminuted / length- unstable fx
  - Complications- refracture after removal, distal femur valgus
- Antegrade femoral nail- age >8-10 y/o or weight >50kg
  - Lateral trochanteric entry preferred (blood supply disruption w/ piriformis entry)
- Open plating/ ex fix also options (ex: damage control orthopaedics)

**What is the indication for operative treatment in a pediatric distal femur metaphyseal fx?**

- Displaced fx
- Tx: closed reduction + fixation (try not to cross physis)
  - Transverse lag screw avoid physis, smooth pins also an option
- Complication: malunion

**What is the indication for operative treatment of a distal femur physeal fx?**

- Displaced fx (nondisplaced SHI + SHII can be tx non-op)
- Tx: closed v ORIF, smooth K-wires if crossing physis
- Complications: growth arrest ~40%, LLD
  - Contralateral epiphysiodesis may be needed

**What is the most common type of patella fx in children?**

- Patella sleeve fx (chondral sleeve of patella separates from main portion of patella)
  - Patella alta may be seen on xrays
- Tx: non-displaced w/o extensor lag- non op, displaced >2mm - operative fixation

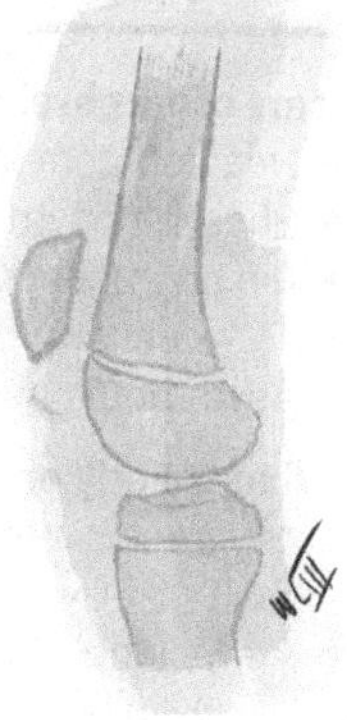

**Figure 8.4: Lateral view of a knee showing a displaced patella sleeve fracture. Note the patella alta.**

**What is the treatment of a displaced tibial spine fx?**

- ORIF + arthroscopic reduction
  - Anterior horn of medial meniscus often entrapped
- PE will be similar to ligamentous injury
- Non displaced or reducible fx can be tx non-op
- Complications: arthrofibrosis, ACL laxity, malunion w/ impingement

**What is the treatment of a displaced (>2mm) tibial tubercle fx?**

- ORIF w/ screws v suture re-attachment
- Complications: compartment syndrome (recurrent ant tib artery), genu recurvatum

**What can be seen after non-operative treatment of pediatric low energy proximal tibial metaphyseal fracture?**

- Genu valgum (Cozen phenomenon)
  - Most resolve spontaneously, no tx needed

Peds 5: 1:15

**What is the typical treatment for a closed tibial shaft fx?**

- Closed reduction + casting
  - WBAT in cast allowed
- Complications: loss of reduction > varus, if tibia +fibula fx > valgus
- Surgical tx w/: open fx, soft tissue injury, polyPeds, unacceptable reduction

**What is the order of distal tibia physis closure?**

- Centrally > posterior>medially> laterally

**What is a Tillaux fx?**

- SH III fx of anterolateral tibial epiphysis
  - Avulsion of AITFL
- Assoc w/ SER injuries
- Tx: closed reduction + CT > if contd displacement ORIF

**What is a triplane fx?**

- SH IV + AL fragment of distal tibia epiphysis + metaphyseal fx
- Tx: similar to Tillaux

**What type of ankle fx has the highest rate of growth arrest?**

- Medial mal SH IV fx, often result in varus LLD

## Pediatric spine

**What are some physical exam findings utilized when evaluating for scoliosis?**

- Head off center
- Shoulder asymmetry
- Rib prominence
- Trunk shift
- Asymmetric abdominal reflexes

Ep: 96 w/ Dr. Landrum

**What is Early onset Scoliosis (EOS)?**

- Scoliosis onset <age 10
- Typically left sided + male predominant*
- Includes: congenital scoliosis, infantile idiopathic scoliosis, juvenile scoliosis, etc

**What are some things on imaging you can use to evaluate scoliosis in young patients?**

- Cobb angle
- Rib vertebral angle distance (RVAD)

**What is the RVAD?**

- Measure of rotation, angle between the vertebrae and take off angle of the ribs

**What is congenital spine deformity due to?**
- Failure of segmentation – bar formation
- Failure of formation- wedge vertebrae, hemivertebrae
- Or mixed (both)
- Assoc w/ congenital anomalies: VACTERL, etc, - get MRI + cardiac echo + renal US

**Which congenital scoliosis deformity has the worst prognosis?**
- Unilateral bar w/ contralateral hemivertebrae

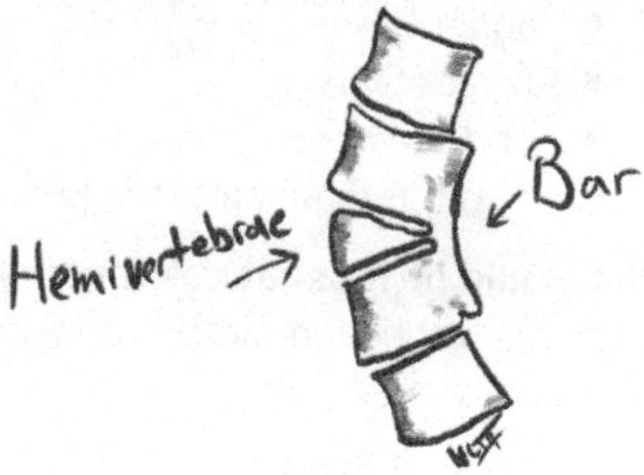


**Figure 8.5: Imaging showing a congenital bar with a contralateral hemivertebrae.**

**What are some operative indications for congenital scoliosis?**
- Progression >10 °
- High risk of progression
- Neuro deficits / declining respiratory function

**What are the operative treatment choices for congenital scoliosis?**
- Unilateral unsegmented bar- in situ arthrodesis (anterior or posterior)
- Segmented hemivertebrae- in situ anterior or A/P arthrodesis or contralateral hemiepiphysiodesis w/ hemiarthrodesis
- Hemivertebrae excision
- Vertebrectomy
- Growing rod constructs- improved results w/ lengthening Q6 months

**What is thoracic insufficiency syndrome (can't support normal respiration) associated with?**
- Idiopathic / congenital scoliosis
- Shortened thorax
- Rib fusions/ aplasia
- Poor growth

**Is congenital kyphosis good or bad?**
- Bad, high risk for neurologic compromise
- Tx: PSF, ASF/PSF

**What are some treatment options for pts w/ congenital scoliosis w/ thoracic insufficiency?**
- VEPTR / MAGEC expandable rods
  - Helps allow lung development
- +/- osteotomy for rib fusions
  - Opening wedge thoracostomy, hemithorax expansion, growth implants across hemithorax

**What are some treatment options for infantile (<3 y/o) idiopathic scoliosis?**
- Cobb <25°, RVAD <20° – observe
- Cobb 25-45°, RVAD >20°- MRI, cast/brace

- Careful w/ multiple anesthesia events
- Cobb >50°- operate (growing rods)
- Thoracic curve most common*

Episode 44 w/ Dr. Cho

**Is female or male incidence of AIS w/ curves worse than 30° more common?**
- Female, 10:1

Peds 7: 1:30

**What are some ways to assess the risk of curve progression in AIS?**
- Age of menarche
- Tanner Stage
- Risser stage
- Sanders stage
- Open triradiate cartilage presence

**Who would be most at risk for curve progression in AIS?**
- Pre menarche female, w/ tanner stage <3, Risser 0, open triradiate cartilage

**What is the Risser stage?**
- Classifies skeletal maturity based on ossification + iliac crest fusion
- Stage 0 – 5 (0= no apophysis, 5= fused apophysis)

**What is the Sanders score based on?**
- Classifies skeletal maturity based on hand xray
- 0-8

**What side curve is most common in AIS?**
- Right sided curve

**What are some indications to obtain an MRI in evaluation of AIS?**
- Left thoracic curve, neurological symptoms, apical kyphosis, rapid curve progression, pain, congenital anomalies

**What are some things you are looking for on MRI when evaluating for AIS?**
- Tethered cord, Chiari malformations, syringomyelia, spinal cord tumor, dysraphism (spina bifida)

**What are some factors that may contribute to curve progression?**
- Younger age (for test growth stops at- boys 16, girls 14)
- Larger curve magnitude
- Less skeletal maturity (Risser 1, sanders 1)
- Thoracic + double curves (opposed to lumbar and single)

**What is the treatment for AIS?**
- Curve <25° + skeletally immature- observe
- Curve 25-40° - skeletally immature- brace
- Curve <40° + skeletally mature- observe
- Curve >50°- operate

**What are some braces used for tx of AIS?**
- CTLSO (curve apex T7 and above)

- TLSO (Curve apex T8 and lower)
- Braces need to be worn about 16-23 hrs daily

**What are some surgical treatment options for AIS?**

- PSF w/ instrumentation
- PSF + ASF (possibly for younger pts w/ extreme curves)
  - +/- osteotomies if needed (ex: Ponte, Smith-Petersen), +/- vertebral column resections
    - See spine section for more spine osteotomy review

**What are some complications after PSF for AIS?**

- Pseudoarthrosis (pain + deformity worsening) – tx: revision PSF +/- grafting
- Delayed infection (C acnes + staph epi)– tx: implant removal + abx (try to keep implant if early infection)

**What are some causes of neuromuscular scoliosis?**

- Spinal muscular atrophy, muscle dystrophy, cerebral palsy, etc

**Is bracing as effective in neuromuscular scoliosis compared to AIS?**

- No

**What is the inheritance of neurofibromatosis?**

- Autosomal dominant
- Spine manifestations common

**What are the types of scoliosis seen in neurofibromatosis?**

- Non-dystrophic, dystrophic

**What are some characteristics of dystrophic neurofibromatosis?**

- Kyphoscoliosis
- Short sharp curves
- Rib pencilling (3 or more consecutive ribs is associated with rapid progression)
- Vertebral scalloping, enlarged foramina

**What is the treatment for dystrophic scoliosis seen in neurofibromatosis?**

- ASF + PSF w/ instrumentation
- Pseudoarthrosis w/ only PSF

**What is a sign of Scheuermann's kyphosis on xray?**

- >5° wedging on 3 consecutive vertebrae
- Schmorl's nodes
- Irregularities in the end plate
- Disc narrowing

**What is the treatment for Scheuermann's kyphosis?**

- 50-70°- bracing ~18 months tx
- >75° / progression/ neuro deficits- PSF w/ instrumentation w/ or w/o anterior release

**What should you be concerned about in a 14 y/o gymnast w/ low back pain and tight hamstrings?**

- Spondylolysis (pars interarticularis stress fx)

**What is the most sensitive test for spondylolysis in pts w/ normal xrays?**

- SPECT

**What is the Meyerding classification for spondylolisthesis?**

- Grading system based on forward slip of superior vertebrae
- Based on quadrants, grade V = Spondyloptosis (100%)

**What is the treatment for spondylolysis?**

- Symptomatic spondylosis + grade I/II spondylolisthesis- lumbosacral orthoses + PT / Activity modification
- Chronic - pars repair, fusion if disc desiccation

**What is the treatment for spondylolisthesis?**

- Non-op (Grade I or II) : PT, activity modification
- Operative: PSF w/ instrumentation (in situ for low slip %, high slip % +/- reduction)
  - Usually L4-S1
  - Careful L5 nerve root injury in L5-S1 slip

**What are the manifestations of Klippel-Feil syndrome?**

- C- spine segmentation failure (decreased ROM), Sprengel deformity, low hairline, scoliosis, short broad neck, torticollis, high scapula + jaw anomalies
- Basilar invagination

**What C-spine abnormalities are associated with down syndrome?**

- Atlanto Occipital hypermobility, atlantoaxial instability
  - Subaxial spine typically not affected

**What are some pediatric conditions where atlantoaxial instability is seen?**

- Down syndrome, Juvenile rheumatoid arthritis, dysplasias
- Tx w/ PSF if ADI >5mm
  - >10mm in down syndrome or symptomatic

**What is the tx of a down syndrome patient with ADI 5<10mm w/o symptoms?**

- Activity modification (ex avoid gymnastics)
- If ADI >5mm w/ symptoms- operative tx

**Can an os-odontoideum cause C1/C2 instability?**

- Yes, the odontoid process is separated from the body of axis
- Tx: if instability ADI >10mm, C1-C2 fusion
  - Limit contact sports

**What are some causes of atlanto-axial rotatory displacement?**

- Upper respiratory infection (Grisel syndrome), torticollis
- CT w/ fine cuts at C1/C2 can help show C1/C2 subluxation

**What is the initial treatment of atlanto-axial rotatory displacement?**

- NSAIDs, rest, soft collar
  - If sxs persist > 1 week- halter traction
  - If sxs persist >1 month- halo or rigid brace. PSF if neurologic involvement continued

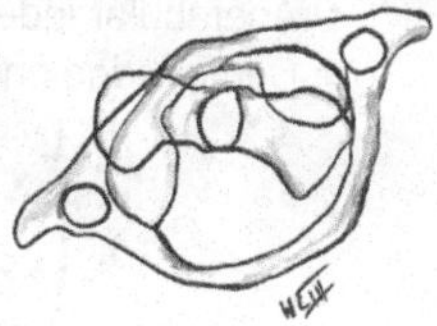

**Figure 8.6: An axial view of C1 and C2, showing atlanto-axial rotary displacement.**

**What are some causes of torticollis?**

- Congenital muscular torticollis, ophthalmologic, vestibular, tumor

**What is the initial treatment of congenital muscular torticollis?**

- Passive stretching
- If failed tx after 1 year- can tx w/ SCM release

**Is C2-3 pseudosubluxation a normal finding in pediatric patients?**

- Yes, it is an incidental finding
- Pay attention to spinal laminal line

**What is considered congenital cervical stenosis & its treatment?**

- Canal diameter <10mm
- Tx: asymptomatic- observe, symptomatic- surgery

# Pediatric hip

**What is the most common disorder of the hip in children?**

- Developmental dysplasia of the hip *DDH)
- Left hip most common
- Multifactorial

**What are the risk factors for DDH?**

Ep: 37 w/ Dr. Schmitz

- Breech presentation*, female, 1st born child, family history
- Intrauterine packaging disorders (ex: congenital knee dislocation, metatarsus adductus, etc)

**What are some physical exam findings seen in DDH?**

- Decreased abduction * sensitive
- Galeazzi test (knee is lower than contralateral knee)
- Ortolani (dislocated hip that is reducible)
- Barlow (reduced hip that is able to be dislocated/subluxed)

**What are some diagnostic imaging tests and findings used to evaluate DDH?**

- 0-6 months old- ultrasound
  - Normal alpha angle at 4-6 weeks- greater than 60° (line along iliac and acetabulum roof)
  - >50% femoral head diameter within acetabulum
- AP pelvis- ossific nucleus appears at 6 months

- Hilgenreiner line- horizontal line through triradiate cartilage
- Perkins line- perpendicular to Hilgenreiner line @ lateral acetabulum edge
- Shenton's line- medial border of femoral neck + superior border of obturator foramen
- Acetabular index- <25° normally, >30° w/ dysplasia
- Center edge angle >25° by age 6 is ideal

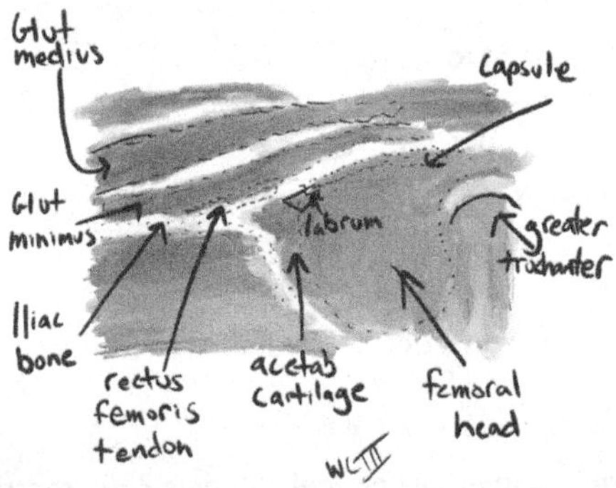


**Figure 8.7: A labeled ultrasound view of a hip. If oriented 90 degrees clockwise, it will look more like a coronal cut of the hip.**

Peds 9: 12:30

### What is the typical treatment of DDH?

- 0-6mo- pavlik harness
- 6-18 mo - closed v open reduction w/ spica casting
  - +/- arthrogram
- >3y/o- open reduction, +/- femoral osteotomy, +/- pelvic osteotomy

### What are some potential complications seen w/ pavlik harness tx?

- Femoral nerve palsy - excessive flexion (anterior straps)
- Osteonecrosis - excessive abduction (posterior straps)
- Pavlik harness disease (posterosuperior acetab rim deformation)- can be seen if hip doesn't reduce within 3-4 weeks, stop harness

### What are some possible blocks to an attempted closed reduction in a 12mo w/ DDH?

- Iliopsoas, adductors, joint capsule, ligamentum teres, pulvinar, transverse acetab ligament, inverted limbus
- Hip arthrogram used to confirm reduction, <5mm medial pooling of dye should be seen if hip reduced

### What is the typical treatment for a unilateral hip dislocation in children up to 10 y/o?

- Open reduction, +/- femoral shortening osteotomy
- Pelvic osteotomy may be needed
- Bilateral dislocation >age 6 - may leave alone

**What are some different types of pelvic reconstructive osteotomies used for DDH?**

- Redirection
  - Single innominate (salter)- hinges on pubic symphysis
  - Triple innominate (steele)- salter + superior/inf rami cuts
  - Ganz PAO- useful in skeletally mature patients w/ closed triradiate cartilage
    - Posterior column intact
- Reshaping (acetabuloplasty)
  - Pemberton, Dega, San Diego osteotomies

**What are some salvage osteotomies for DDH?**

- Chiari + shelf osteotomies
- These procedures rely on fibrocartilaginous metaplasia of interposed capsule

**What is the operative treatment for congenital coxa vara?**

- Indication: neck shaft angle 90° or less
- Valgus osteotomy

**What is idiopathic AVN of the proximal femur epiphysis?**

- Legg-Calve Perthes disease
- Leads to an aspherical femoral head
- More common in boys age 4-8
  - Presentation <6 y/o assoc w/ better prognosis
- May present w/ a limp and pain

**What are the stages of Perthes?**

- Initial -irritable hip
- Fragmentation - inc hip pain, segmental ossific nucleus collapse on xray
- Reossification- reparative, vascularity restored
- Residual- remodeling, minimal pain

**What does the Herring lateral pillar classification look at?**

- % loss of height
- A- none, C- >50% loss of height

**What is the treatment of Legg Calve-Perthes disease?**

- Supportive (+/- casting or bracing- goal is to contain femoral head)
- Femoral / pelvic osteotomies for later disease (Herring B, B/C)

**What is the typical presentation of a patient with a slipped capital femoral epiphysis (SCFE)?**

- Adolescent obese (or thin) male with a limp
- Hip / knee pain, obligate ER of the hip
  - Stable: they can ambulate
  - Unstable: unable to ambulate

Ep 32 w/ Dr. Gonzales

**Through what zone does SCFE happen?**
- Hypertrophic zone
- Femoral neck is displaced anteriorly and ER

**What is a radiographic clue that there is a SCFE?**
- Klein's line (tangential line to superior femoral neck border) does not intersect the proximal femoral epiphyses (it normally should)
- Also: widening of physis, blurring of proximal metaphysis
- Lateral xrays of the hip are sensitive to detect SCFE

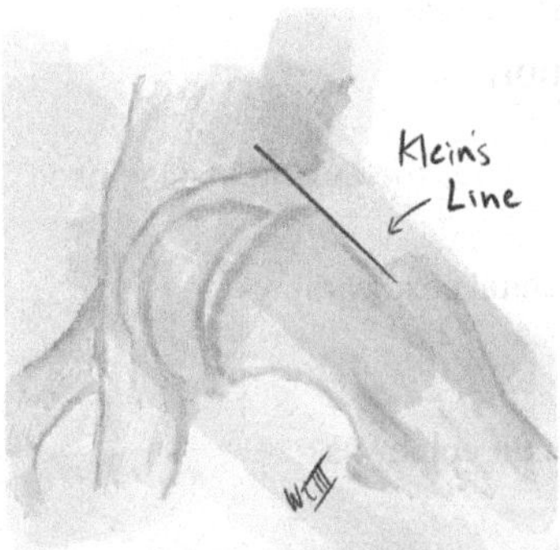


**Figure 8.8: A frog leg lateral of the left hip showing a SCFE. You can note Klein's line does not intersect the proximal femoral epiphyses.**

**What is the treatment for SCFE?**
- In situ pinning
  - 6.5 or larger screw, center center + perpendicular to physis
  - Other tx as well are but are controversial including: intracapsular hematoma decompression,open reduction, surgical hip dislocation
- w/u for endocrine abnormalities if <10 y/o

**What are some instances with pinning bilateral hips in pts w/ SCFE is indicated (prophylactic)?**
- Endocrinopathies (ex: renal osteodystrophy, thyroid disorders)
- Open triradiate cartilage/ young <10 y/o

**What are some complications seen w/ SCFE?**
- Chondrolysis (hardware penetration)
- Impingement w/ residual deformity
- Osteonecrosis

## Pediatric Foot

**(See foot and ankle section for similar topics covered)**

Ep 41 w/ Dr. Gantsoudes

**What is the deformity seen in clubfoot?**
- Hindfoot equinus + varus, midfoot + forefoot adduction and cavus
- Navicular is subluxed medially + plantar on talus

**What gene plays a role in clubfoot?**
- PITX 1- TBX 4 transcriptional pathway (assoc w/ hindfoot formation)

Peds 11: 5:00

**What are some conditions clubfoot is associated with?**
- Arthrogryposis, myelomeningocele, amniotic band syndrome, diastrophic dysplasia
  - More difficult to treat in these conditions

**What is the treatment for clubfoot?**

- Ponseti casting
- Fix cavus, adductus, varus, then equinus last (percutaneous achilles tenotomy)
- Foot abduction orthosis used after casting
  - Brace compliance is assoc w/ better outcomes*
- Recurrence: repeat manipulation + bracing
  - Posteromedial release if necessary

**What is the treatment of choice for a patient w/ a hx of club foot now with dynamic supination?**

- Anterior tibialis to lateral cuneiform transfer
- Pts are weight bearing on lateral foot due to the supination during swing phase

**What xray do you get to view and eval for congenital vertical talus?**

- Lateral xray in plantar flexion
- 1st MT axis is above talus (navicular not yet ossified)

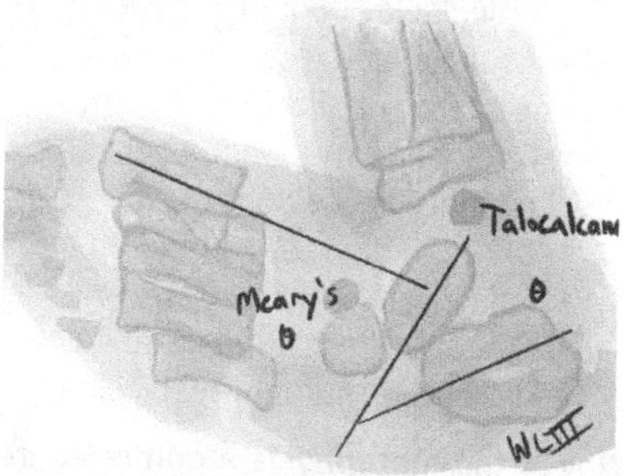


**Figure 8.9: A lateral view of a pediatric ankle, showing a congenital vertical talus.**

**What is the treatment for congenital vertical talus?**

- Reverse Ponseti method casting
- Reduction of dorsal navicular dislocation on talus> foot stretched into plantarflexion + inversion> release + pinning of TN joint + achilles tenotomy
- 50% are due to genetic or neuromuscular causes

**What is the cause and treatment of calcaneovalgus foot?**

- Hyperdorsiflexion of foot due to intrauterine positioning
- Tx: observe, stretching (if anything)
  - Tarsal coalition, pes planovalgus, cavovarus feet covered in FA section

# Infections

**How can a child with a musculoskeletal infection present?**

- Limp, refusal to bear weight, recent URI, febrile, skin warmth, TTP, joint held in a position than maximizes joint volume (hip in FABER)
- Inc: CBC, ESR, CRP

**Ideally when should blood cultures and joint synovial analysis be performed?**

- Before antibiotics start if pt is clinically ok

- Send analysis for PCR in pts <5 y/o (*Kingella*)

**What imaging is useful and what are you looking for when evaluating for pediatric MSK infection?**

- Xray: if septic arthritis- joint effusion; if osteomyelitis- at 1 week new periosteal bone formation + osteolysis
- Ultrasound- may identify subperiosteal abscess
- MRI w/ + w/o contrast: abscesses, myositis, effusion, osteomyelitis (edema)
- Technetium 99 bone scan- may show areas of multifocal infection

**What are some differential diagnoses for suspected pediatric MSK infection (septic arthritis/ osteomyelitis)?**

- Septic arthritis- cell count >50k
- Toxic synovitis- cell count 5-15k
- Juvenile idiopathic arthritis- autoimmune, rash, fever x2 weeks, polyarticular, cell count 15-80k
- Acute leukemia- anemia/ thrombocytopenia/ neutropenia in 80% pts, immature leukocytes on smear
- Osteosarcoma - metaphyseal lesion w/ mixed lytic + sclerotic components, more normal labs
- Chondroblastoma- localized tenderness, well demarcated epiphyseal lytic lesion
- Metastatic neuroblastoma- elevated homovanillic acid or vanillylmandelic acid, metaphyseal lesion

**Why is the metaphysis a common area for infection in acute hematogenous osteomyelitis?**

- Slower capillary blood flow allows bacteria to exit vessel walls

**What is the most common pathogen in pediatric MSK infection?**

- *Staphylococcus aureus*
  - <1 y/o consider GBS
  - 1-5 y/o consider *K. kingae*, *Strep pneumoniae*

**What makes MRSA different from MSSA?**

- mecA gene is transferred to S aureus > penicillin-binding protein w/ low affinity for beta-lactam abx
- w/ MRSA: inc hospital stay, inc risk DVT, more soft tissue destruction
  - Panton-Valentine leukocidin (PVL) cytotoxin assoc w/ more severe infections

**What are some other organisms that cause pediatric MSK infections?**

- *K. kingae* (<4, PCR test)
- *Tuberculosis* (acid fast bacilli)
- *Borrelia burgdorferi* (Lyme disease, erythema migrans, reactive arthritis, cardiac arrhythmia, ELISA test for antibodies, confirm w/ Western blot)

- *N gonorrhoeae* (sexually active, adolescents, culture on chocolate blood agar)
- *Candida* + coccidioides (fungi)

**What are the indications for operative tx in pediatric MSk infections?**

- Abscess formation, septic arthritis, failure to respond to non-op treatment (abx)
- If pts get I&D and get worse 3 days after, repeat MRI to assess for any osteo

## Neuromuscular Disease

**What is cerebral palsy?**

- A static encephalopathy due to brain injury by damage, defectiveness, or illness
- Leads to peripheral manifestations (contractures, etc)

**What are risk factors for CP?**

- Brain ischemia/ hemorrhage, low birth weight, TORCH infections, prematurity

**What is a positive predictive factor for walking in kids with CP?**

- Standing + sitting independently by 2 y/o

**What is the physiologic classification of CP?**

- Spastic- inc tone or rigidity w/ rapid stretching- most often benefit from ortho intervention*
- Dyskinetic/ choreoathetoid- involuntary movements + dystonia (seen less often)
- Ataxia - decreased balance + coordination
- Mixed- spasticity + dyskinesia

**What is the Gross Motor and Functional Classification System?**

- A system to assess level of funcion
  - I- walks indoors/outdoors
  - II-limited on uneven surfaces
  - III- walker/wheelchair required for long distances
  - IV- mostly wheelchair/walker dependent
  - V- no independent mobility, wheelchair bound, poor head control

**What is the anatomic classification of cerebral palsy?**

- Quadriplegia - 4 limbs affected
- Whole body- four limbs + bulbar problems (swallowing)
- Hemiplegia- one side of body
- Diplegia - lower extremity>UE
  - Most often assoc w/ prematurity, periventricular leukomalacia, low birth weight

**What is spasticity?**

- Velocity dependent increase in muscle tone

**What are some non-surgical treatment options for CP?**

- PT- address gait
- OT- address fine motor function
- Speech therapy- for kids w/ bulbar involvement
- Splint/casting- contractures/ spasticity
- Bracing- AFO's, KAFOs (knee ankle foot orthroses)
- Medications

**What are some medications used for treatment of CP and their MOA?**

- Baclofen- GABA agonist- decreases release of excitatory neurotransmitters
  - Oral- may need to adjust dose
  - Intrathecal- given w/ pump, requires less sedation (used w/ non ambulators)
- Botulinum toxin- block presynaptic release of acetylcholine at NM junction
- Diazepam

**What are some complications associated w/ baclofen?**

- Withdrawal sxs- febrile, spasticity increase, rhabdomyolysis
- Wound problems

**What does selective dorsal rhizotomy do?**

- Decreases spasticity by severing dorsal nerve rootlets between L1 and S1
- Useful in 3-8 y/o w/ spastic diplegia w/ GMFCS I/II
- Complications: scoliosis, spondylolisthesis, hip subluxation

**Where is the hip wear in the acetabulum in CP patients with hip subluxation?**

- Posterosuperior
- Evaluate hips using the Reimer migration percentage

**What is crouch gait seen in CP?**

- Hip flexion, knee flexion, ankle dorsiflexion
- Tx:
  - Non op- ground reaction AFO
  - Op:psoas/ hamstring lengthening, foot/femur osteotomies

**What is the treatment for foot deformities seen in CP? (ex: equinovalgus/ varus, planovalgus, hallux valgus)**

- Bracing 1st
- Flexible deformity- soft tissue
- Rigid deformity- bony procedure

**What tendon transfers could you do for a CP patient with an flexible equinovarus foot?**

- Hindfoot varus- split post tib

- Dynamic supination in swing- split tib ant
- (achilles lengthening for equinus)

**What are the surgical treatment options for CP patients w/ hip subluxation >50%?**

- <8 y/o w/ <60% subluxation- adductor tenotomy, iliopsoas release
- <8 y/o w/ >60% subluxation- varus femoral osteotomy +/- pelvic osteotomy (Dega or San Diego)
- > 8 y/o w/ >40% subluxation- varus femur osteotomy +/- pelvic osteotomy (Dega or San Diego)
- Bilateral non ambulatory- bilateral proximal femur osteotomy

**What are some treatment options for a symptomatic failed hip recon or hip arthritis in a CP patient?**

- Subtroch valgus osteotomy + femoral head resection, proximal femur resection + interposition arthroplasty, prosthetic arthroplasty

**Does bracing typically help stop progression in CP patients with scoliosis?**

- No, spinal fusion for curves >50°
  - Higher complication rate

**What is myelomeningocele?**

- Protrusion of dura + spinal cord due to failure of neural fold closure
- Initial tx: closure +/- VP shunt if hydrocephalus or chiari malformation
- Many have a latex allergy

**What should you do in a patient w/ a hx of myelomeningocele closure now w/ inc spasticity + scoliosis?**

- Repeat MRI (recurrent hydrocephalus, VP shunt malformation, syrinx, tethered cord)

**What is the classification of myelomeningocele based on?**

- Lowest intact functional neurological level
- Ex: L4- has intact knee extension/ankle dorsiflexion, ambulates, tx w/ AFO (no intact ankle plantarflexion)

**What is the management for hip subluxation in patients w/ myelomeningocele?**

- Observation if this occurs at mid lumbar level or proximal
  - Assoc w/ a high recurrence rate
- Possible operative tx if unilateral dislocation in ambulator w/ low-level lesion

**How do patients w/ a hx of a myelomeningocele present w/ a fx?**

- Hot, red swollen leg
- Get xrays, splint

**What are some types of muscular dystrophies?**

- Duchenne (DMD), becker, facioscapulohumeral, myotonic, limb-girdle

**Peds 13: 18:30**

**What is the inheritance of DMD + some manifestations?**

- X linked recessive- absent dystrophin

- + gower sign (uses hands to rise from floor), toe walking, calf pseudo-hypertrophy, inc lumbar lordosis
- Elevated CK levels

**What is a medication that can be used to treat DMD?**

- Corticosteroid therapy- Deflazacort
  - Decreases risk of scoliosis development
  - High risk of complications + steroid side effects

**Does bracing help in DMD patients with scoliosis?**

- No, may require surgery due to pulmonary complications
- PSF if > 30° + do before FVC <35%
  - Pts may get anesthesia induced rhabdomyolysis

**What is the inheritance for Becker muscular dystrophy?**

- X linked recessive, lower dystrophin, later onset than DMD

**What is the inheritance of spinal muscular atrophy and its manifestations?**

- Autosomal recessive- survival motor neuron I mutation on chromosome 5q
- Proximal limb, trunk, bulbar weakness, tongue fasciculations, scoliosis, hip subluxation

**What are some treatment options for SMA?**

- Nusinersen (Spinraza)- inc functional survival motor neuron SMN protein
- Gene therapy

**What is the inheritance and manifestations of Charcot-Marie-Tooth Disease type I?**

- Autosomal dominant, duplication of peripheral myelin protein 22 gene on chromosome 17
- Absent reflexes, distal intrinsic muscle weakness (see F/A section for foot manifestations)

**What condition is noted by multiple rigid joints with static contractures?**

- Arthrogryposis multiplex congenita

**What condition is noted by ataxia, areflexia, weakness and a positive extensor plantar response?**

- Friedrich ataxia
- Cardiomyopathy, diabetes, and deafness common
- Mutation is repetition of GAA in FXN gene on chromosome 9q13

## Limb growth + Congenital Deformities

**What limb length discrepancy (LLD) length is typically tolerated?**

- Up to 2 cm (no tx of shoe lift is symptoms)
- <2cm may lead to back + hip pain

**At what ages do we assume (for test) growth ends?**

- 14 y/o girls
- 16 y/o boys

**How many mm of growth is contributed from the different parts of the lower extremity?**

- Proximal femur -3mm
- Distal femur- 9mm
- Proximal tibia- 6mm
- Distal tibia- 5mm

**What are some treatment options for a predicted LLD?**

- <2 cm- shoe lift
- 2-5 cm- contralateral epiphysiodesis, shortening (skeletally mature)
- >5-6 cm - limb lengthening (osteotomy, ex fix, IMN)

**How long does physiologic varus and valgus go on for?**

- Varus ~ 2 years
- Valgus 5-6 years

**What is the most common cause of pathologic genu varum?**

- Tibia vara (Blount disease)
  - Infants- excessive medial pressure> physis + epiphysis osteochondrosis>physeal bar
  - Adolescent - varus thrust> inhibition of medial physeal growth (Hueter- Volkman principle

**What do you assess on xrays for blount disease?**

- Metaphyseal- diaphyseal angle
  - <10°- 95% chance bowing resolves
  - >16°- 95% chance bowing progresses

**What is the treatment for Blount disease?**

- Infantile: 2-3 y/o + mild disease- bracing
- Infantile: >3y/o - severe disease- surgical overcorrection - proximal tibia osteotomy + bar resection if present
- Adolescent blount: 15-18 mo growth remain, hemiepiphysiodesis (proximal lateral tibia)
  - Severe deformity- proximal tibia osteotomy

**What is the tx of genu valgum?**

- Observe most, shouldn't increase after 7 y/o
- Operative options: hemiepiphysiodesis, varus producing osteotomy

**What is the typical treatment for femoral anteversion and internal tibial torsion (measure prone)?**

- Non-op, patient education
- Operative options: derotational osteotomy if >8 and severe deformity

**What are the types of tibial bowing and their associations?**

- Anterolateral bowing- neurofibromatosis
- Posteromedial bowing- calcaneal valgus foot
- Anteromedial bowing- fibular deficiency

Peds 15: 3:00

**What is the typical treatment for the different types of tibial bowing?**

- AL- brace (clamshell orthosis)
  - If pseudoarthrosis develops- IMN, bone transport, grafting
- PM- monitor, may develop LLD down the line (avg 4cm)
- AM- amputation if foot nonfunctional, LLD 10%- engthen, LLD >30% amputation

**What gene is longitudinal femoral deficiency associated with?**

- Sonic hedgehog gene

**What is proximal femoral focal deficiency) associated with?**

- Deficient cruciate ligaments, fibular hemimelia, absent lateral rays
- Tx: projected LLD <20cm- lengthening, LLD>20cm - amputation + prosthesis vs Van Ness rotationplasty (ankle converted to functional knee)

**What is fibular deficiency associated with?**

- Femoral deficiency, cruciate ligament deficiency, coxa vara, genu valgum, ball & socket ankle joint, tarsal coalition, absent rays

**What is the only lower limb deficiency w/ a defined inheritance pattern?**

- Tibial deficiency- autosomal dominant
  - Tx dependent on knee function
    - If present> BKA or syme
    - If none> knee disarticulation

**What is associated with congenital dislocation of the knee?**

- DDH + clubfoot
- Tx: stretching followed by casting
- Address knee prior to hip if DDH is present

**What is the treatment for congenital patellar dislocation?**

- Lateral release + realignment

**What is the difference between Osgood-Schlatter and Sinding-Larsen Johanson syndrome?**

- Osgood schlatter- tibial tubercle
- Sinding- Larsen- inferior pole of patella
- Tx: symptomatic tx

**What is the best view to diagnose osteochondritis dessicans?**

- Notch view, MRI good to evaluate extent
- Tx: open physis- non-op, limit activities
  - Operate- skeletally mature + cartilage disruption, lesion >2cm

## Upper extremity deformities

**A disruption in what signal leads to transverse deficiency of the upper extremity?**

- AER (responsible for proximal/distal orientation during development)

**What is the most common congenital anomaly of the elbow?**

- Congenital elbow dislocation
- Radial head is dome shaped,
- Tx: observe in kid (asymptomatic), if adult + symptomatic consider radial head resection

**Disruption of what gene product leads to radial longitudinal deficiency syndrome?**

- ZPA or Sonic hedgehog
- Failure to form radial side of forearm, writs + hand
- Tx options: stretching, centralization, ex fix distraction, ulnar osteotomy, thumb reconstruction
  - Dont do if elbow contracture or older patient (compensated)

**What syndromes are assoc w/ radial longitudinal deficiency?**

- VACTERL, Holt-Oral - cardiac defects, thrombocytopenia, fanconi's anemia
- Get CBC, echo, renal US, chromosomal karyotyping to screen for assoc syndromes

**Is hypoplastic thumb considered a part of radial deficiency?**

- Yes, its assoc w/ the same conditions

**What is the treatment for hypoplastic thumb?**

- If CMC stable> reconstruction
- If CMC unstable> index pollicization

**What is the tx for trigger thumb?**

- Spontaneously resolve 30-65%, A1 pulley release

**What is seen in Sprengel's deformity?**

- Failure of scapular descent, high small scapula, diminished abduction, UE anomalies
- Assoc w/ Klippel- Feil syndrome
- Tx: observe, woodward procedure (distal advancement)

**What are some UE deformity conditions due to failure of differentiation?**

- Radioulnar synostosis- limited ROM but typically functionally ok, hand pronated (Sx if bilateral)
- Syndactyly- apoptosis failure, assoc w/ Poland (absent sternal pec major) + Apert's + Carpenter's syndrome- tx: release digits
- Symphalangism- failure of differentiation of IP joint- observe
- Camptodactyly- digital flexion contracture
- Clinodactyly- digital angulation

- Delta phalanx- physis not perpendicular to long axis

**What is the tx of preaxial polydactyly (thumb)?**

- Surgical reconstruction, RCL ligament reconstruction, + thumb realignment

**What is postaxial polydactyly?**

- Duplication of ulnar most digit
- Autosomal dominant, more common in african americans
- Tx options: excision/ suture ligation, reconstruction

**What are some risk factors for brachial plexus birth palsy?**

- Macrosomia, shoulder dystocia, multiparous pregnancy
- Erbs palsy- C5-C6 +/- C7- better prognosis- waiters tip
- C8-T1- assoc w/ horner's- poor prognosis- claw hand
- Worst prognosis: preganglionic lesion
- Biceps return by 2 months- better prognosis*

## Syndromes & Dysplasias

Peds 17: 1:15

**What is the most common chromosomal disorder and some of its manifestations?**

- Down syndrome
- Atlantoaxial instability, inc SCFE risk, hip + patellar instability

**What condition is noted in a patient w/ blue sclera, hearing loss, and a hx of multiple fx?**

- Osteogenesis imperfecta, COL1A or IA2 mutation (glycine substitution)
- Inc risk malignant hyperthermia
- Tx: bisphosphonates used to dec fx incidence

**What is the most common skeletal dysplasia and what characterizes it (including etiology)?**

- Achondroplasia
- Rhizomelic limbs, genu varum, decreasing interpediculate distance from L1-L5, foramen magnum stenosis, thoracolumbar kyphosis, frontal bossing
- FGFR3 mutation, autosomal dominant, defect in endochondral bone formation (proliferative zone)

**What are some other conditions that FRFR3 is mutated?**

- Achondroplasia, hypochondroplasia, thanatophoric dysplasia
- Remember it's a mutation in the RECEPTOR

**What is the gene defect seen in cleidocranial dysplasia?**

- CBFA1 (defect in intramembranous ossification)
  - Absent clavicles, etc

**What are the treatments for some of the manifestations of achondroplasia?**

- Genu varum- observe, osteotomy if needed + symptomatic + progression
- Foramen magnum stenosis- screen infants (may result in sudden death)
- Thoracolumbar kyphosis- most resolves w/ walking, PSF curve >50°

**What is the difference between achondroplasia + pseudoachondroplasia?**

- Normal facial appearance, severe limb malalignment, odontoid hypoplasia, (both have rhizomelic limbs)
- Mutation: COMP (cartilage oligomeric protein)

**What condition characterized by cauliflower ear, hitchhiker thumb, cleft palate, w/ short stature and rhizomelic limbs?**

- Diastrophic dysplasia (DTDST- sulfate transporter) gene mutation
- Autosomal recessive
- May also have clubfoot + other MSK manifestations

**What characterizes multiple epiphyseal dysplasia and what is the gene mutation?**

- Abnormal epiphysis ossification
- COMP, COL9A2
- May have short stature, hip resemble perthes but are bilateral + simultaneous

**What condition is noted by multiple joint dislocations (hips, knees, shoulder, radial head, etc)?**

- Larsen syndrome
- Autosomal dominant
- May also have clubfoot and cervical kyphosis (screen c spine)

**What is the mode of inheritance for the mucopolysaccharidoses?**

- Autosomal recessive
- EXCEPT for Hunter syndrome - X linked recessive
- Multiple manifestations: inc carpal tunnel syndrome, limb malalignment, proportionate dwarfism

**Morquio syndrome results in an accumulation of what substance?**

- Keratin sulfate
- Pts also have odontoid hypoplasia, hip dysplasia, other MSK abnormalities
- Get c-spine xrays

**What condition would you be concerned about in a 2 y/o w/ long bone bowing, metaphyseal cupping, and increased physeal width?**

- Rickets

**What are the types of inheritance for familial hypophosphatemic rickets?**

- X linked dominant- PHEX mutation
- Autosomal dominant- FGF-23 mutation

- Autosomal recessive- dentin matrix protein I mutation

**What is the defect seen in hypophosphatasia?**

- Defect in alkaline phosphatase
- Low alkaline phosphatase + high urinary phosphoethanolamine

**What condition would you be concerned about in a patient with anterolateral tibia bowing, hemihypertrophy, and scoliosis?**

- Neurofibromatosis, autosomal dominant
- NF1 gene mutation
- Also cafe- au-lait macules, optic gliomas + other manifestations

**What condition would you be concerned about in a 15M w/ pectus excavatum, acetabuli protrusio, scoliosis, long digits, and flatfeet?**

- Marfans, Fibrillin- 1
- Increase TGF-b
- Autosomal dominant

**What would you be concerned about in a pt with hyperelastic skin, ligamentous laxity, and poor wound healing?**

- Ehlers danlos syndrome, 90% due to type V collagen disorders
- Aortic root dilation

## Podcast episodes for a deeper dive

- Episode 12 w/ Dr. Weiss: Intro to supracondylar humerus fractures https://naileditortho.com/suprahumerus/
- Episode 22 w/ Dr Payares Lizano: Intro to Cerebral Palsy https://naileditortho.com/cerebralpalsy/
- Episode 32 w/ Dr. Gonzales https://naileditortho.com/32-pediatric-hip-pain-w-dr-gonzales/
- Episode 34 w/ Dr. Heffernan: Pediatric femur fractures https://naileditortho.com/pedsfemur/
  Video: https://youtu.be/b_ni2Pm9u6c
- Episode 37 w/ Dr. Schmitz: Developmental dysplasia of the hip https://naileditortho.com/ddh/
- Episode 41 w/ Dr. Gantsoudes: Clubfoot https://naileditortho.com/clubfoot/
- Episode 44 w/ Dr. Cho: Adolescent Idiopathic Scoliosis https://naileditortho.com/ais/
  Video: https://www.youtube.com/watch?v=x5-tut6-zUg
- Episode 94 w/ Dr. Gibbons: Pediatric Upper Extremity Peds https://naileditortho.com/pedsfractures/
  Video: https://youtu.be/c9eWsvfDKF4
- Episode 96 w/ Dr. Landrum: Early Onset Scoliosis https://www.naileditortho.com/eos

# NOTES

# NOTES

# PATHOLOGY CHAPTER 9

## Overview + treatment principles

**Remember to review imaging for this section!**

**What are some important aspects of the history to note when evaluating an oncologic patient?**

- Age
- Pain (night pain better w/ NSAIDS- osteoid osteoma, pathologic fx, painless- many soft tissue sarcomas)
- Presence of a mass
- Rate of growth (rapid may suggest malignancy)
- Family history (ex: neurofibromatosis)
- Hx of trauma (myositis ossificans)

**What are some questions you should ask when evaluating xrays in tumor patients?**

- Location? (epiphysis, metaphysis, diaphysis, flat bone, spine)
- What is the tumor doing to the bone?
  - Erosion, lysis, expanding cortex
- What is bone doing to the tumor?
  - Rim of calcium/bone more likely to be slow growing tumor as bone has had time to contain it
  - Onion skinning - bone multiple attempts to contain tumor but tumor keeps breaking through and expanding, seen classically in Ewings
  - Codman's triangle - lifting of the periosteum and calcification, seen classically in osteosarcoma
- What is the lesion matrix?
  - Lytic, blastic, both

**What are some common epiphyseal tumors?**

- Adults: clear cell chondrosarcoma, mets, myeloma, lymphoma
- Children: chondroblastoma, eosinophilic granuloma, giant cell tumor

**What are some common metaphyseal tumors?**

- Metastases (adults), osteosarcoma (adolescents), chondrosarcoma, giant cell tumor (can extend to epiphysis)

**What are some common diaphyseal tumors?**

- A- Adamantinoma
- E- Eosinophilic granuloma
- I- Infection - not technically tumor, but always considered in differential
  - Some teach that you should culture every biopsy, and biopsy every culture

- O- Osteoid osteoma (OO)/ Osteoblastoma (OB)
- U- Ewing's (U-wings)
- Y- fibrous dYsplasia, lYmphoma, mYeloma

**What are some common bone tumors in kids?**

- 0-5 y/o: langerhans cell histiocytosis, metastatic disease (neuro-blastoma, rhabdomyosarcoma), leukemia
- 5-10: Ewing's
- 11-18: osteosarcoma, ewing sarcoma

**What are locations within the bone where tumors can occur?**

- Central (ex: enchondroma, bone cysts)
- Eccentric (ex: GCT, chondrosarcoma, osteosarcoma)
- Cortical (ex:NOF, osteoid osteoma, adamantinoma, brodie's abscess)
- Juxtacortical - (ex: periosteal chondrosarcoma, parosteal osteosarcoma)

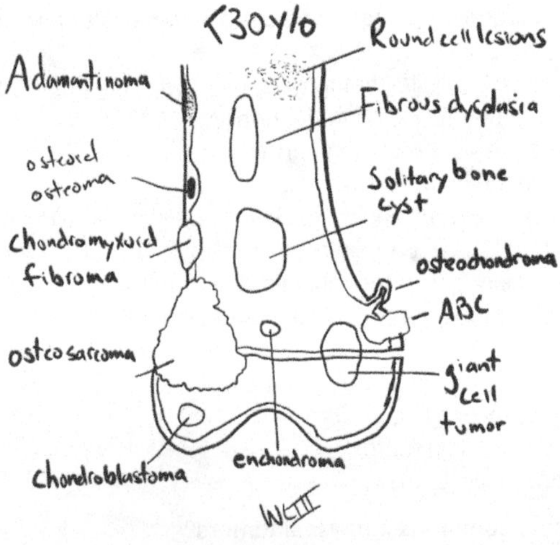


**Figure 9.1: An image showing common places for tumors in patients <30 y/o. ABC- Aneurysmal bone cyst**

**What are some common spine tumors?**

- Anterior elements- GCT, mets, osteosarcoma
- Posterior elements- ABC, OO/OB, osteochondroma

**What are some types of appearances of tumors on xray as they interact w/ the bone?**

- Geographic - sharp borders + zone of transition
  - Usually benign, more sclerosis- less active area
- Moth eaten- less well defined
- Larger zone of transition from normal -> abnormal

- Permeative- can't make out borders, more malignant
  - Can't delineate where tumor begins/ ends

**How do tumors that have a cartilage matrix grow?**

- In a lobular/ ball like manner
- Calcification occurs around the periphery- rings and arcs appearance on xray
- Dedifferentiation on xray- ex: ring + arc calcifications next to a lytic bone lesion

**How do bone forming tumors / ossification look like on xrays?**

- Cloud like, fluffy, marble like
- Soft tissue mass w/ mineralization + forming bone- think osteosarcoma

**What are some tumors where you may see internal trabeculations on xray?**

- GCT, nonossifying fibroma, hemangioma
- Residual trabeculae or new bone formation due to adjacent tumor

**What are some examples of periosteal reactions seen w/ tumors?**

- Continuous - periosteal reaction never broken, solid
- Interrupted- worrisome patterns
- Perpendicular - hair on end
- Divergent - sunburst
- Lamellated - onion skinning
- Codman triangle

**What is a clue you can use to differentiate periosteal reaction between infection + Ewings?**

- Infection / Langerhans cell histiocytosis- single thick layer of periosteal reaction- more likely to be benign
- Ewing sarcoma- lamellated (onion skinning) periosteal reaction- more likely to be malignant

**What are some other things you can note on xrays in different tumors?**

- Endosteal scalloping- chondrosarcoma
- Punched out lesions- myeloma, Langerhans Cell Histiocytosis
- Ground glass appearance- fibrous dysplasia

**What are some other modalities that can be obtained to help diagnose and stage tumors?**

- CT scan (good for osteoid osteoma)
- MRI entire bone involved- eval soft tissue mass (T1- eval anatomy, T2- eval pathology)
- Whole body Tc99 bone scan
- 18F- FDH- glucose transported intracellularly
- PET (useful in lymphomas)
- CT chest - evaluate for metastases
- Labs

**What are the different types of biopsy?**

- Needle biopsy (can be used to confirm suspected diagnosis)
    - Fine needle aspiration- aspirates tumor cells
    - Core needle aspiration- larger needle, core of tissue removed
- Open incisional biopsy (more accurate than needle biopsy, but requires trip to OR)
- Excisional biopsy (remove mass in its entirety and then send to pathology)

**What are some incisional biopsy principles?**

- Same incision as planned resection
    - Core needle biopsy has a lower chance of recurrence within the biopsy tract if the biopsy tract is NOT removed. Example, if the interventional radiologist performing biopsy does core needle not in your planned incision line, only ~2% of tumors recur at the biopsy tract, so low chance of tumor contamination with core needle.
- Longitudinal incisions (transverse for clavicle)
- Avoid critical structures
- Biopsy soft tissue component of tumor
- Intramuscular approach - only contaminate singe muscle rather than multiple
- Hemostasis

**What are some of the different types of resection margins?**

- Radical - resecting entire compartment
    - Not commonly done anymore now that neoadjuvant radiation is more of a standard of care
- Wide- cuff of normal tissue, no tumor cells (standard teaching is 1.5-2 cm cuff of tissue, but many tumor surgeons get closer than this)
    - Most sarcomas are removed in this manner
- Marginal- cut through the reactive zone, some tumor cells may be present (essentially only taking tumor out, leaving minimal to no cuff of healthy tissues)
    - Common for lipomas
- Intralesional- cut inside the lesion
    - GCT, ABC, symptomatic enchondroma/low grade chondrosarcoma

**What are some different treatment options for benign bone tumors?**

- Observation
- Aspiration + injection (UBC, Eosinophilic granuloma)
- Curettage w/ burr (GCT, chondroblastoma, ABC, UBC)
- Surgical adjuvants (for tumors w/ local recurrence)
    - Phenol (coagulates proteins)
    - Liquid nitrogen (freezes tissue)
    - Argon beam coagulation, hydrogen peroxide
- + Defect reconstruction

- Methylmethacrylate
- Bone grafting
- Excision / resection

**What are some different treatment options for malignant bone tumors?**

- Limb salvage v amputation
- Wide resection alone (chondrosarcoma, adamantinoma, parosteal osteosarcoma, low grade intramedullary osteosarcoma)
- Chemotherapy (kills micrometastases)
  - Osteosarcoma, Ewing's sarcoma, malignant fibrous histiocytoma
- Radiation therapy
  - Ewing sarcoma, primary lymphoma of bone

**What are some treatment options for benign soft tissue tumors?**

- Observation
- Excision (intralesional or marginal)- intramuscular lipoma
- Wide resection (lesions w/ local recurrence)- extra abdominal desmoid tumor, atypical lipomatous tumors

**What are some different treatment options for malignant soft tissue tumors?**

- Wide resection + external beam irradiation- decreases local recurrence
- No consensus on neoadjuvant versus adjuvant as standard of care
  - Neoadjuvant has less overall radiation and smaller field, but increased risk of skin issues and wound healing
  - Adjuvant radiation has more radiation as the surgical wound bed is larger than the tumor itself, but risk of late complications and secondary radiation induced sarcoma formation

**What are some complications seen w/ pre-op external beam irradiation?**

- Higher risk of wound healing complications
- Post- op irradiation assoc w/ higher rates fibrosis

**Do most slow growing tumors respond to chemotherapy?**

- No, chemotherapy relies on high cellular turnover to be effective

## Benign bone forming lesions

**What is the Enneking classification of benign bone tumors?**

- 1- inactive / latent (ex: enchondroma)
- 2- active (ex: chondroblastoma, ABC, GCT)
- 3- aggressive (GCT, ABC)

**What is the Enneking classification of malignant bone tumors?**

- I- low grade
  - IA- intracompartmental
  - IB- extracompartmental
- II- high grade

Ep 52 w/ Dr. Porter & Dr. Hodo

- IIA- intracompartmental
- IIB- extracompartmental*
- III- Metastatic disease

**What are some benign bone producing lesions?**

- Enostosis (bone island/ mature lamellar bone in canal)
- Osteoma (same but on cortex or outside bone)
- Osteoid osteoma
- Osteoblastoma

**What should you be concerned for in a patient <30 w/ night pain relief by NSAIDS?**

- Osteoid osteoma- produces high levels of PGE2
- Seen on CT best, misdiagnosed as a stress fx (geographic, eccentric)
  - Sclerotic rim with radiolucent nidus
- Can cause secondary scoliosis + paraspinal pain (if located in spine- posterior)

**What does osteoid osteoma look like in histology?**

- Woven bone w/ rimming osteoblasts
- No pleomorphism

**What is the treatment for osteoid osteoma?**

- NSAIDs
- Excision (en bloc or curettage)
- Radiofrequency ablation (but not in spine or near NV bundle)

**What are some differences seen in osteoblastoma that make it different from OO?**

- Lesion >2.0cm (same histology)
- Tx w/ intralesional resection / curettage +/- grafting
- Posterior spine elements common

**What are some benign lesions commonly found in posterior spine elements?**

- ABC, osteoblastoma, osteoid osteoma

## Malignant bone forming tumors

**What are some precursor cells that form different type of malignant tumors?**

- Parenchymal - organs- ex: carcinomas
- Hematopoietic - lymphoid/ marrow- ex: myeloma, leukemia
- Mesenchymal - connective tissues- ex: sarcoma

**What is the stem cell precursor for osteosarcoma (OS)?**

- Mesenchymal

**What is osteosarcoma?**

- Cancerous spindle cell tumor derived from mesenchymal stem cell precursor that **produces immature woven bone/ osteoid**

**What are some different types of osteosarcomas?**

- Intramedullary- conventional
- Juxtacortical/surface- Parosteal, periosteal, high grade surface
- Telangiectatic
- Secondary - Paget's

**Are all of the osteosarcomas high grade?**

- Most of them except:
- Parosteal osteosarcoma and well differentiated low grade OS
  - Chemo doesn't work on these

**What are some predisposing conditions to osteosarcoma?**

- Pagets disease, radiation osteitis, familial retinoblastoma syndrome (Rb), Li-Frameni syndrome (p53)
- + more

**What will an osteosarcoma in a patient with pre-existing Paget's look like in histology?**

- Malignant osteoblasts within pagetoid bone
- Worse prognosis than high grade osteosarcoma

**How does conventional osteosarcoma present?**

- Age <30 or >60
- Pain
- May feel mass, especially for parosteal osteosarcoma in posterior distal femur

**What is the most common site for conventional osteosarcoma?**

- Distal femur, lungs are common met site
- Presence of skip metastases in same bone- poor prognosis

**What are the studies used to stage osteosarcoma if there is a concern on xray?**

- MRI of the extremity, CT of lungs, whole body bone scan, biopsy

**What does conventional osteosarcoma look like on xray?**

- Metaphyseal, mixed lytic/destructive aggressive intramedullary bone producing lesion (cloudy), permeative
  - Can be lytic or blastic, sclerosis represents calcified osteoid
- Codman triangle, "sunburst" periosteal reaction

**What do you find in histology with conventional osteosarcoma?**

- High grade anaplasia, poorly arranged osseous trabeculae, atypical spindle cells

**What is the treatment for conventional osteosarcoma?**

- Chemotherapy (MAP therapy- Methotrexate, Adriamycin, Platin)

- Surgery- wide resection / limb salvage
- Post-op chemo

**What are some other chemotherapeutic drugs used to treat osteosarcoma?**

- Etoposide, ifosfamide (can be used in relapse cases, as well as 3 drug regimen)

**Which chemotherapy drug is associated with cardiotoxicity?**

- Doxorubicin (usually get echo pre and post treatment)
- Cisplatin is assoc w/ renal failure, neuropathy + ototoxicity

**Do patients tend to have a better prognosis w/ a higher or lower % necrosis w/ chemotherapy (Huvos grade)?**

- Better with grade III (91-99%) and grade IV (100%) tumor necrosis

**What is periosteal osteosarcoma and what will you see on imaging/ histology and its tx?**

- Chondroblastic tumor that produces osteoid or bone
- Arises from inner layer of periosteum
- Xrays: diaphyseal lesion, hair on end/ sunburst appearance, tibia common
- Histology: lobules of cartilage w/ malignant spindle cells, osteoid production
- Tx: chemo + wide resection/ limb salvage

**What is parosteal osteosarcoma and its characteristics on imaging + its tx?**

- Low grade well differentiated fibroblastic tumor producing osteoid
  - Comes from periosteum outer layer
- Xray: posterior distal femur common, exophytic mass, centrally radiodense + peripherally radiolucent (cartilaginous lobules/fibrous tissue)
- Histo: osseous trabeculae w/ minimal atypical spindle cells
- Tx: wide resection (not chemo)

**What is a way to tell the difference between parosteal osteosarcoma vs osteochondroma?**

- Cortex typically intact w/ parosteal osteosarcoma

**What is a way to tell the difference between parosteal osteosarcoma and high grade surface osteosarcoma?**

- Intramedullary tumor extension w/ high grade surface/ high grade osteosarcoma

**How does telangiectatic osteosarcoma present in imaging and histology?**

- Xray: metaphyseal, lytic lesion, permeative margins, +/- codman triangle
- MRI: fluid filled levels on MRI
- Histology: scant osteoid, malignant cells w/ hyperchromatic atypical nuclei

- Tx: chemo + resect

**How can you tell the difference between an ABC and telangiectatic osteosarcoma?**

- ABC: Osteoid production w/ benign appearing cells + vascular lakes
- Telangiectatic osteosarcoma- **malignant osteoid production** + vascular lakes

**What does fibrosarcoma of bone look like under histology?**

- Numerous spindle cells in a herringbone pattern, mitotic activity

# Benign cartilage forming lesions

**What are some different types of benign cartilage tumors?**

- Enchondroma, osteochondroma, chondroblastoma, chondromyxofibroma, periosteal chondroma

**How does an enchondroma present and what is seen on imaging?**

- Many times an incidental finding
- Imaging:calcified rings+ arcs or punctate calcification seen around metaphysis, intramedullary
- Histo: acellular, ground glass matrix (due to GAG staining), lacunae (more cellular in hand)
- Tx: observe, 1% malignant transformation rate

**What does a bone infarct look like on xray?**

- Rising smoke, may be assoc w/ underlying etiology (Ex: sickle cell, alcohol use)

**What is the most common tumor in the hands/feet?**

- Enchondroma, can occur w/ fx
- May have more aggressive appearance (even on histology)

**What condition is noted where there are multiple enchondromas/ enchondromatosis?**

- Ollier's disease, may affect limb and lead to deformities
- Higher risk of malignant transformation to chondrosarcoma (5-50%)

**What condition is noted with multiple enchondromas and hemangiomas?**

- Mafucci's syndrome, may see calcified phleboliths
- Assoc w/ high risk of malignant vascular tumors

**What tumor is noted w/ outgrowth from the bone w/ a cartilaginous cap?**

- Osteochondroma
- Xray: corticomedullary continuity +/- calcification of cartilage cap (ring + arc)
- Histo: hyaline cartilage over medullary bone
- Tx: observe, excise if symptomatic, 1% risk transforms to chondrosarcoma

**What is the inheritance pattern and mutation seen in multiple hereditary exostoses (MHE)?**

- Autosomal dominant
- EXT1 or EXT2 gene mutation, assoc w/ decrease in heparin sulfate

**What malignant tumor can an osteochondroma transform into?**

- Low grade chondrosarcoma
- Transformation can also be seen in MHE

**What should you be thinking w/ epiphyseal lesions (common tumors)?**

- Skeletally immature- chondroblastoma
- Skeletally mature- giant cell tumor, clear cell chondrosarcoma (femoral head)

**How does a chondroblastoma present and what is seen on imaging?**

- Mild pain in skeletally immature patient
- Xray: geographic lytic lesion in epiphysis, surrounding edema common on MRI

**What are some findings on histology for chondroblastoma?**

- "Chicken-wire" calcifications, " fried egg" cell appearance, +/- secondary ABC
- Tx: curettage + bone graft +/- local adjuvant
- 2-% local recurrence rate

**Where is a common place for a chondroblastoma to metastasize ?**

- Lungs, 2% risk
  - GCT and clear cell chondrosarcoma met to the lung as well

**How does a chondromyxofibroma present and what can be seen on imaging?**

- Pain, proximal tibia common, aggressive lesion
- Xray: eccentric geographic metaphyseal lesion, +/- indolent sclerotic medullary border + expansive exterior border
- Histo: myxoid tissue,fibrous + chondroid tissue w/ stellate cells, +/-giant cells
- Tx: curettage excision + bone grafting (high recurrence)

## Malignant cartilage forming tumors

**What are some different types of malignant cartilage tumors?**

- Chondrosarcoma
  - Primary- conventional, dedifferentiated, clear cell, mesenchymal, periosteal
  - secondary - preexisting enchondroma, osteochondroma, Ollier's, Paget's, etc

**How does conventional chondrosarcoma present and what is seen on imaging?**

- Pain w/ or w/o mass, more common in males, age 40+, common in femur/ scapula
- Xray: metaphysis or diaphysis, ring + arc calcifications, endosteal scalloping
    - Low grade: uniform calcifications, subtle cortical thickening, high grade- large non-calcified areas, irregular margins, cortical destruction
- MRI: bright on T2 due to GAGs in cartilage (holds water)

**What is seen in histology in conventional chondrosarcoma?**

- Chondroid ground glass matrix, inc cellularity, binucleate cells, +/- pre-existing trabecular bone entrapment
    - Degree of the above determines grade

**What is the treatment of chondrosarcoma?**

- Stage w/ chest CT or Xray
- Limb sparing surgery, radical resection

**What is a de-differentiated chondrosarcoma and what will you see on imaging?**

- Low grade chondrosarcoma + high grade non chondral spindle sarcoma
- Xray: biphasic, one area looks like chondrosarcoma, other is dedifferentiated component
- Histo: low grade cartilage component w/ high grade spindle cell component
- Tx: wide resection

**How does clear cell chondrosarcoma present and what can you see on imaging?**

- Age 20-40 +/- pain, femoral head common
- Xray: lytic epiphyseal lesion, expansile
- Histo: large clear cells w/ abundant cytoplasm, pleomorphism
    - + S-100, PAS positive (a lot of glycogen)
- Tx: wide resection

# Benign fibrous/ histiocytic tumors

**What are some benign fibrous / histiocytic tumors?**

- Nonossifying fibroma, fibrous dysplasia, osteofibrous dysplasia, langerhans cell histiocytosis/ eosinophilic granuloma

**What does non-ossifying fibroma look like on imaging?**

- Xray: eccentric, lytic, metaphyseal, "bubbly", tibia common
- Histo: spindle shaped fibroblast in whorled/storiform pattern, giant cells, hemosiderin

- Tx: observation, symptomatic- curettage + bone graft
- Multiple lesions- Jaffe-Campanacci syndrome

**What are the conditions associated w/ Jaffe- Campanacci syndrome?**

- Cafe au lait, hypogonadism/cryptorchidism, cognitive delay, multiple NOF

**What is fibrous dysplasia and what does it look like on imaging?**

- Developmental abnormality w/ fibro-osseous tissue proliferation in bone, <30 y/o
- Xray: ground glass appearance
- Histology: spindle cells, irregular curvilinear trabeculae of woven bone- chinese characters, no rimming osteoblasts
- Tx: curettage if symptomatic, if fx: intramedullary device is useful (plastic-ish bone)

**When fixing a fx in a patient with fibrous dysplasia, what type of graft should be used?**

- Allograft (autograft bone still has fibrous dysplasia)

**What is the gene affected in fibrous dysplasia?**

- GNAS 1 gene mutation
- Also high expression of FGF 23

**What condition is noted by polyostotic fibrous dysplasia, cafe-au-lait (coast of main), precocious puberty, and endocrine abnormalities?**

- McCune-Albright syndrome

**What condition is noted by polyostotic fibrous dysplasia and soft tissue myxomas?**

- Mazabraud

**What does osteofibrous dysplasia look like on imaging?**

- Multiloculated intracortical lucencies, <20 y/o
  - Anterior tibia cortex common +/- tibial bowing
- Histo: fibroblast like spindle cells, scattered trabeculae of bone w/ rimming osteoblasts
- Tx: observe, excise if symptomatic

**What is the difference between fibrous dysplasia and osteofibrous dysplasia in histology?**

- Rimming osteoblasts are seen in osteofibrous dysplasia

**What is another lesion commonly seen in the tibia diaphysis in addition to osteofibrous dysplasia?**

- Adamantinoma
  - Histo: biphasic, EMA + cytokeratin
  - Tx w/ wide excision, lung mets present 25% cases

**What is the difference between osteofibrous dysplasia and adamantinoma in histology?**

- Adamantinoma- nests of epithelial cells in fibrous stroma

**What is Langerhans cell histiocytosis (Eosinophilic granuloma histiocytosis)?**
- Neoplastic proliferation of langerhans cells, a spectrum of diseases
- **Age 5-15**
- Xray: "Punched out" lesion, vertebra plana
- Histo: histiocyte w/ grooved nucleus, birbeck granules, CD-1a +, S-100+

**What are some clinical variants of LCH?**
- Hand-Schuller-Christian disease- destructive skeletal lesion, exophthalmos, diabetes
- Letterer Siwe disease- fatal, develops in 1st year

**What are some common tumors seen in the sacrum?**
- Chordoma, GCT, ABC, sarcoma

## Cystic/Other benign bone tumors

**What are some types of cystic benign bone tumors?**
- Aneurysmal bone cyst, unicameral bone cyst

**What is an aneurysmal bone cyst and how does it present?**
- Tumor w/ cystic blood filled cavities w/ walls of spindle cells, reactive osteoid + giant cells
- Seen in skeletally immature patients
- Xray: metaphyseal, eccentric (or central/ parosteal), geographic lytic lesion, can be expansile
    - Tumor width can be wider than physis
- MRI: fluid filled levels w/ surrounding edema
- Histo: giant cells w/ spindle cells/ fibrous tissue

**What is the treatment for ABC?**
- Intralesional curettage + bone grafting, +/- adjuvant

**What is another lesion that can look similar to an ABC?**
- Telangiectatic osteosarcoma (forms malignant osteoid)

**What is a unicameral bone cyst and how does it present?**
- Fluid containing lesion, seen in pts <20
- Xray: metaphyseal lytic lesion, geographic, mildly expansile, +/- pathologic fx
    - Fallen leaf sign (fallen fragment)
    - Tumor width typically not wider than physis
- Histo: straw colored fluid filled cyst
- Tx: aspiration/ steroid injection (DBX also), curettage + bone grafting

**What are the xray and histology findings seen in giant cell tumor?**
- Xray: Meta-epiphyseal lytic bone lesion, geographic, aggressive
    - Common in distal radius
- Histo: abundant giant cells +/- secondary ABC formation

- Tx: intralesional curettage +/- local adjuvant

**What medications have been used in treatment of giant cell tumors?**

- Denosumab, mAb to RANK L
    - Controversial, may increase recurrence

## Other malignant bone tumors

Ep 20 w/ Dr. Domson

**What are the most common causes of lytic bone lesions in adults?**

- Mets, mets, mets
- Myeloma, lymphoma

**What are the most common metastatic carcinomas?**

- Breast, lung, prostate

**What are some common sites of metastasis?**

- Vertebrae, ribs, pelvis, femur

**What is the physiology behind osteolytic metastases?**

- Tumor cells + TGF-b > inc PTHrP + IL 1 production> decrease osteoprotegerin + increase RANK L> inc osteoclast production> repeat cycle

**What should you be concerned about in an oncology patient with nausea, constipation, confusion, and arrhythmia?**

- Hypercalcemia of malignancy (in addition to many other things that can cause the above symptoms)
- Tx: fluids, EKG, check labs

**What tests should be ordered in a patient with a suspected lytic bone lesion?**

- Labs: CBC, SPEP, UPEP, SMA-7
- Chest xray, CT chest, CT abdomen/Pelvis, whole body bone scan, biopsy

**What type of primary cancer should you think about in a patient with a blastic instead of a lytic bone lesion?**

- Prostate, carcinoma mets

**What does adenocarcinoma look like on histo?**

- Organoid growth pattern (nests / glands)
    - Squamous cell carcinoma- makes keratin
    - Adenocarcinoma- makes glands
    - Renal cell carcinoma- may have clear cells
    - Prostate carcinoma- invades between trabeculae of mature bone
- Staining: epithelial membrane antigen (EMA), cytokeratin

**What conditions stain for cytokeratin or EMA?**

- Epithelioid sarcoma
- Biphasic synovial sarcoma
- Adamantinoma

- Chordoma
- Metastatic carcinoma

**What is a way to determine the risk of a pathologic fracture in an 76F w/ a lytic bone lesion and thigh pain?**

- Mirels score, 9+ = 33% risk of fracture

**What is a procedure you should consider doing before operating on a patient with renal cell carcinoma mets to the bone?**

- Embolization, high risk for bleeding
- Also w/ bladder carcinoma

**Is radiation therapy used in patients with metastatic carcinoma?**

- Yes, relieve pain and can slow tumor growth in most lesions
- 30Gy typically

**What are some tumors that are highly radiosensitive?**

- Myeloma, lymphoma

**What are some indications to operate on adult patients w/ a metastatic bone lesion?**

- Fracture, fracture/paralysis prevention, spinal compression, pain

**What is the treatment for post-radiation sarcoma?**

- Chemo + surgery + chemo
- Typically high grade + seen at least 3 years after previous radiation

**How will a chordoma (malignant tumor of notochord origin) present on the test typically?**

- Pelvis lesion (can be anywhere in spine), bright on MRI, sxs assoc w/ involved nerve root
- Histo: physaliferous cells (bubbly cytoplasm), myxoid matrix, T-Brachyury stain, S100 +
- Tx: radiation + wide excision, high recurrence

## Hematopoietic Bone tumors

**What are some different types of hematopoietic bone tumors?**

- Lymphoma, multiple myeloma, solitary plasmacytoma

**What is the presentation of lymphoma in adults and its characteristics?**

- Age 50+
- Xray: permeative appearance
- MRI: intramedullary mass w/ soft tissue extension, intervening cortex relatively maintained
    - Get PET/CT, CD20+, CD 45+, LCA (leukocyte common antigen)
- Tx: chemo, radiation (very sensitive) +/- surgery

**What is the most common cancer in kids?**

- Leukemia (acute lymphoblastic most common)

**What is multiple myeloma and what are its characteristics?**

- Monoclonal malignancy of plasma cells
- Labs: SPEP, UPEP, inc calcium, CBC, BUN, Cr
- Xray: punched out lytic lesion, diffuse osteopenia
  - Bone scans typically negative (cytokines impair osteoblast), PET/ MRI/ skeletal survey
- Histo: eccentric clock face nucleus, atypical plasma cells, CD56+
- Tx: radiation, surgery for impending fx

**What are some other monoclonal gammopathies?**

- Plasmacytoma, multiple myeloma, MGUS, amyloidosis, etc

**What is a solitary plasmacytoma?**

- Single focus of bone destruction w/ clonal plasma cells (v multiple in myeloma)
- No M proteins, no other bone marrow involvement, tx: radiation or surgery
- May progress to multiple myeloma

## Small round blue cell tumors

**What are some different small round blue cell tumors?**

- Ewing sarcoma (CD99), Lymphoma (CD20+, CD45+), Rhabdomyosarcoma (desmin +, Myogenin +), osteomyelitis, small cell osteosarcoma, metastatic neuroblastoma, langerhans cell histiocytosis (CD1a), alveolar rhabdomyosarcoma

**What are common stains seen in bone tumors?**

- CD 20 B cells (B-cell lymphoma)
- CD45 Leukocytes (lymphoma, leukemia)
- CD138 Plasma cells (multiple myeloma)
- CD1a Langerhans cells
- CD99 Ewing's sarcoma

**What should you note in a pediatric patient w/a pelvic tumor that stains CD20+?**

- Lymphoma, B cell lymphoma

**What is Ewing Sarcoma and how does it present?**

- Round cell tumor w/ varying degrees of neuroectodermal differentiation (PNET)
- Seen in kids (<20)
- Xray: diaphyseal, lytic, permeative, onion skin periosteal reaction
- MRI: marrow involvement + soft tissue mass
- Histo: high grade, small round blue cells, pseudorosettes, prominent nuclei, CD99+, FLI1+
- Tx: pre op chemo, local control (radiation/ surgery), post-op chemo

**What tests should you order for staging of Ewing sarcoma?**

- MRI primary site, chest CT, technetium bone scan PET scan, bone marrow biopsy, biopsy

**What is the most common translocation commonly seen in ewing sarcoma?**

- EWS- FLI1, t11:22
- EWS- ERG t21:22 is 2nd most common

**What is the chemotherapy regimen used in treatment of Ewing sarcoma?**

- 5 drug regimen: vincristine, doxorubicin, cyclophosphamide, ifosfamide, etoposide

**What are some favorable prognostic factors for Ewing Sarcoma?**

- Younger age <10, distal extremity (pelvis is worse), tumor volume <100mL, good response to chemo before resection

## Benign soft tissue tumors

**What are some nerve sheath tumors?**

- Schwannoma - composed of schwann cells
- Neurofibroma- arising within the nerves

**What are some characteristics of a schwannoma?**

- Arises on flexor surfaces, schwannomatosis assoc w/ NF2
- MRI: rests on top of nerve
- Histo: antoni A (more cellular)+ antoni B (less cellular) areas

**What is a way to tell a neurofibroma from a schwannoma on imaging?**

- Neurofibroma is in continuity with the nerve

**What condition are neurofibromas associated with?**

- NF1, can undergo malignant transformation to malignant peripheral nerve sheath tumor
- Histo: S100 positive
- Tx: marginal excision if painful

**What are some characteristics of a giant cell tumor of tendon sheath (tenosynovial giant cell tumor)?**

- Common hand tumor, also seen in foot, knee
- Histo: similar to PVNS, foamy macrophages w/ hemosiderin
- Imaging: may erode into the bone on MRI
- Tx: marginal excision

**What tumor should you have on your mind that is a painful mass in the foot that gets worse during the day and can vary in size?**

- Hemangioma/ vascular malformation
- Imaging: xray- phleboliths
- Histo: blood vessels
- Tx: excision v embolization, sclerotherapy

**How does a lipoma present on MRI?**

- Mimics fat on all sequences
- T1- isointense to subcutaneous fat
- Fat suppression T2- uniform suppression
- Tx: marginal excision

**What is a stain you can use to differentiate lipoma vs atypical lipomatous tumor?**

- MDM2+ amplification
- MRI: thickened enhancing septae

**How does an elastofibroma present?**

- Painless mass, commonly sub scapular + deep to serratus anterior
- Histo: elastin
- Tx: observe, excise if symptomatic

**What benign, but locally aggressive tumor is associated w/ pain and more irregular borders on MRI?**

- Extra abdominal desmoid tumor/ aggressive fibromatosis
- High local recurrence rate ~50%
- Histo: bland, beta catenin +
- Tx: no consensus

**What is another benign soft tissue tumor that has more of a bland appearance on histology but can mimic sarcoma on MRI?**

- Intramuscular myxoma- biopsy

## Soft tissue sarcomas

**What are the three general types of histology and their appearance?**

- Carcinoma - nests of cells that form glands
- Hematopoietic tumor- little stroma, discohesive, round blue cells
- Sarcoma- dense stroma w/ spindle/cigar shaped cells

**What are some signs of a sarcoma in histology?**

- Loss of polarity (loss of cell architecture)
- Abnormal nuclear morphology (hyperchromatism, pyknosis- inc nuclear/cytoplasmic ratio)
- Pleomorphism (size/shape variation)
- Numerous mitoses
- Tumor giant cells, areas of necrosis

**What is cell metaplasia?**

- Reversible substitution of one type of fully differentiated cell for another one within a given tissue

**Review normal histological appearance of bone + cartilage + bone marrow**

**How are soft tissue tumors classified?**

- By histology according to predominant cell type

- Ex: fibrous, smooth muscle, synovial, cartilage, nerve sheath, etc

**What are some characteristics of a soft tissue tumor that is a concern for malignancy?**

- Deep, firm, large >5 cm, non-mobile (stage w/ CT chest)

**What studies do you get for staging soft tissue sarcomas (STS)?**

- MRI of compartment (T1, Fat-suppressed T2, STIR, gadolinium), lung CT, biopsy
  - CT C/A/P- myxoid liposarcoma
  - Sentinel node biopsy- epithelioid

**What are some predisposing factors for STS?**

- NF-1 - MPNST
- Radiation - high grade STS
- Stewart-treves - angiosarcoma
- Gardner's familial polyposis- low grade fibrosarcoma

**How are soft tissue sarcomas typically treated?**

- Radiation + wide excision(chemo is controversial)
  - Radiation dec local recurrence but not survival (50k Gy pre op, 60k post op)
  - Photons -create free radicals

**Can a secondary malignancy happen after radiation therapy?**

- Yes, latency period of 3 years + tumor should be different than original

**Is pre-op or post-op radiation associated w/ higher wound complications?**

- Pre op (post op assoc w/ fibrosis)

**What are some tumors where targeted therapy w/ disease specific inhibitors may be effective?**

- Chondrosarcoma - IDH1/2
- PVNS- CSF1R

**Which pediatric soft tissue sarcomas are chemotherapy indicated?**

- Rhabdomyosarcoma, extraskeletal Ewing sarcoma

**What should you do if an outside surgeon excised a soft tissue mass found to be a sarcoma with inadequate margins?**

- MRI, radiation, wide re-excision

**What are some soft tissue sarcomas that have mineralization on xray?**

- Synovial sarcoma, extraskeletal osteosarcoma

**What are some soft tissue sarcomas that metastasize to the lymph nodes?**

- SCARE (i'm scared !)
- Synovial sarcoma, Clear cell sarcoma, Angiosarcoma, Rhabdomyosarcoma, Epithelioid sarcoma
- Remember most common mets are to the lungs... but these can also go to the lymph nodes

**What are some common translocations seen in soft tissue sarcomas?**

- Ewing's/PNET 11;22
- Myxoid liposarcoma 12'16
- Synovial sarcoma X;18
- Alveolar rhabdomyosarcoma 2;13
- Clear cell sarcoma 12;22

**What are some common immunohistochemical stains seen w/ orthopaedic oncology?**

- S-100- nerve tissue +chondrocyte + skeletal muscle - MPNST
- Vimentin - mesenchymal tissue- sarcoma
- Actin (SMA)- smooth muscle- leiomyosarcoma
- Epithelial membrane antigen (EMA)- epithelium- synovial sarcoma, epithelioid sarcoma
- Keratin- epithelium + mesothelium- carcinoma, synovial sarcoma
- CD99- PNET- Ewing

**What is the most common soft tissue sarcoma in kids?**

- Rhabdomyosarcoma (common in head & neck)
- t(2;13), PAX-FKHR, desmin +, myogenin +
- Responsive to chemo!

**What is the most common soft tissue sarcoma of the foot?**

- Synovial sarcoma
  - Also seen in periarticular region

**What are some histology characteristics of synovial sarcoma?**

- Monophasic v biphasic
  - Biphasic- composed of epithelial cells + spindle cells
  - EMA +. Keratin +

**What is the translocation seen in synovial sarcoma?**

- t(X;18) SYT/SSX

**What condition is malignant peripheral nerve sheath tumor associated with?**

- NF1 (S100+)
  - Spindle cells in a whirling pattern on histo

**Which cutaneous STS can be assoc w/ chronic vascular stasis or lymphedema?**

- Angiosarcoma (lymph node mets)
- Histo: epithelioid nests, spindle cells, vascular channels

**What are some of the subtypes of liposarcoma?**

- Well differentiated: MDM2+
- Myxoid: t(12;16), bone mets, >5% round cell= high grade
- Round cell
- Dedifferentiated

**What is a characteristic finding on MRI of dedifferentiated liposarcoma?**

- Normal fat next to non-fatty area (high grade sarcoma)
- Histo: similar appearance (high grade spindle cell next to lower grade fat component)

**What type of sarcoma is made from smooth muscle cells?**

- Leiomyosarcoma (Smooth muscle actin +)
  - Arises near vessels in extremity
- Histo: spindle cells intersecting at 90°
- CT pelvis to rule out mets (MC in uterus)

**Which sarcoma is characterized by a "herringbone pattern" on histology?**

- Fibrosarcoma

**What tumor was previously known as MFH?**

- Undifferentiated pleomorphic sarcoma (no distinguishing features)
- Xray: lytic destructive lesion w/ variable periosteal rxn (not forming bone)
- Histo: Bizarre giant cells + spindle cells, chronic inflammatory cells

**What is the difference between extra-skeletal Ewing sarcoma (PNET) and Ewing sarcoma?**

- Its extra-skeletal ... otherwise is same as skeletal Ewing
  - t(11;22) FL1

## Synovial proliferative disorders

**What are some synovial proliferative diseases?**

- Pigmented villonodular synovitis (tenosynovial giant cell tumor tendon sheath), synovial chondromatosis

**What are the symptoms assoc w/ PVNS?**

- Recurrent bloody effusions (MC in knee)> hemosiderin staining> erosive arthritis
- Histo: synovial cells, giant cells, histiocytes, hemosiderin stain

**What is the treatment for PVNS?**

- Nodular- complete excision
- Diffuse- complete synovectomy
- CSF1R (receptor inhibitor)

**What happens in synovial chondromatosis?**

- Metaplastic change of synovial tissue > cartilage nodules
- Xray: mineralized nodules + rice bodies
- Tx: excision + synovectomy

**What should you be concerned about in a patient w/ a wrist mass that transilluminates?**

- Ganglion cyst
- MRI: low signal on T1, high signal on T2, peripheral enhancement w/ contrast

## Episodes for a Deeper Dive:

Episode 20 w/ Dr. Domson: Workup of a Lytic Lesion https://naileditortho.com/lyticlesions/

Episode 52 w/ Dr Porter & Dr. Hodo: Intro to Oncology Staging & Grading https://naileditortho.com/oncstaging/

Episode 73 w/ Dr. Balach: Soft Tissue Sarcomas https://naileditortho.com/soft-tissuesarcoma/ Video: https://youtu.be/xqeAk1JBLK0

# NOTES

# NOTES

# STATISTICS CHAPTER 10

**This section is by no way, shape, or form all of the information you need to know about statistics, but just a general overview of some concepts. Further reading will likely be required to understand the vast world of statistics.**

**What is the difference between a retrospective and a prospective study?**

- Retrospective - looking back in time and evaluating
- Prospective- group of individuals followed into the future

**What are some of the different types of studies?**

- Case report - individual patient, unique situation
- Case series- retrospective analysis of a group of patients, no comparative
- Case-control- retrospective comparison of a group of patients with similar conditions, odds ratio
- Cross sectional- single time point sampling a population
- Cohort- prospectively comparing patients w/ similar conditions
- Experimental - randomized control trial- prospectively following groups randomized to treatment, determines causality
- Systematic review- methodical review of previously published studies
- Meta analysis- systematic review + utilizing statistics to combine results

**What are the different levels of a study?**

- Level 1- randomized controlled trial or meta-analysis
- Level 2- cohort study (prospective) or RCT w/ 80% follow up
- Level 3- case-control study (retrospective)
- Level 4- case series, cross sectional
- Level 5- expert opinion

**What are the FDA phases of research?**

- Phase I- focus on safety and proper dose
- Phase II- focus on effectiveness and side effects, common phase for device/drug failure*
- Phase III- compares new treatment to existing treatment
- Phase IV- treatment is approved and available, observation of long term effects

**What is the incidence of disease?**

- New cases of disease over a certain time period
- Ex: 75,000 tibia fractures / year

**What is the disease prevalence?**

- Number of existing cases in a population
- Ex: right now 3/10 people in your class have rabies - 30%
- Measured in cross sectional studies

**What is relative risk?**

- Risk of a health event among one group w/ the risk v another
- Incidence (risk) of exposure / incidence (risk) of unexposed
- Obtained in cohort studies

**What does a relative risk of 1 indicate?**

- No association
- Ex: risk of skin cancer in exposed .7 / risk of skin cancer in non-exposed .7 = 1
- Relative risk >1, may be casual
- Ex: risk of skin cancer in exposed is 1 / risk of skin cancer in non-exposed .5 = 2
- RR <1, may be protective

**What happens if the confidence interval for relative risk includes 1?**

- No significant difference between the two groups

**Is relative risk obtained in prospective or retrospective studies?**

- Prospective

**Is the odds ratio obtained in prospective or retrospective studies?**

- Retrospective, in case control studies
- Odds ratio- probability event will occur / probability event will not occur

**What does an odds ratio >1 signify?**

- Odds of exposure among case patients are greater than the odds of exposure among the control.. Exposure may be risk factor for disease

**What are some different types of bias that occur before a study begins?**

- Selection bias- error in choosing individuals to take part in a study
- Channeling - drug with similar indications are given to patients with prognostic differences

**What are some different types of bias that occur during a study?**

- Hawthorne effect- subjects altering behavior because they know they are being watched (ex: junior resident closes skin differently while attending stands and watches)
- Interviewer - trying to get specific answers from interviewee that will support hypothesis
- Recall- participants don't accurately remember an event or forget details
- Detection- systematic differences between groups in how outcomes are determined, blinding outcome assessors may decrease risk
- Performance- procedures may not be performed in a similar way

**What is categorical vs continuous data?**

- Continuous - data that can take virtually any value, ex: height, weight, any numerical value
- Categorical data- information presented according to its division

into certain groups, its a way of sorting + presenting information in a report

**What are some examples of continuous and categorical data?**

- Continuous - blood pressure, height, age
- Categorical- male/female, blood group

**What statistical tests do you use for categorical data?**

- Chi- square or fisher's exact
- Fisher's exact - small groups

**What are some statistical tests you can use for normally distributed continuous data?**

- T- test - use if 2 groups
- ANOVA- use if 3+ groups
- Regression analysis- to predict outcomes
- Pearson correlation coefficient - use to determine relationships
- For NON normally distributed data.. There are a multitude of tests

**What is the sensitivity of a test?**

- Ability to designate an individual with disease as positive
- True positives/ true positives + false negatives = true positives / total patients w/ disease

**What is the positive predictive value?**

- Likelihood a person with a positive has the disease
- TP/ TP + FP

**What is the specificity of a test?**

- People who test negative for a disease who do not have the disease
- True negatives / true negatives + false positive = true negatives / total patients without disease

**What is the negative predictive value?**

- Likelihood that a person w/ a negative result does not have the disease
- TN/ TN+FN

**Crybaby Syndrome**

| | Raging Crybaby | Not Raging Crybaby |
|---|---|---|
| **Positive** | 50 TP | 10 FP |
| **Negative** | 20 FN | 5 TN |

**Sensitivity = 50/50+20 = TP/TP + FN**
**Specifity = 5/5+10 = TN/TN+FP**
**PPV = 50/50+10= TP/TP+FP**
**NPV = 5/5+20= TN/TN+FP**

**Table 10.1**

**What is a type I (alpha) error?**

- Saying an association exists when it doesn't, i.e.- false positive error
- The same as- rejecting the null hypothesis when it is true
- Willing to accept this only 5% of the time (hence $p<.05$)

**What is a type II (beta) error?**

- Saying there is no association when there actually is, i.e- false negative error
- The same as- accepting the null hypothesis when it is false
- Willing to accept this 20% of the time

**What is the power of a study?**

- 1- beta = power
- So if beta is .2, 1 - 0.2 = 0.8 or 80% chance that a type II error did not occur

**What happens to the chances of making a type II error as power increases?**

- Beta, or the chance of making a type II error will decrease as power increases

**Does a $p<.0001$ mean that there is a clinical significance ?**

- No it means that the chance of the result being due to error is <.05 %, so statistically significant, but may not be clinically significant

**What can be used to determine clinical significance?**

- Minimal clinically important difference

# NOTES

# NOTES

**Thank you for using our podcast companion book. We hope that this helps you ace your OITE and board exams. Make sure you are subscribed to the podcast and to our email list so you don't miss out on projects we will release in the future!**

Made in the USA
Monee, IL
13 September 2026

62981970R00187